Health
LAW
& Medical
ETHICS
for Healthcare Professionals

James F. Allen Jr., RN, BSN, MBA/HCM, JD

PEARSON

Boston   Columbus   Indianapolis   New York   San Francisco   Upper Saddle River
Amsterdam   Cape Town   Dubai   London   Madrid   Milan   Munich   Paris   Montreal   Toronto
Delhi   Mexico City   São Paulo   Sydney   Hong Kong   Seoul   Singapore   Taipei   Tokyo

Publisher: Julie Alexander
Editor-in-Chief: Mark Cohen
Executive Editor: Joan Gill
Development Editor: Melissa Kerian
Editorial Assistant: Mary Ellen Ruitenberg
Director of Marketing: David Gesell
Executive Marketing Manager: Katrin Beacom
Marketing Specialist: Michael Sirinides
Managing Production Editor: Patrick Walsh
Production Liaison: Julie Boddorf
Manufacturing Manager: Ilene Sanford
Art Director: Mary Siener
Media Producer: Amy Peltier
Media Project Manager: Lorena Cerisano
Full-Service Project Management: PreMediaGlobal, Inc.
Composition: PreMediaGlobal, Inc.
Printer/Binder: Courier/Kendalville
Cover Printer: Lehigh-Phoenix Color/Hagerstown

What are the laws that govern healthcare? The laws that govern healthcare are varied and complex. Chapters 3–7 will help you learn what those laws are.

What do I do when faced with an ethical dilemma? This text provides lots of information to help you deal with ethical decisions. Chapters 8 and 9 will help you learn what to do when faced with an ethical dilemma.

Do I have any legal or ethical responsibilites? There are situations that arise in healthcare that you will need to know what the legal and ethical ramifications are. Chapters 10–13 will help you learn what those responsibilites are.

Cover image: Stephen Cobum/Shutterstock Images

Credits and acknowledgments borrowed from other sources and reproduced, with permission, in this textbook appear on the appropriate page within text.

Notice: The material in this textbook contains the most current information about the topics at the time of publication. This text is not meant to be used in lieu of qualified legal advice for situations that arise in either one's professional practice or personal life. An attorney should always be consulted for legal advice. Since laws for healthcare professionals vary from state to state, it is always wise to consult specific laws within one's state of practice.

Library of Congress Cataloging in Publication Data:
Allen, James F.
  Health law and medical ethics for healthcare professionals / James F. Allen Jr.
      p. cm.
  Includes index.
  ISBN-13: 978-0-13-502799-8 (alk. paper)
  ISBN-10: 0-13-502799-3 (alk. paper)
  ISBN-13: 978-0-13-284039-2 (ebook)
I. Title.
[DNLM: 1. Ethics, Clinical. 2. Bioethical Issues. 3. Legislation, Medical. WB 60]
  174.2—dc23
                      2011037882

ISBN-10: 0135027993
ISBN-13: 9780135027998

10 9 8 7 6 5 4 3 2 1

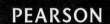

DEDICATION

I would not be the person that I am today, without the help and support of many others. It is to them, that I dedicate this text.

First, I dedicate this text to my parents, Rev. James Allen and Mrs. Jean W. Allen, who have supported me through good times and bad. Without them, I would not be the person I am today.

Second, I dedicate this text to all the patients and clients I have cared for throughout my career. I appreciate you letting me help you and take care of you; but more importantly allowing me to learn from you. Without you, I would not have become the professional I am today.

Third, I dedicate this text to Joan Berry, Director of Community Health Services Education at Lansing Community College in Lansing, Michigan. Without her guidance and support, I would not be the instructor I am today.

Fourth, I dedicate this text to all of my students, past, present, and future. Through the experiences that I have shared with you and learned from you, I was able to become the teacher I am today.

Fifth, I dedicate this text to Mark Cohen, Editor in Chief at Pearson Health Science. He provided support, direction, and guidance throughout many of the projects that we have worked on together, including this text. Without his dedication to professionalism and infectious enthusiasm I would not be the author I am today, nor written this text for you.

Contents in Brief

Preface

Chapter Content

When writing this text, great care was taken to provide as much consistency throughout the chapters as possible. To that end, each chapter has a similar layout and design to help you navigate this text and each chapter.

Chapter Openers

Latin Phrase
The law is full of Latin phrases that are used in legal writing and court proceedings, or to identify concepts. Each chapter starts with a Latin phrase, followed by a brief explanation of why that Latin phrase is relevant to the chapter. These Latin phrases also serve as a starting point for readers to understand what concepts are going to be discussed in each chapter.

Measure Your Progress
Each chapter starts with a list of the nine objectives that are used to guide you through the main goals for each chapter.

Key Terms
For each chapter, we have identified the nine key terms that are essential to the topics discussed in each chapter. The terms that were chosen identify the most important and relevant terms in the chapter.

Professional Highlight
There are many different and varied careers within the healthcare field. All of the topics that we discuss in this text can relate to specific career choices within healthcare. The professional highlight feature found at the beginning of each chapter includes information from select professionals who rely on the information in each chapter to perform their duties. These highlights demonstrate why the information is relevant and how it can be used in the real world.

Introduction Question
We start each chapter with a question. The questions we chose are modeled after actual questions asked by students who were taking a health law and medical ethics class. Starting each chapter with a question will engage you, by allowing you to take an active role in learning the material presented in the chapter that follows.

---

1 Introduction to Law

Change is inevitable. Change has been a part of the history of America from the very beginning. Our ancestors fought in the Revolutionary War because they wanted change; change from an oppressive tyranny to a democratic form of government. Our founding fathers knew that even after the war, change was inevitable. When they wrote the U.S. Constitution, they included mechanisms that allowed the law to be changed. The law would be able to adapt, grow, and change as society adapted, grew, and changed. In this chapter, we will discuss the origins of the law and the legal system used in the United States and some of the legal mechanisms that are used to incorporate change.

MEASURE YOUR PROGRESS: LEARNING OBJECTIVES
After studying this chapter, you will be able to:

- List three general areas that are used to understand the development of law.
- Explain what the purpose of law has on society.
- List the five principles of law and provide an example of each.
- Give an example of the three different types of law writing.
- Describe what the original U.S. Constitutions accomplished.
- Provide a list of the three branches of U.S. government.
- Determine what unique powers are provided to each of the three branches of the government.
- Explain what the common law is and how it is used in the United States.
- Explain the concept of checks and balances that are written into the Constitution.

KEY TERMS
apodictic
autonomy
casuistry
common law
jurisprudence
law
parens patriae
precedence
sovereign

mutatis mutandis

{ With those things changed which needed to be changed.

PROFESSIONAL HIGHLIGHT
Sarah is an ombudsman who represents the interests of the elderly who reside within her state. She works closely with nursing home administrators, long-term-care facilities, outreach programs, and elected officials to ensure that the services and support that elderly citizens need are provided for. Part of Sarah's job involves investigating complaints, writing reports, and working with the appropriate governmental officials and agencies to resolve issues. To accomplish her goal, Sarah needs to have a thorough understanding of what the law is.

The law is not intentionally written to be confusing or hard to understand. Instead, it is a result of the complex society that we live in. When the law was first developed, it was written to provide a list of instructions for us to follow so that we would know how to act and what was expected of us. However, as society grew and became more complex, so did the law. In order to provide better instructions for a changing society, the law had to evolve to meet those changes. Nevertheless, as complex as the law appears, it is founded in some basic principles that will make it easier to understand.

Think about the human body and all of the different cells, organs, and systems that the body has and how each system works together. Part of your healthcare education will include learning about the different body systems (known as anatomy) and how the body works (known as physiology). You will also learn about diseases, when the body systems do not work properly or how they respond to certain conditions, like injuries or infections (known as patho-

Why is the law so confusing and hard to understand?

Chapter Material

Court Case/Ethics Case

Actual court cases and actual ethical case studies can be a great way to understand the material, to show that it has real life application and to demonstrate how that information is used in the real world. Each chapter has four court cases or ethical case studies (except for the chapters 1, 2, 7, and 8, which introduce the topics of law and ethics). The court cases presented in this text use the F.I.R.E. approach (Facts, Issue, Rule, Emphasis).

> **Court Case**
> **Marbury v. Madison**
> 5 U.S. (1 Cranch) 137 (1803)
> United States Supreme Court
>
> **FACTS:** Article 3 of the United States Constitution, created the federal judicial branch, which included the United States Supreme Court. For the most part, the United States Supreme Court only provides appellate review (reviewing decisions made by other courts). But, there are a few rare circumstances where lawsuits can be filed directly in the United States Supreme Court.
>
> At one point, Congress wanted to increase the number and type of cases that could be filed in the United States Supreme Court. To do so, Congress passed the Judiciary Act of 1789. After that law was enacted, Marbury, who had a legal dispute with Madison, filed his lawsuit directly in the United States Supreme Court. The problem that the Supreme Court struggled with in this case, was whether they had the authority to accept an original lawsuit? Because the Constitution detailed what the authority of the Judicial branch was, did Congress have the right to change that authority?
>
> **ISSUE:** What happens when a law passed by Congress conflicts with the Constitution? At issue in this case was the powers al-
>
> located to each of the three branches. While the legislature is granted with the authority to create laws, the judicial branch is provided with the power to interpret laws. The problem that this case presented was whether the judiciary could use their power of interpretation to determine that a law created by congress was unconstitutional?
>
> **RULE:** "It is emphatically the province and duty of the Judicial Department [the judicial branch] to say what the law is. Those who apply the rule to particular cases must, of necessity, expound and interpret that rule. If two laws conflict with each other, the Courts must decide on the operation of each."
>
> **EMPHASIS:** This case is significant because for the first time the U.S. Supreme Court overturned a law *created* by Congress by ruling that the Judiciary Act was unconstitutional. Congress cannot change the Constitution by creating a new law. The Constitution can only be changed by following the amendment process that is outlined in the Constitution. The court ruled that Congress, in creating the Judiciary Act, created an illegal law. The importance of this case, for our present purposes, demonstrates what the powers of the different branches of the federal government are and how the checks and balances are used.

> **FACTS:** The facts of a court case or ethical study provides the foundational information for the case, such as what events occurred that caused a lawsuit or are important in how the lawsuit was decided.
>
> **ISSUE:** The issue found in a case is the question that the courts or study is trying to address. It specifically identifies what each case is trying to decide.
>
> **RULE:** The rule found in each case is how the court decided the issue, or what the results of the ethical case study were.
>
> **EMPHASIS:** This section answers the questions, "Why am I reading this case; and what does it have to do with me or the content in the chapter?" The court and ethics cases are used to demonstrate how the case relates to the information that has been presented in the text. It also shows the reader how the case, and the rulings made, impact the topic presented in the chapter.

Because of how court cases are published, the final disposition of some cases is not known. When the information is available, it will be presented in the court or ethics case. While the author has spent a lot of time researching issues and has taken great care to ascertain final results, regrettably, the ultimate outcome of some cases is not available to the general public.

Special Features

Besides the content that can be found in each chapter, there is additional information that can be found throughout the text. These special features are content specific, so information may appear in some chapters, but not all.

Concept Application

If you have ever read a section of text and wondered what it had to do with what you are learning, this feature is for you! Some of the topics discussed in health law and medical ethics can be complex or difficult to understand. This feature provides commonly known examples of the topics being presented, or demonstrates the relevance that topics have to healthcare professionals.

Concept Connection

There are many topics in health law and medical ethics that are dependent on each other. In order to understand one topic fully, you have to have an appreciation or understanding of another topic. And sometimes, certain topics do not make complete sense until other topics are reviewed. This feature addresses those problems by linking concepts that have either been discussed already or will be discussed in future sections.

Legal Alert!

While the study of health law is important, there are times when information is especially important and needs to be highlighted. Sometimes that information specifically informs the reader what they can or cannot do. Other times, it corrects common mistakes or misconceptions about the law. This feature highlights those situations.

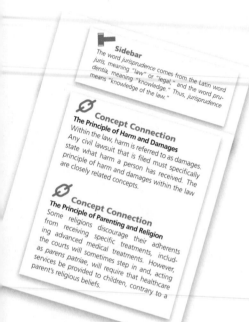

Sidebar

Attorneys and judges use sidebars to discuss issues outside of the earshot of the jury. When interesting, fun, and sometimes anecdotal information borders on issues presented in the text, this feature will highlight that information. It can be looked at as a mini-break in the material, making it more manageable and fun to learn.

The Ethics of Law/The Law of Ethics

Not all legal decisions are ethical; and not all ethical decisions are necessarily legal. When those situations arise, they are identified in this feature. This feature is presented in the form of thought-provoking questions that can be used to generate discussions or as critical thinking exercises.

Understanding Your State/Understanding Your Profession

The majority of healthcare laws are written at the state level. There are times when each state can set their own requirements and write their own laws regarding certain healthcare topics. While there is some commonality between states, some major differences exist as well. In order for readers to understand the state-specific laws that apply to them, this feature directs the reader to the Companion Website, where readers can click on their state and find their state-specific information. In addition, there are times when certain information is different between healthcare professionals as well. That information will also be contained on the Companion Website, where readers can check out the information that relates to their chosen career.

Beyond The Scope

The law can be very complex sometimes. There are times when exceptions to exceptions to exceptions exist or areas of the law that are much more involved and convoluted than what can be covered in an introductory text. When issues are presented that are beyond the scope of this text, this feature will direct readers to outside resources where they can gain more information about a topic if they so choose.

Chapter Endings

Cross-Examination–End of Chapter Exercises

At the end of each chapter, you will find a mix of the traditional questions found in textbooks. One difference is the combination of true/false and fill-in-the-blank questions in the Make FALSE Statements TRUE section. Each chapter also includes modified multiple choice questions, called circle exercise, to test your knowledge of certain concepts. There is also a matching question section where you are asked to match up the key terms and definitions provided in each chapter.

Deliberations: Critical Thinking Questions

Each chapter contains five discussion questions for readers to consider. They present information or situations that can generate thought-provoking discussions.

Closing Arguments: Case Analysis

Each chapter has one case analysis that asks the readers to put themselves in the position of another and address issues that have been presented in the chapter. The case analysis can be used to fine tune some of the critical thinking skills that are essential to working in the healthcare profession.

The Briefcase

The Briefcase is a brief overview of the material presented in the chapter. Using the course objectives found at the beginning of each chapter, The Briefcase provides a quick summary of the material present within the chapter to help you accomplish the objectives listed.

A Note from the Author

When I set out to write this text, the main focus was on the student and the student's perspective. While some find the topic of health law dry, dull, and boring, it does not necessarily have to be. If the material can be presented in a fun and interesting way, it can help make a dry topic interesting and even a boring topic exciting. In creating this text, we took great care to look at law and ethics from the student's perspective. We hope that we have put together a text that will benefit you.

One of the first approaches we took was to identify the information people entering the healthcare profession need to know about health law and medical ethics. We chose content with that specific purpose in mind, to give an entry-level healthcare professional the relevant and pertinent information they need to enter the healthcare profession. While the topic of health law and medical ethics is always evolving, and advanced study is sometimes needed, the basic principles will remain the same.

With the content determined, the next thing we looked at was how to present that content. We wanted to use a writing style and develop a design of the text to help make the topic fun and interesting to learn. To achieve that goal, we used a conversational style of writing that will actively engage you as you are reading through the text. In addition, the design team, working closely with the author, has come up with an imaginative and visually stimulating design. The combination of writing style and visual design, we hope, will make this text interesting and fun to read and learn.

A Commitment to Accuracy

Part of the reason I wrote this text was to make sure that readers were getting the right information. While the use of mnemonics and other tips and tricks that are found in other resources can help students learn, their use sometimes changes the emphasis of a law or alters how the law is interpreted and applied. I draw on my 30-plus years of education and experience to provide accurate and complete information throughout this text.

James F. Allen Jr., RN, BSN, MBA/HCM, JD

About The Author

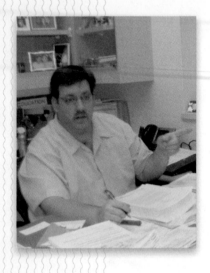

James F. Allen Jr., RN, BSN, MBA/HCM, JD, has worn many hats throughout his long and varied career. Jim, as he prefers to be called, was first introduced to the medical field when he joined the U.S. Army out of high school. He served his country by working as a flight medic on helicopter ambulances. When his tour of duty was over, Jim returned home and started working for an ambulance service and as a nursing assistant in the local emergency room. After graduating from the nursing program, and earning his RN (Registered Nurse) license, Jim started working in the Intensive Care Unit.

Never turning down an opportunity to learn, Jim worked in many different departments throughout the hospital, including both patient care and non-patient care areas. Jim later returned to school earning his BSN (Bachelor's of Science in Nursing) degree. During this same time period, friends of Jim, who were attorneys, started asking him about his opinion on medical/legal cases they were working on. Realizing that this was an opportunity, Jim opened his own legal nurse consulting business. Jim decided to return to school and earned his MBA/HCM (Masters of Business Administration/Health Care Management) degree to help him manage his consulting business. Even though Jim worked as a consultant, he never gave up his love of medicine and taking care of patients. He continued to work part time at various units throughout the hospital until a car accident caused injuries making it impossible for him to continue to provide bed-side nursing care. Never letting anything stand in his way, Jim decided that if a career change was necessary, that he was going to go to law school and continue his medical/legal career. Jim moved across the country to attend law school and earned his JD (Juris Doctorate) degree.

While attending law school, Jim worked as a Nursing Supervisor at the local hospital. Because of his love for education, one of his colleagues suggested that he apply to the local community college. He has been teaching classes ever since. Currently Jim teaches classes in the Community Health Services Education Department at Lansing Community College, including Health Law and Ethics, Medical Terminology, Pathophysiology, and Pharmacology.

Just prior to graduating from law school Jim went to work for Legal Services, a non-profit organization that provides free legal advice and representation to senior citizens and persons of low income.

While Jim's primary focus today is on teaching and writing, he still provides medical/legal consulting services as well. Jim also guest lectures and speaks at professional conferences around the country discussing various health law and medical ethic topics. Jim is also the co-author of *Medical Language STAT!* with Susan Turley.

Acknowledgments

Writing a textbook is not a one-person job. There are many people who either worked on this text or made this text possible, and the author would like to acknowledge them. While it can be difficult to come up with a complete list, hoping that you do not forget someone who has contributed to this project, where to start is not difficult.

Melissa Kerian (Development Editor): While the developmental editor's job is to help develop the text and manuscript, there is much more involved than most realize when looking at a text. The contribution that Melissa has made to this project is evident on every page. She has been a valuable resource, paid meticulous attention to detail, and contributed exhaustive time and energy to make this text possible. Without Melissa's dedication, professionalism, and unique abilities, this project would have been much more difficult. The author cannot thank her enough as developmental editor, support person, and friend.

Joan Gill (Executive Editor): The job of executive editor is multi-faceted. While some think that the job of editor is that of a proofreader, it is so much more. Joan provided guidance, insight, and direction throughout the writing and development of this text. Her dedication to writing, publishing, and the healthcare profession guided this project throughout the lengthy and involved journey a textbook takes.

Mary Siener (Designer): While the work of putting together a text is difficult and complex, Mary had perhaps one of the more challenging and difficult tasks, which she accomplished brilliantly. In writing this text, we wanted to take on a different and unique approach not seen in other health law and medical ethics text. We challenged Mary to come up with a completely different and radical design to make this text distinct from the others. You may have noticed when you first picked up this book and flipped through the pages that this text is different from others. You can thank Mary for that. Her creativity, artistic abilities, and dedication to this project make this text stand out.

Haylee Schwenk (Production Editor) and Julie Boddorf (Production Liaison): With all the work provided by others, Haylee and Julie were tasked with putting everything together. While the production team provides the paint, and the author the color, it is Haylee and Julie who paint the picture. The text that you are viewing is a direct result of their working tirelessly to put together the final product for you.

Susan Turley: Susan is not only a best-selling author, but a friend and confidant who provided much information, support, and encouragement throughout the writing process. Although we co-authored a supplemental text together, I was a first-time author writing this text on my own, and she answered every question about the writing process and how authoring a textbook works. While Susan's contributions to this text cannot be seen on the written pages, her contribution has an enormous impact on this text.

Besides the people to whom this text is dedicated, the list of acknowledgments would not be complete without mentioning the friendship and support of my dog-walking group. On almost daily walks, they listened about the text and discussed it with me. But most importantly, they provided support and friendship throughout the writing of this text. For that, the author wishes to recognize and acknowledge the support of: Kim and Ed Wesoloski (and their dogs Maggie Mae, Hoppy Girl, and Shirley Sue); Peggy Billig and Gary Tuma (and their dogs Bowen and Fiona); and Greg DeKubber (and his dogs Mr. Peepers, Daphne, Bella, and Lord Sheva).

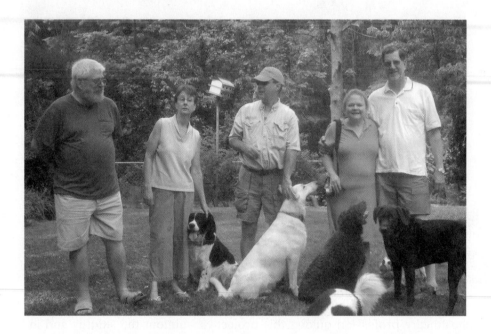

Reviewers

Table of Contents

PART 1 HEALTH LAW

Why do I have to study the law first? I've always found ethics to be more fun and interesting.

Both the study of law and ethics is an important part of your healthcare career. While ethics can be more fun to study than the law, there is an important reason the law is discussed first. Part of the ethical decision-making process includes considering all of the alternatives. For example, what are the legal consequences of your ethical decision? Without a full understanding of what the law is and how it is applied, you will not have all of the information that you need to make a sound ethical decision.

The law is concerned with "... *doing what is right*;" while ethics is concerned with "... *doing the right thing*." As we will see throughout this text, not all legal decisions are ethical and not all ethical decisions are legal.

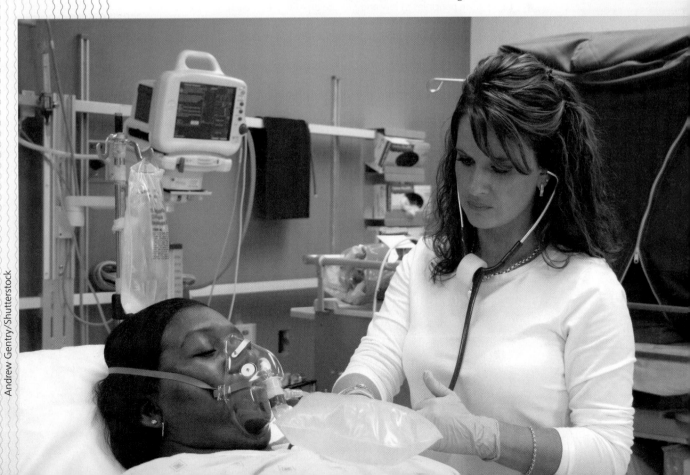

Andrew Gentry/Shutterstock

1 Introduction to Law

Change is inevitable. Change has been a part of the history of America from the very beginning. Our ancestors fought in the Revolutionary War because they wanted change; change from an oppressive tyranny to a democratic form of government. Our founding fathers knew that even after the war, change was inevitable. When they wrote the U.S. Constitution, they included mechanisms that allowed the law to be changed. The law would be able to adapt, grow, and change as society adapted, grew, and changed. In this chapter, we will discuss the origins of the law and the legal system used in the United States and some of the legal mechanisms that are used to incorporate change.

MEASURE YOUR PROGRESS: LEARNING OBJECTIVES

After studying this chapter, you will be able to:

- List three general areas that are used to understand the development of law.

- Explain what the purpose of law has on society.

- List the five principles of law and provide an example of each.

- Give an example of the three different types of law writing.

- Describe what the original U.S. Constitutions accomplished.

- Provide a list of the three branches of U.S. government.

- Determine what unique powers are provided to each of the three branches of the government.

- Explain what the common law is and how it is used in the United States.

- Explain the concept of checks and balances that are written into the Constitution.

KEY TERMS

apodictic

autonomy

casuistry

common law

jurisprudence

law

parens patriae

precedence

sovereign

PROFESSIONAL HIGHLIGHT

Sarah is an ombudsman who represents the interests of the elderly who reside within her state. She works closely with nursing home administrators, long-term-care facilities, outreach programs, and elected officials to ensure that the services and support that elderly citizens need are provided for. Part of Sarah's job involves investigating complaints, writing reports, and working with the appropriate governmental officials and agencies to resolve issues. To accomplish her goal, Sarah needs to have a thorough understanding of what the law is.

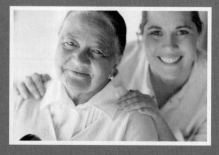

Yuri Arcurs / Shutterstock

The law is not intentionally written to be confusing or hard to understand. Instead, it is a result of the complex society that we live in. When the law was first developed, it was written to provide a list of instructions for us to follow so that we would know how to act and what was expected of us. However, as society grew and became more complex, so did the law. In order to provide better instructions for a changing society, the law had to evolve to meet those changes. Nevertheless, as complex as the law appears, it is founded in some basic principles that will make it easier to understand.

Think about the human body and all of the different cells, organs, and systems that the body has and how each system works together. Part of your healthcare education will include learning about the different body systems (known as anatomy) and how the body works (known as physiology). You will also learn about diseases, when the body systems do not work properly or how they respond to certain conditions, like injuries or infections (known as pathophysiology). Learning about the law is not much different. We start by looking at the different structures of law (the anatomy) and how the law works (the physiology). Then we can learn about what happens when the legal anatomy and physiology does not work as it is supposed to (the pathophysiology). The science and study of the law is known as **jurisprudence**.

In order to understand our current laws and legal system, it is necessary to explore a little bit of the history of law. But instead of reviewing all of ancient history, we can focus on three different subject areas to provide the foundation that we need:

1. the purpose of law

2. the writing of law

3. the structure of law

The Purpose of Law

Each of the body systems has a unique purpose. The cardiovascular system delivers blood to all of the tissue in the body; the skeletal system provides support for the body and offers protection for some body organs. The law is very similar, as each law serves some type of purpose, whether it provides services to all of its citizens or protects citizens from harm.

The law is not that much different from the rules that you grew up with as a child. Parents institute rules for a variety of different reasons: "Do not run with scissors" in order to protect you from injury; "Do not hit your brother" to maintain family order and keep the peace; "Say 'please and thank you'" to demonstrate what type of behavior is acceptable or appropriate. Like family rules, society also needs rules to live by in order for it to function smoothly. A rule developed by society is called a **law**.

Although it may not always be apparent, every law serves some purpose. The purpose of a law can be identified by determining what the law is trying to achieve. There are five principles of law:

1. The Harm Principle (see Fig. 1-1)

2. The Parent Principle

3. The Morality Principle

4. The Donation Principle

5. The Static Principle

Why is the law so confusing and hard to understand?

jurisprudence: the theory, philosophy, science, or study of the law

Sidebar

The word *jurisprudence* comes from the Latin word *juris*, meaning "law" or "legal," and the word *prudentia*, meaning "knowledge." Thus, *jurisprudence* means "knowledge of the law."

law: standards of conduct or a system of rules established by an authority

Fig. 1-1. Helmet laws help protect members of society from serious harm.

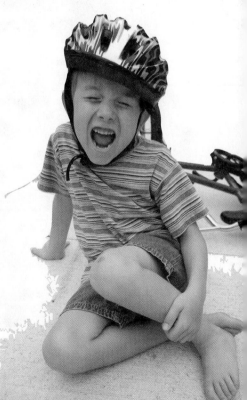

Suzanne Tucker/Shutterstock

The Harm Principle

Some of the laws that are written focus on the principle of harm. Any time that a person inflicts harm on another, the person causing the harm should be held responsible for harm they have inflicted. Without laws that focus on harm, the strong members of society would overtake the weak members.

Examples of laws based on the principle of harm include criminal laws and tort laws. Negligence is a type of tort law.

The Parent Principle

There are times the government, when enacting laws, takes on the role of a parent. When the government takes on this role, it is referred to as *parens patriae* (see Fig. 1-2).

The focus of laws categorized by the Parent Principle are written so that we do not harm ourselves. For example, a parent may institute a curfew so that children are not subject to some of the dangers that can occur at night. Acting as a parent, lawmakers occasionally have to make difficult and sometimes unpopular decisions. But they do so with the intent of keeping society (the government's "children") from harm. Some of the most complex ethical issues that you will face in healthcare are derived from laws based on the principle of parenting.

Examples of laws based on the principle of parenting include public health laws and laws related to drug use.

The Morality Principle

Often based on religious beliefs, the principle of morality focuses on the type of behavior society has determined to be right or correct. A law categorized on the principle of morality informs us what behavior society allows, and by contrast, what type of behavior society will not tolerate. Morality-based laws are usually the focus of controversy, because they are dictating what is right and what is wrong. Examples of laws written on the principle of morality include late-term or partial birth abortion laws or laws related to cloning.

parens patriae: Latin for "father of the people" a legal concept whereby the government takes on the role of parent

Fig. 1-2. A coin with an image of Caesar and the words *parens patriae*. Caesar was often referred to as the father of the people. Courtesy of Australian Center for Ancient Numismatic Studies.

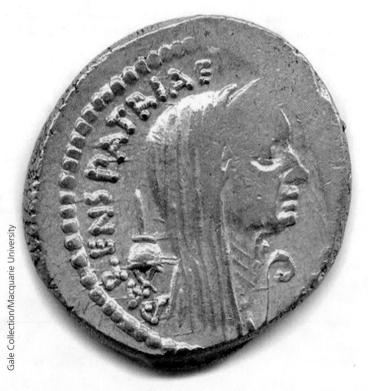

> **⌀ Concept Connection**
> **The Principle of Harm and Damages**
> Within the law, harm is referred to as damages. Any civil lawsuit that is filed must specifically state what harm a person has received. The principle of harm and damages within the law are closely related concepts.

> **⌀ Concept Connection**
> **The Principle of Parenting and Religion**
> Some religions discourage their adherents from receiving specific treatments, including advanced medical treatments. However, the courts will sometimes step in and, acting as *parens patriae*, will require that healthcare services be provided to children, contrary to a parent's religious beliefs.

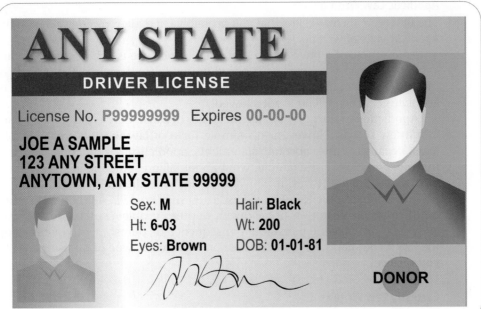

Fig.1-3. Many states have passed laws allowing drivers to indicate whether they are an organ donor on their driver's license. This type of law is an example of the Donation Principle.

The Donation Principle

The principle of donation focuses on helping the less fortunate members of society. Laws founded in the Donation Principle are written to provide help to the less fortunate members of society or members who are in need. Examples of laws based on the principle of donation include low-income housing laws, welfare programs, and disability laws (see also Fig. 1-3).

The Static Principle

Static principle laws focus on keeping the status quo within society. The laws contained in this category include the rules used to help society function. Examples of laws written under the static principle include administrative laws and laws relating to licensing and credentials.

How the Law Is Written

The healthcare industry is highly regulated, with a lot of rules and laws that must be followed. Laws are like instructions, as they tell us what we need to do or what we cannot do. If you have ever tried to assemble a piece of furniture or bake a cake, following the instructions or the recipe will help you achieve that goal. If you have ever tried to do those things without reading the instructions, you have probably run into problems. The law is very similar, without reading it and understanding it, you will probably run into problems.

Part of the reason the law appears confusing and difficult to understand is because of how laws are written. But once you understand how the law is written, you will be able to understand the legal instructions that you need to know. There are three different styles of law writing:

- apodictic law writing
- casuistry law writing
- definitional law writing

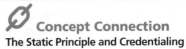

Concept Connection
The Static Principle and Credentialing
Depending on the type of health profession and the state that you live in, there are requirements for obtaining certain credentials, such as licensure or certification. The laws related to credentialing are an example of Static Principle laws.

Apodictic Law Writing

The first type of written law that you probably encountered was written in the **apodictic** style of writing.

An example of a law written in the apodictic style is "Thou shall not kill." While the purpose of this law is based on the harm principle, the writing of the law is done in the apodictic style. Apodictic law writing uses statements of absolute certainty: killing is not allowed!

Apodictic laws are pretty easy to write, because they typically only contain a few words. However, this simple form of law writing creates problems. Because of their absolute statements, apodictic laws do not leave room for interpretation. For example, what about killing someone in self-defense; what about killing in war; is allowing someone to die (euthanasia) an act of killing? Under apodictic laws such as "Thou shall not kill," all killing—no matter the form or reason—is not allowed. Another problem with apodictic laws is they do not provide a result (a consequence or punishment) for breaking the law. What happens if you do kill someone, what type of punishment will you receive?

Casuistry Law Writing

The oldest surviving example of a written law comes from Ur-Nammu, who reigned over the Sumerian dynasty (located in what is now Iraq) from 2112 to 2095 BC. The laws of Ur-Nammu are important, not only because of their historical survival but because they were written in the **casuistry** method of law writing.

Casuistry written laws not only inform us of what the law is, but also what the result is for breaking the law. Casuistry laws are written using a simple formula; if this occurs (the condition), then that happens (the result or punishment). To understand how casuistry written laws work, look at an example of one of Ur-Nammu's laws:

If you strike and kill a slave, the slave's wife must go free.

To demonstrate the casuistry style: *If you strike and kill a slave* (the condition), *the slave's wife must go free* (the result). Once the condition occurs, we now know what the result is going to be. Therefore, casuistry written laws provide the consequence or punishment that apodictic laws lacked. In addition, casuistry written laws are more specific because they tell exactly when the law applies. But that specificity can create additional problems.

Because of how casuistry laws are written, we would need a law specifying each conceivable incident. Returning to our example, we would need separate casuistry written laws to determine when killing in self-defense applies; whether killing in war is allowed; and still another stating whether allowing someone to die constitutes a killing. To combat the overwhelming number of laws that are needed with the casuistry style of law writing, definitional laws were created to provide one law that would cover a variety of different situations.

Definitional Law Writing

Definitional written laws are similar to casuistry written laws because they also contain conditions and results. But unlike casuistry written laws that apply to only one scenario, definitional laws can apply to many different situations. Definitional laws are very similar to a definition found in a dictionary. We look up definitions to find out what words mean. But in doing so, we can also tell whether something meets a definition or not. For example, oranges, bananas, and strawberries are fruits, but what about a tomato? While we commonly think of a tomato as a vegetable, is it a fruit? The scientific definition of fruit

apodictic: pertaining to an expression or statement of absolute certainty

casuistry: a method of reasoning or legal analysis using conditions and results

is "any part of an edible plant that is derived from a flower." To determine whether something is a fruit or not, we only need to look at the definition and apply that definition. Is a tomato an *edible plant*? Yes it is, so that part of the definition applies. Is it *from a flower*? Yes, so that part of the definition applies as well. By definition, a tomato is a fruit. This process is the essential component of definitional law writing. With definitional law writing, we can create one definition to cover a variety of different situations (unlike what occurs with casuistry law writing). For example, look at the common law definition of murder:

Murder is the unlawful killing of another person, with malice aforethought.

To determine whether someone has committed murder or not, we only need to look at the definition of the law to find out. Returning to our examples, what happens if you kill someone in self-defense; is that murder? Because a killing performed in self-defense is not malice aforethought (thinking about it ahead of time), it does not meet the definition of murder.

The Structure of Law

Once the laws are written, the next step is to provide a mechanism for the application of the law. The structure of law includes all of the mechanisms that are utilized to apply the law. For example, who has the authority to write laws, what courts are, and who decides how the law is enforced.

A review of history does not provide much information about when the first courts were created or who the first judges were. Instead of providing an exhaustive journey through ancient history, we can start our discussion about the structure of law by looking at how it was formed in the United States.

The U.S. Constitution

After winning their freedom in the Revolutionary War, representatives of the colonies gathered together in what history would call the Constitutional Convention. The goal of this historical meeting was to develop a new form of government for the **sovereign** nation.

The U.S. Constitution, created by the Constitutional Convention, is the same one that we use today, but it has been amended 27 times over the years. The original constitution, written by our founding fathers, accomplished three different goals:

1. It limited government power to protect individual liberties (the preamble).

2. It established the federal government by creating and allocating powers to three branches:
   - Legislative Branch
   - Executive Branch
   - Judicial Branch

3. It determined the relationship between the federal government and state governments.

> **Concept Connection**
>
> **Definitional Law Writing and Legal Analysis**
>
> The process of using a law's definition is referred to as performing a legal analysis. Lawyers, judges, and courts use this definitional approach to perform a legal analysis to determine, for example, if a person has committed negligence.

sovereign: having independent and supreme power and authority

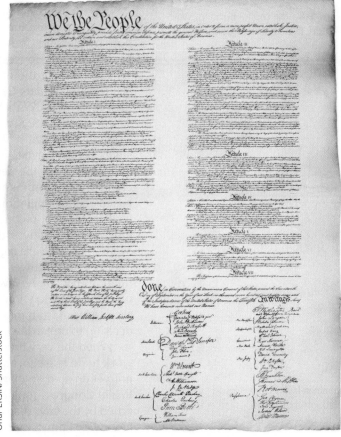

Onur ERSIN/Shutterstock

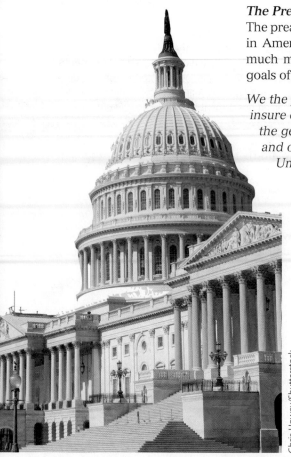

Fig. 1-4. The capitol building, Washington, D.C., home to Congress.

common law: law developed by judges through court decisions rather than through a legislature

The Preamble

The preamble to the Constitution is perhaps one of the most famous sentences in American history. Although often viewed as an introduction, it provides much more. The preamble states the fundamental purpose, principles, and goals of the Constitution.

We the people, in order to form a more perfect union, establish Justice, insure domestic Tranquility, provide for the common defence, promote the general Welfare, and secure the Blessings of Liberty to ourselves and our Posterity, do ordain and establish this Constitution for the United States of America.

The Federal Government

After winning their freedom in the Revolutionary War, the drafters of the original Constitution set out to establish a government for the newly created nation. In doing so, they did not want to create a government where power resided in only one individual, such as the oppressive monarchy they had fought hard to escape. To accomplish that goal, the drafters created a federal government that consisted of three different branches, with each branch being allocated distinct and unique powers.

Article 1 Establishes the Legislative Branch

Article 1 of the U.S. Constitution created the legislative branch of the federal government. The legislative branch was designed so that the people would be represented in government. One of the first problems that the original drafters encountered, however, was how that representation should be provided? Some thought that representation should be provided by state, while others wanted representation to be based on population. The Constitution satisfied both by creating Congress, a legislative branch containing two chambers: the Senate and the House of Representatives (see Fig. 1-4).

To represent the people by state, each state elects two representatives to send to the Senate. Senators are charged with representing the interests of the entire state. With 50 states in the United States, there are 100 Senators serving in the U.S. Senate today. By providing representation by state, smaller, less populated states like Delaware have a say equal to larger, more populated states like California.

To represent the people by population, the House of Representatives was created. More commonly referred to as "the House," representatives are elected based on the population, which is determined by the decennial (every ten years) census. More populous sections of the country, like New York City, will have more representatives than less populated sections of the country, like rural Montana. There are currently 435 members in the House of Representatives.

The unique power granted to the legislative branch by the Constitution is the power to *create* laws. The legislative branch, as representative of the people, has sole discretion in determining which laws will be created. While it can receive input from many different sources as to which laws to create, the final decision to create laws rests solely with Congress.

When the very first members of Congress were sworn in, they had a lot of work to do in a short amount of time. But even though the first Congress had not yet created any laws, it did not mean that the country was without laws. While Congress took on the task of creating laws, the country was still governed by the laws that were in place prior to passing of the Constitution. Those laws were known as the **common law**.

Chris Howey/Shutterstock

Sidebar

You will hear different words used to describe laws, such as *legislation, statutes, ordinances,* or *acts*. While each term has some slightly different meanings and nuances, each essentially means the same thing—a law passed by a governmental body that has the authority to create laws.

Sidebar

The origins of common law have both civil and criminal aspects. Today, in the United States only some aspects of civil common law remain. The courts have specifically ruled that criminal common laws can no longer be utilized or applied.

Concept Application
Common Law

Under the common law, if a man and woman live together for an established period of time (typically seven years or more) they can be granted the same rights and privileges as a married couple, even though they are not married. While common law marriage has all but been replaced in every state, there are times when the courts may recognize a man and a women as common law spouses.

Understanding Your State

To find out who represents you in the Senate and the House of Representatives, check out the map of the United States on the companion website.

While the common law still exists today, it is rarely used. Most of the common laws have all been replaced by legislatively *created* laws. Today, the common law is only used when no legislative laws cover a particular problem or the current laws are found to be inadequate.

Article 2 Establishes the Executive Branch

Article 2 of the U.S. Constitution created the executive branch, which is held by the President of the United States. When the executive branch was first proposed at the Constitutional Convention, many were concerned about duplicating the position of the king. Some believed that it was not necessary to have an executive branch of government. However, it was ultimately decided that a person needed to be responsible for carrying out the day-to-day operations of the country. To accomplish this goal, the executive branch of the federal government was allocated the power to *execute* laws.

After a law is enacted, the President takes the necessary steps to ensure that the law is executed properly. For example, if Congress enacts a law related to health care, the President, with assistance from the Department of Health and Human Services (HHS), will take on the responsibility of ensuring that the law is carried out.

Article 3 Establishes the Judicial Branch

Article 3 of the U.S. Constitution created the judicial branch (see Fig. 1-5). The judicial branch functions to settle disputes about the law and to make sure that both the government and society adhere to the law. To provide the necessary means to ensure the application of law, the judicial branch is allocated with the power to *interpret* the law. This power of interpretation is not arbitrary. The judicial branch does not get to decide which laws it feels like upholding, while ignoring others. Instead, the judiciary must follow established rules when interpreting the law. To understand those rules, we have to return to the discussion concerning the common law.

Prior to the development of the common law, court decisions were based on what result would best serve the king or emperor. Instead of having different courts issuing different rulings, judges started to rely on decisions that had already been made by other judges in other courts. Judges would use these past decisions to help them decide current disputes, which provided consistency among the different court rulings. This process continued to evolve over the years until there was a *common*

VanHart/Shutterstock

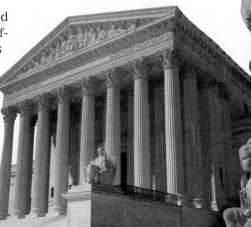

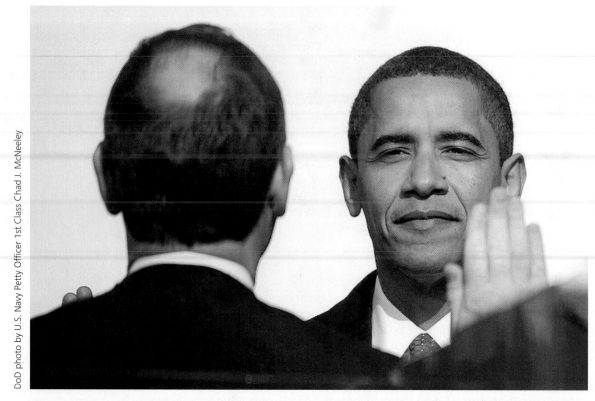

DoD photo by U.S. Navy Petty Officer 1st Class Chad J. McNeeley

Fig. 1-5. Chief Justice John Roberts administers the oath of office to Barak Obama during the 56th Presidential Inauguration Ceremony, Washington, D.C., on January 20, 2009.

precedence: a decision by a court made in the past that is used to determine the outcome of a current court case

way of deciding disputes that all courts could use—hence the development of the common law. The core principle used in developing the common law is the concept of **precedence**.

Once a court *interprets* the law a certain way, all inferior courts are then required to follow that interpretation. For example, when the U.S. Supreme Court interprets a law, all courts within the United States are required to follow that interpretation because the U.S. Supreme Court is superior to all other courts.

Checks and Balances
One of the reasons this country fought for its freedom was to escape the tyranny of an oppressive king. When our new government was created, the founding fathers wanted to ensure that no one branch became more powerful than the other two. To ensure that no one branch overused their unique powers, a system of checks and balances was written into the Constitution. (See Figs. 1-6 and 1-7.)

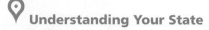

Concept Connection
Precedence and Court Structure
The concepts of interpretation and precedence are dependent on the court structure. Since only inferior courts are required to follow a superior court's interpretation, we have to have knowledge about the court structure and what superior and inferior courts are. The answer to that question can be found by reviewing the concept of court structure.

Understanding Your State
To find out the court structure for your state, check out the map of the United States on the companion website.

Checks

The check portion of the checks and balances system makes sure that a branch's power does not become too strong *before* its power is used. For example, the legislature is provided with the power to create laws, but in order to keep that power in check, the executive is given the opportunity to veto a law that has been created by the legislature. The veto power of the executive ensures that the legislature does not become too powerful in creating laws.

Balance

The balance portion of the checks and balances system makes sure that a branch's power does not become too strong *after* its power has been used. For example, if the legislature creates a law, the judiciary can declare that law unconstitutional. The interpretation power of the judicial branch ensures that the legislature does not become too powerful *after* the law has been created.

Article 4 Determines the Relationship Between the Federal Government and State Governments.

Each individual state in the United States has a system of government that is separate from the federal government. All states have:

- a state legislature that *creates* state laws (each with a House of Representatives and a Senate),

- a state executive (called a governor) that *executes* the laws, and

- a state judiciary that *interprets* the law.

Article 4 of the U.S. Constitution determines how the two systems of government (the federal government and the state government) coexist. Article 4 says that each state is free to operate independently, as a sovereign entity, as long as its actions and laws are not contrary to federal laws and do not interfere with another state's autonomy.

The rules and regulations that govern healthcare are a perfect example of how each state operates autonomously while coexisting with the federal government system. The healthcare industry is highly regulated, at both the federal and the state level. The federal government enacts rules and regulations for the healthcare industry, typically providing minimal standards that each state needs to follow. However, if a state wants to require more stringent rules, it has the freedom, or autonomy, to enact those laws.

Throughout this text, many of the subjects that we will be discussing are state-law specific, which

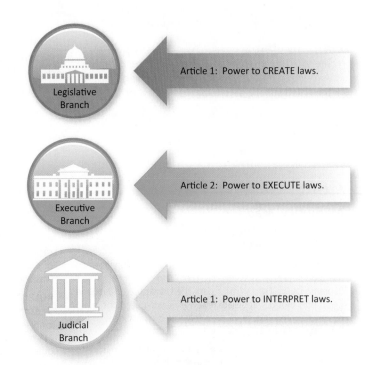

Fig. 1-6. In creating the government, the Constitution gave each branch specific powers that are not shared by the other two branches.

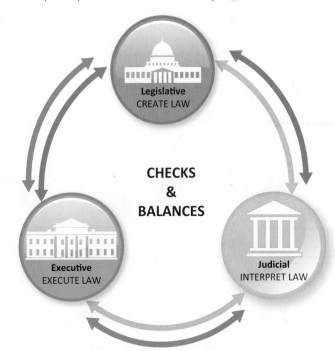

Fig. 1-7. The checks and balances system is an integral part of our democracy. It ensures that no one branch becomes more powerful than the other two.

---

autonomy: being independent, making your own decisions; the right of self-governance

Sidebar

The word *autonomy* comes from the Greek words *auto*, meaning "self," and *nomos*, meaning "law." Translated literally, *autonomy* means "law of self."

means that each state may have a separate law. While there are many similarities among the states' laws, there are also some very important differences. When these subjects are presented, the reader will be directed to the companion website, where information can be located regarding state-specific laws.

Court Case

Marbury v. Madison

5 U.S. (1 Cranch) 137 (1803)
United States Supreme Court

FACTS: Article 3 of the United States Constitution, created the federal judicial branch, which included the United States Supreme Court. For the most part, the United States Supreme Court only provides appellate review (reviewing decisions made by other courts). But, there are a few rare circumstances where lawsuits can be filed directly in the United States Supreme Court.

At one point, Congress wanted to increase the number and type of cases that could be filed in the United States Supreme Court. To do so, Congress passed the Judiciary Act of 1789. After that law was enacted, Marbury, who had a legal dispute with Madison, filed his lawsuit directly in the United States Supreme Court. The problem that the Supreme Court struggled with in this case, was whether they had the authority to accept an original lawsuit? Because the Constitution detailed what the authority of the Judicial branch was, did Congress have the right to change that authority?

ISSUE: What happens when a law passed by Congress conflicts with the Constitution? At issue in this case was the powers al-

located to each of the three branches. While the legislature is granted with the authority to create laws, the judicial branch is provided with the power to interpret laws. The problem that this case presented was whether the judiciary could use their power of interpretation to determine that a law created by congress was unconstitutional?

RULE: "It is emphatically the province and duty of the Judicial Department [the judicial branch] to say what the law is. Those who apply the rule to particular cases must, of necessity, expound and interpret that rule. If two laws conflict with each other, the Courts must decide on the operation of each."

EMPHASIS: This case is significant because for the first time the U.S. Supreme Court overturned a law *created* by Congress by ruling that the Judiciary Act was unconstitutional. Congress cannot change the Constitution by creating a new law. The Constitution can only be changed by following the amendment process that is outlined in the Constitution. The court ruled that Congress, in creating the Judiciary Act, created an illegal law. The importance of this case, for our present purposes, demonstrates what the powers of the different branches of the federal government are and how the checks and balances are used.

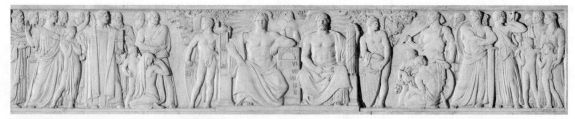

Photograph by Franz Jantzen, Collection of the Supreme Court of the United States

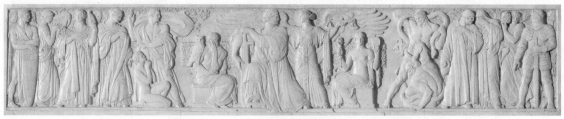

Photograph by Franz Jantzen, Collection of the Supreme Court of the United States

Make FALSE statements TRUE.

Rewrite the false statements below by replacing the bolded, italicized, and underlined word(s) to make it a true statement.

1. A rule developed by a society is called ***jurisprudence***.

   _____

2. An example of the laws based on the principle of harm includes ***the licensing of healthcare***.

   _____

3. Each individual state can operate ***sovereignly*** by making its own decisions and exercising the right of self-governance.

   _____

4. The people of the country are represented in government by the ***executive*** branch.

   _____

5. To analyze the checks and balances written into the Constitution, you have to look at how the other branches influence the ***jurisprudence*** of a branch.

   _____

Circle Exercise

Circle the correct word from the choices given.

1. The concept of law and government (**did not originate**, **originated**) in the United States.

2. The harm principle focuses on not allowing us to harm (**others**, **ourselves**; **the less fortunate**).

3. Some of the most complex ethical issues that you will face in the healthcare arena are derived from laws that are based on the (**Donation**, **Harm**, **Parent**) Principle.

4. Abortion laws and laws related to cloning are examples of laws written in the (**Donation**, **Harm**, **Morality**) Principle.

5. A law using results and conditions is an example of (**apodictic**, **casuistry**, **legislation**) laws.

Matching

Match the numbered term to its lettered definition.

1. _____ apodictic

2. _____ autonomy

3. _____ casuistry

4. _____ common law

5. _____ jurisprudence

6. _____ law

7. _____ *parens patriae*

8. _____ precedence

9. _____ sovereign

A. a decision by a court made in the past that is used to determine the outcome of a current court case

B. a method of reasoning or legal analysis using conditions and results

C. being independent, making your own decisions; the right of self-governance

D. having independent and supreme power and authority

E. Latin for "father of the people" a legal concept whereby the government

F. law developed by judges through court decisions rather than through a legislature

G. pertaining to an expression or statement of absolute certainty

H. standards of conduct or a system of rules established by an authority the theory, philosophy, science, or study of the law

Deliberations: Critical Thinking Questions

Question 1: The drafters of the U.S. Constitution originally intended for the executive branch to be the weakest of the three branches of the federal government. Do you think that still holds true today? Explain your answer.

Question 2: Some analysts have said that the judicial branch of the federal government is the strongest of the three branches. Do you think that is true? Explain your answer.

Question 3: After reviewing the principles listed for the purpose of law, which category do you think most of the laws in the United States fall under? Explain your answer.

Question 4: There are no examples of medical-specific laws in ancient history. In fact, the earliest laws relating to healthcare were not written until the early nineteenth century. Why do you think that is?

Question 5: Review the course syllabus that your instructor gave you; try to find an example of instructions that are written in the apodictic or casuistry style of law writing. Which instructions do you think are easier to write? Which do you think are easier to follow? Explain your answer.

Closing Arguments: Case Analysis

The state in which you reside does not require massage therapists to be licensed. The professional organizations that govern the massage therapy profession want to change that—by enacting a law that requires all massage therapist be licensed. Representatives of these organizations come to your school to get some ideas about how to proceed.

Question 1: Any change in the profession's requirements is going to require that a law be written. Which branch of the state government would you advise the professional organizations to contact to help them with their endeavor?

Question 2: The insurance industry is concerned about massage therapists becoming licensed, because they fear that they will have to start paying for these types of services. If they wanted to counter the professional organizations' movements, which branch of the state government might the insurance industry contact?

Question 3: Are the people of your state involved in this decision, either directly or indirectly? Explain your answer.

The Briefcase

This section repeats the objectives from the beginning of the chapter and provides a summary of the important concepts for each objective. Use this section as a quick review and to check your understanding of the chapter's key points.

Objective 1: List three general areas that are used to understand the development of law.
- the purpose of law
- the writing of law
- the structure of law

Objective 2: Explain what the purpose of law has on society
- to protect society from injury
- to keep the peace in society
- to determine what behavior is acceptable and what is not

Objective 3: List the five principles of law and provide an example of each.
- Harm Principle—does not allow us to hurt others
- Parenting Principle—does not allow us to hurt ourselves
- Morality Principle—what society will and will not tolerate
- Donation Principle—provides for the less fortunate of society
- Static Principle—maintains the status quo within society

Objective 4: Give an example of the three different types of law writing style.
- apodictic—simple, absolute statements. *Thou shall not kill.*
- casuistry—uses conditions and results. *If you strike and kill a married slave, the slave's wife must go free.*
- definitional—uses definition forms. *Murder is the unlawful killing done with malice aforethought.*

Objective 5: Describe what the original U.S. Constitution accomplished.

1. It limited government power to protect individual liberties (the preamble)
2. It established the federal government by creating and allocating powers to three branches (Articles 1, 2, and 3)
3. It determined the relationship between the federal government and state governments (Article 4).

Objective 6: Provide a list of the three branches of U.S. government.

- legislative branch (Article 1) Congress and House of Representatives
- executive—(Article 2) President of the United States
- judicial (Article 3) U.S. Supreme Court

Objective 7: Determine what unique powers are provided to each of the three branches of the government

- legislative – power to create laws
- executive – power to execute the law
- judicial – power to interpret the law

Objective 8: Explain what the common law is and how it is used in the United States

- The law used prior to formation of the country.
- The United States only allows the use of civil common laws.
- Based on precedence
- Common laws are used when no law exists or the law is inadequate to cover a situation.

Objective 9: Explain the concept of checks and balances that are written into the Constitution.

- ensures no branch is more powerful than the other two
- provides a system of checks on a branch's power before it is used
- provides a system of balances on a branch's power after it is used

Maximize Your Success with the Companion Website

The companion website to this textbook contains materials that can help you better understand the concepts presented in this chapter. Go to www.myhealthprofessionskit.com and click "Chapter 1."

Web Links

- sample quizzes
- related web links
- learning games
- and more…

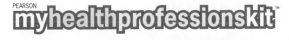

2 How the Law Works

The law can be confusing to read, comprehend, and analyze, especially when you first start taking an in-depth look at the written law. The complexity of the law demonstrates that the law is not concerned with trivial matters but instead involves complex issues and disputes. These complex situations only make the interpretation of the law more difficult to process and understand. In this chapter, we will review the process involved for understanding how the law actually works, look at how to analyze the law, and explain the steps involved in how the law is applied.

MEASURE YOUR PROGRESS: LEARNING OBJECTIVES

After studying this chapter, you will be able to:

- Describe the difference between criminal laws and civil laws.

- Give an example of how a civil law subcategory can impact healthcare.

- List the steps involved in a legal analysis.

- Identify who the parties are in a lawsuit.

- List the steps involved in a civil lawsuit.

- Provide an explanation of what jurisdiction gives a court of law.

- Explain what interrogatories and depositions are and how they are used.

- Describe the different types of proof and when they are used.

- Compare and contrast the different alternative dispute resolution methods.

KEY TERMS

arbitration

civil law

defendant

deposition

interrogatories

jurisdiction

mediation

perjury

plaintiff

The law is not concerned with trivial matters.

de minimus non curat lex

PROFESSIONAL HIGHLIGHT

Barbara is a medical malpractice attorney who was a nurse before attending law school. Combining her medical and legal education, she is able to understand how the law works. Barbara would not be able to help her clients through the legal process a lawsuit involves without a thorough understanding of how the law works.

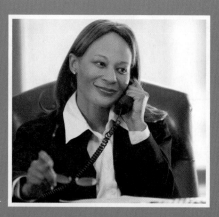

Sportstock/Shutterstock

Laws fall into two main categories; criminal laws and civil laws. While most of the laws that relate to your work as a healthcare professional are civil laws, there are some criminal laws that you will be responsible for knowing about as well.

Criminal Law

Due to the popularity of television courtroom dramas, most are familiar with the crime and punishment aspect of the law. But how do we know what actions or omissions constitute a crime?

The legislature is provided with the power to *create* laws. This power includes determining which laws will be created; and in contrast, which laws will not be created. In addition to deciding what laws to create, the legislature also decides what laws will be criminal laws and what laws will be civil laws. Any law that includes as punishment, the possibility of the offender being sent to jail or prison is classified as a crime. Therefore, when creating a law, if the legislature wants to make that law a criminal law, they include as punishment the possibility of jail or prison time (see Fig. 2-1).

When the legislature writes the punishment portion of a criminal law, another consideration they have to entertain is how severe the punishment for breaking the law is going to be; a felony or a misdemeanor. The difference between a felony and a misdemeanor is how long a person can be incarcerated and where a person will serve his or her sentence.

- Felony: A felony is any crime that is punishable by serving *more than* one year in prison or jail.

- Misdemeanor: A misdemeanor is a crime that is punishable by paying a fine and/or serving *no more than* one year in jail.

Because the legislature has the sole power to create laws, it also has the power to determine whether crimes are going to be classified as a misdemeanor or a felony. The determination is made when Congress writes the punishment portion of a criminal law.

One more aspect of criminal law is worth noting. As a citizen, you cannot sue a person for breaking a criminal law. Criminal charges can only be brought by a prosecutor, an attorney who works in the district attorney's office. Prosecutors have sole discretion on who will be charged with a crime and what crimes that person will be charged with. While individual citizens cannot bring criminal charges against another citizen, what they can do is press charges. Pressing charges is an official request by a citizen to the District Attorney's office that a prosecutor charge someone with a crime. However, because of prosecutorial discretion, the final decision of who gets charged and with what rests solely with the prosecutor's office.

Even though private citizens cannot bring criminal charges against another citizen, that does not mean that they are out of options. Private citizens can file a civil lawsuit against another citizen.

> I have heard of crimes and criminal law, but those aren't the types of law I'm going to encounter; there are other types of law that govern healthcare, right?

Concept Connection
Criminal Law and Casuistry Written Law
What criminal laws are, and how they are written, are a good example of casuistry law writing. Criminal laws include a condition (what the crime is) and what the result is (the punishment, jail or prison).

Concept Connection
Crime and Mandatory Reporting
There are times when a healthcare worker is required by law to report information or situations to governmental authority. For example, some healthcare workers are required by law to report suspicions of child abuse. A healthcare worker who is required to report and fails to report suspected abuse can be charged with a misdemeanor.

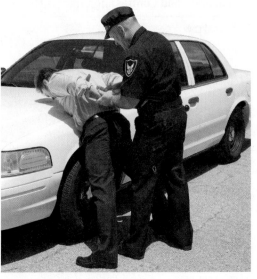

Fig. 2-1. A policeman arrests a suspected criminal. As representatives of the people in government, the legislature will write criminal laws that help ensure societal order is maintained; an example of The Harm Principle.

Lisa F. Young/Shutterstock

Civil Law

While criminal laws are a part of working in healthcare, most of the laws that you will encounter as a healthcare professional are civil laws.

As individuals, we exist and interact with other members of society every day. Sometimes those interactions do not go as smoothly as we would like. When conflicts between individuals arise, the courts can be asked to intervene to settle those conflicts. But asking for the courts to intervene is not as simple as going to the court house and asking for a judge. The only way to get the courts involved in settling a dispute between individuals is to file a lawsuit.

While there are many similarities between criminal laws and civil laws, there are also some important differences. Table 2-1 shows the similarities and differences between criminal laws and civil laws.

Included in the two main categories of law, criminal law and civil law, are multiple subcategories, some of which have a direct impact on healthcare. Table 2-2 provides a list of the most common subcategories of law with healthcare examples.

Legal Analysis

With an understanding of what the law is, the next step is to actually start applying the law. In order to apply the law, the first step that we have to take is to perform a legal analysis. A legal analysis is the process of breaking down the law into its component parts in order to identify what the requirements of the law are. The definitional style of law writing helps us to achieve that goal, because we can look at the law as a definition. But why is performing a legal analysis an important step?

Suppose that you hear on the news that a man was beaten outside a bar last night and is now in a coma. A person of interest has been detained by police and is currently being questioned by detectives. Would you initially think that the person they arrested committed assault or maybe even attempted murder? If you did, it is a common reaction, looking at the result first to determine whether a person is guilty or not of breaking the law. However, that is not how the law works. Instead, the law does the exact opposite. In order to determine whether a person is guilty or not, the law looks at the person's action first, before it even considers the result. To understand why, we have to look at how

TABLE 2-1

Comparing and Contrasting Criminal Law and Civil Law

Criminal Law	Civil Law
Written by the legislature.	Written by the legislature.
Exists in the common law, but is no longer used. All criminal laws must be written into codified law in order to be applied.	Exists in the common law, but is only used if no written law exists to cover the specific situation or if the written law is deemed unconstitutional or ineffective by the courts.
Based on the Harm Principle category of law.	Based on the Harm Principle category of law.
The focus is on maintaining order in society.	The focus is on maintaining order between individuals.
Determines what actions society will not tolerate.	Determines what interactions are inappropriate between individuals.
Court proceedings start with the filing of criminal charges by the prosecutor.	Court proceedings start with the filing of a lawsuit by an individual.
Criminal charges can only be brought by the government (prosecutor).	A civil lawsuit is brought by an individual.
Provides punishment to offenders through monetary fines and/or imprisonment.	Provides for a monetary award only. Imprisonment is not allowed.

TABLE 2-2

Types of Law and Their Effects on Healthcare

Type of Law	Healthcare Examples
Administrative Law	• Administrative agencies grant licenses and set rules for the delivery of healthcare. • Government agencies, which are covered by administrative law, provide disability payments which healthcare plays an essential role in.
Alternative Dispute Resolution Law	• The use of alternatives to trial is becoming more popular, and in some cases is required.
Bankruptcy, Debtor, and Credit Law	• Patients sometimes go into debt accumulating medical bills. Overwhelming medical expenses is currently the leading cause for bankruptcies in the United States.
Business Law	• Just like any major corporation, healthcare is a business. There are specific laws concerning how businesses are run, whether they are for-profit, not-for-profit, or nonprofit entities.
Constitutional Law	• Every aspect of law has some roots in Constitutional law—whether it is how laws are enacted or determining if someone's civil rights have been violated.
Contract Law	• The formation and application of contracts is commonplace in any business. Healthcare institutions sign contracts almost every day, such as contracts with insurance companies so they can seek reimbursement. • Healthcare employees deal with contracts every day as well. Consent forms and authorizations for treatment are contracts.
Criminal Law	• There are situations when a healthcare employee can be charged with a crime. • As a healthcare provider, if we care for a patient that has committed a crime there are times when we must report that crime to governmental officials (Abuse, Rape, Battery, etc.).
Employment/Labor Law	• Healthcare institutions need to know about the laws related to the labor force they employ. • Many healthcare workers belong to a union. How unions operate fall under labor law.
Family Law	• Family law can influence which parent has authority to provide consent for a child's operation or procedures. • Some aspects of family law can dictate which family member can speak for patients who may be unable to speak for themselves, such as patients who are in a coma and need further care.
Real Property Law	• Property law governs land that some healthcare institutions own, but also covers leasing, rental property, and landlord-tenant issues.
Taxation Law	• Even nonprofit hospitals must be aware of tax law and file a tax return. Knowing the taxation laws is an important aspect of operating any business, whether it is a for profit, not for profit, or nonprofit business.
Tort Law	• The law of torts regards the different types of harms and/or damages that one citizen can inflict on another citizen. An example of a tort is negligence.
Wills, Estates, and Trust Law	• Wills, estates, and trust law covers advance directives and who can make end-of-life decisions for someone who may be incapacitated.

Gunnar Pippel/Shutterstock

the law performs a legal analysis. The three, specific steps involved in performing a legal analysis are:

1. identifying the law's elements
2. applying the facts to the law
3. determining the outcome

Legal Analysis Step 1: Identifying the Law's Elements

The first step in performing a legal analysis is to determine what the law's elements are. Definitional law writing makes this step relatively easy. What the law calls elements are the items or requirements that make up a definition of a law. To demonstrate the concept of elements, and how the definition of a law correlates to those elements, take a look at an actual law; the common law of assault.

"A person who intentionally threatens another with physical harm is guilty of assault."

After reading this law, ask yourself; what does this specific law require in order for someone to be guilty of assault? The answer is the items that make up the definition. Two factors in the law of assault define the law:

1. the notion of intentional threat against another
2. the notion of physical harm

These definitional items are also the legal elements that are used in a legal analysis. By reading the law, and identifying the definitional requirements, you can also identify what the elements of the law are. The conditions determining the law of assault are:

1. *intentionally threatens another*
2. *the threat is of physical harm*

Having identified the elements of the law, we can proceed to the next step in a legal analysis; applying the elements of the law to the events that have occurred.

Legal Analysis Step 2: Applying the Facts to the Law

The second step in the legal analysis is applying the facts to the law. The *facts* that we are referring are what happened to cause the analysis. Consider the following scenario to explain this concept:

Scenario

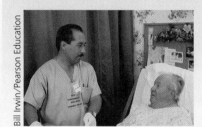

Bill Irwin/Pearson Education

Ned is a nursing assistant is working in a nursing home. Mr. Jones is convalescing in the nursing home after hip replacement surgery. Because of his surgery, he has strict orders to be on complete bed rest, and is not allowed out of bed for any reason. During the night,

Mr. Jones becomes disorientated and tries to climb out of bed. Ned puts him back into bed and comforts him until he falls asleep. A few minutes later, when walking by the room, Ned noticed Mr. Jones trying to crawl out of bed again. Ned takes a pair of restraints from the supply room into Mr. Jones' room. He shows the restraints to him and says "If you do not stay in bed I'm going to have to restrain you."

Has Ned committed assault upon Mr. Jones?

Now that we have a scenario, we can apply the facts to the law. To answer the question of whether Ned has committed assault, we turn to the law's elements of assault that we identified in Step 1:

1. *intentionally threatens another*
2. *the threat is of physical harm.*

But how do we use those elements to apply the law? The easiest way to accomplish this is to turn each element into a simple yes or no question.

1. Was there an *intentional threat of another*? Yes or no?
2. Was the threat of *physical harm*? Yes or no?

By using the scenario to answer these element questions, you are applying the facts (scenario) to the law of assault.

1. Was there *intentional threatening of another?* (Yes or No) After reviewing the scenario above, make a determination of whether there was an *intentional threat of another?* If you said yes, then this element (definition) of the law has been satisfied. If you said no, then this element (definition) has not been satisfied.

2. Was the threat of *physical harm?* (Yes or No) After reviewing the scenario make a determination of whether there was a *threat of physical harm?* If you said yes, then this element (definition) has been satisfied. If you said no, then this element (definition) has not been satisfied.

There are reasons we form the elements into yes or no questions. First, by keeping things simple, we can make the legal analysis easier. But second, and perhaps more important, by using simple yes-or-no questions, it's possible to avoid some of the common pitfalls that can occur in performing a legal analysis—the "should have, would have, could have" arguments that can easily interfere with and alter a legal analysis.

Shoulda, Woulda, Coulda

When you first read the scenario above, did you catch yourself thinking: "Ned *should have* called the doctor first" or maybe, "If they *would have* hired a patient safety sitter the problem might have been avoided altogether," or even considered that "Ned could have stayed with Mr. Jones and asked someone else to call the doctor." While these are all legitimate reactions, they do not address the legal elements of whether assault has occurred or not.

To determine whether someone has broken the law, we can only use what actually happened, not what should have happened, what would have happened if..., or what could have happened. Can Ned be guilty of committing assault because he should have called the doctor first? Since calling the doctor first is not included in the definition of the law of assault, we cannot use that as a determining factor in deciding Ned's guilt. Likewise, we cannot find Ned guilty of assault based on if he would have or he could have reasoning, as they are not part of the definition of the law of assault.

It may seem obvious, but to demonstrate the concept, the law of assault does not say: Anyone who should have called the doctor first before they intentionally threatened another with physical harm is guilty of assault. If we add considerations to the legal analysis, we are adding to the definition of the law as well; something we cannot do. The only way that we can determine if the law has been broken is to use the definition (elements) of the law that is being analyzed.

Think of it this way: If we were allowed to use coulda, woulda, shoulda questions when performing a legal analysis, we would always be able to come up with a "should have, would have, or could have" for every situation. That would mean that every person would be found guilty, in any instance under consideration, of breaking any law that he or she was accused of.

Legal Analysis Step 3: Determine the Outcome

The final step in a legal analysis is determining the outcome, or whether a person's actions have satisfied the requirements of the law. In order for a person to be guilty of assault, how many things (elements) have to happen? The answer is two, there has to be:

1. an intentional threat of another, and

2. a threat of physical harm.

Because the law of assault has two elements, both of those elements have to be satisfied in order for a person to be guilty of assault. If *all of the elements* of a law have been satisfied, the person has broken the law. If *one of the elements* has *not* been satisfied, then the definition of the law has not been satisfied, and

✔ **Concept Application**

Legal Analysis—Determining the Outcome

After the skeletal remains of 2-year old Caylee Anthony were discovered, her mother Casey Anthony was charged with first-degree murder. Many who watched the story, and the trial that followed, thought that Casey murdered her daughter. When Casey was found not guilty, the verdict shocked many who had followed the trial. One jury member was quoted as saying "everybody agreed if we were going fully on feelings and emotions, she was done." The jury members who talked to the media agreed, the legal definition of murder had not been proven in court. While they did not believe that she was totally innocent, they could not find her guilty of murder based on emotions alone. Instead, they based their decision on the definition of murder and whether the evidence provided had proved that definition—which, they felt, it had not.

the law's requirements have not been satisfied. Meaning, for example, a person cannot be guilty of assault by only intentionally threatening another person. If that threat is not also of physical harm, then assault has not occurred.

Many people believe that when something goes wrong, somebody has to be guilty of something. But as we saw at the beginning of this section, you do not look at the result first. Instead, you go through the steps of a legal analysis and see if a particular law fits.

So what happens if a particular law does not apply? Does that mean the person gets off? No, not necessarily. If one particular law does not fit a situation, the person is not guilty of only that particular law. That does not mean that other laws might not apply to the situation. If one law's requirements do not apply to a situation, one can move on to another law and perform another legal analysis to see if that law fits. If that particular law does not fit, one can then move on to yet another law and another to see what laws, if any, laws apply.

While the law does not look at the result first, attorneys and judges will sometimes look at the result to determine which law they are going to analyze. Lawyers are well versed in the law and have a good idea of what laws might apply. Instead of analyzing every single law that has ever been written, lawyers use their education, knowledge, and experience to help them decide which law, or laws, they are going to analyze. Now that we have considered how a legal analysis is performed, we can look at the result of the scenario that we used in our analysis. (If you came up with a different result than what is provided below, do not worry. Right now we only want to understand the concept of how a legal analysis is performed. Later in this chapter, you will see how different people might come up with different results.)

Example Result: Ned is likely to be found guilty of assault because both of the elements for assault have been satisfied.

Explanation: 1) Was there an intentional threat of another? Yes, Ned threatened Mr. Jones by saying, "*If you do not stay in bed I'm going to have to restrain you.*" Being tied up or restrained can be very threatening, especially to an elderly, confused individual. 2) Was the threat of physical harm? Yes, even though there was no actual physical harm, there was a *threat* of physical harm, being restrained. Being restrained can cause physical harm because it restricts movement, which can lead to sore joints and muscles, and the beginning stages of bed sores. The restraints themselves can cause bruises and pain if not applied correctly or checked often.

NOTE: The law of assault does not require *actual* harm, only the *threat of* harm. Actual harm is an element of battery, something that commonly goes with assault. But assault and battery are two different laws that need to be analyzed separately. This emphasizes why you need to perform a legal analysis of each law separately. (You will be provided with an opportunity to apply the law of battery in the exercises at the end of this chapter.)

A Civil Lawsuit

⊘ **Concept Connection**

Legal Analysis and Negligence

It is important to understand the concept of performing a legal analysis because it is used with any law, criminal proceeding, or civil lawsuit. For example, in order to determine if someone is negligent, you have to perform a legal analysis first.

Now that we have reviewed the process involved in a legal analysis, you might be asking yourself, why that is important? Making a determination of whether someone has broken the law is one of the first things an attorney will do before filing a lawsuit. If a person has not broken the law, then there is no basis for a lawsuit. But if the attorney, after performing a legal analysis, determines that the law has been broken, he or she might proceed with the filing of a lawsuit. For example, if a patient thinks he or she has been the victim of an act of negligence by a healthcare worker, one of the first things an attorney is going to do is perform a legal analysis of the law of negligence.

The rules and regulations regarding lawsuits range from the requirements for filing a lawsuit all the way up to how a jury trial is handled and the appeals process. All of the rules for each step in the lawsuit process are outlined in a procedure manual called *The Rules of Civil Procedure*. Before we get into an explanation of how a lawsuit works its way through the court system, we should first identify the parties. The person who brings the lawsuit is known as the **plaintiff**.

For example, if a patient believes that a healthcare worker has committed negligence and wants to file a lawsuit, the patient would be the plaintiff. The person who is being sued is known as the **defendant**.

A defendant is the person who is *defending* himself or herself against the allegations that have been made in a lawsuit. Using our healthcare negligence example, the healthcare worker would be the defendant.

Now that we have identified the parties involved in a lawsuit, we can proceed with the steps involved in filing a lawsuit. There are six major steps that a lawsuit takes:

1. A Wrong or Injury Occurs
2. The Wrong or Injury Is Discovered
3. The Lawsuit Is Filed
4. The Involved Parties Are Notified (Notice/Service of Process)
5. A Pretrial Conference Occurs
6. The Lawsuit Proceeds to Trial

A Civil Lawsuit: Step 1—A Wrong or Injury Occurs

The first step in civil litigation is the occurrence of an injury or a wrong that the court will recognize. While this step may seem obvious, it is important to note in understanding how lawsuits develop. Wrongs against people are committed every day, even in the healthcare arena. But just because wrongs are committed, does not mean that they will always lead to a lawsuit. Sometimes people may *think* that a wrong has occurred and may even attempt to file a lawsuit. But unless there is a *court recognized* harm, a lawsuit will not be successful. (This is another reason attorneys will perform a legal analysis before they actually file a lawsuit. If no law has been broken, then there is no reason to file a lawsuit.)

A Civil Lawsuit: Step 2—The Wrong or Injury Is Discovered

Crimes are committed every day in our country that the police do not always discover. The same holds true on the civil law side. People can commit wrongs against another person without the person ever discovering that they have been harmed. For example, a surgical instrument that is left in a patient may go undiscovered by both the healthcare staff and the patient (see Fig. 2-2). Only after the mistake has been discovered can a lawsuit be filed. This distinction is important, because without discovery of the mistake, no one knows that a mistake has been made. If no one knows that a harm has been committed, then a lawsuit cannot be filed.

A Civil Lawsuit: Step 3—The Lawsuit is Filed

A person who has been harmed and wants to involve the courts in addressing his or her injuries needs to file a lawsuit. The filing of the lawsuit itself not only

plaintiff: the party who brings a civil claim of wrongdoing against another party; or, in criminal prosecutions, the state, district, or federal government

defendant: the person accused of wrongdoing in a civil case; or the person charges with a crime in criminal prosecutions

 Concept Application

Civil Procedure—Court Citation

If you have ever seen a case referred to as Smith v. Jones, typically the plaintiff's name is listed first and the defendant's name is listed second. Using a healthcare example, the court case citation would appear as *Patient v. Healthcare Worker*. But, there are exceptions to this rule. In some appellate courts, the name of the party who filed the appeal will appear first in the court citation. For example, if a healthcare worker files an appeal, that appeal might be cited as *Healthcare Worker v. Patient*, even though the healthcare worker was the defendant in the original trial.

 Concept Connection

Wrong Committed and Damages

The rules of civil procedure require that any lawsuit that is filed contain statement(s) indicating what damages a person has received. This requirement ensures that all lawsuits are based on some wrong occurring. Lawsuits cannot be brought on principle alone.

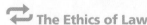 **The Ethics of Law**

A Wrong or Injury Occurs

Should a person who makes a mistake or commits a wrong against another member of society be legally required to notify the other party? If you accidently hit a parked car on the street, you may be legally required to notify the person of the accident by leaving a note. But in the healthcare setting what happens if you make a medical mistake?

- Should a healthcare worker be legally required to inform the patient that a medical mistake was made?

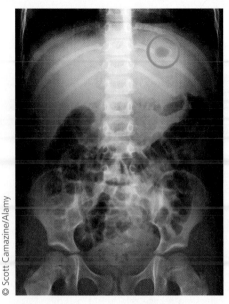

Fig. 2-2. Post-operative X-rays have become common practice following surgical procedures to identify any retained equipment or sponges.

© Scott Camazine/Alamy

jurisdiction: the authority provided to a court to preside (exercise authority) over specific legal matters

Fig. 2-3. The bronze entrance to the United States Supreme Court. In order for a lawsuit to enter these doors, the court must have jurisdiction.

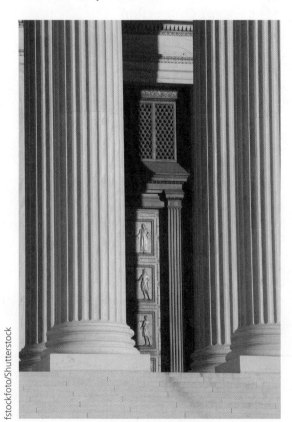

fstockfoto/Shutterstock

activates the judicial system but also serves as the foundation for all legal proceedings that will follow. But with all of the different courts that are available—city, county, district, state, federal, and specialty courts—how does a person know which court to file the lawsuit in?

Even though there are many different courts in the judicial system, the plaintiff cannot just choose any court he or she would like to choose. Instead, lawsuits can only be filed in a court that has jurisdiction (see Fig. 2-3).

Each court in the American judicial system has very specific jurisdiction. The jurisdictional requirements come from the laws that created that court. Jurisdiction gives the court authority to:

- **hear a case** because it has authority over the parties involved in the lawsuit (known as *personal jurisdiction*);

- **decide the issues** being presented the lawsuit because it has the authority over the law that is the subject of the lawsuit (known as *subject matter jurisdiction*);

- **make a decision** and rulings that interpret the law (as it is provided with the power to interpret the law); and

- **enforce the application of law** by providing remedies or punishments (such as contempt of court, issuing arrest warrants, or injunctions).

 Concept Connection

Discovery of Harm and Statute of Limitations

There are limits as to when a civil lawsuit can be filed, referred to as the Statute of Limitations. The discovery of the harm may alter the normal Statute of Limitation requirements.

 Beyond the Scope

The U.S. Constitution and other laws determine what jurisdiction each specific court has. When a law is written that creates a court, it will also include language outlining the jurisdiction of that court. For example, the U.S Constitution not only created the U.S. Supreme Court, but it also provided it with specific jurisdiction. With all of the different courts in the country, the exact jurisdictional requirements for each specific court are beyond the scope of this text, but it is important to note that courts do have limitations on what lawsuits they are able to address.

 The Ethics of Law

Filing a Civil Lawsuit

Any person can file a civil lawsuit against another person, at any time, for any reason. The only requirements that are needed to *file* a lawsuit are the completion of the paperwork and the payment of the filing fee. While there is no guarantee that the lawsuit will survive the legal process, the courts do not believe in hindering a person's ability to file a lawsuit.

- Should there be a limitation on whether a person is allowed to file a lawsuit or not?

Once the plaintiff has determined which court to file his or her lawsuit in, the next step is to complete all of the appropriate paperwork and file it with the court clerk. The plaintiff will take all the required paperwork to the court clerk. The court clerk will then process the paperwork and will hand back copies to the plaintiff. At this point the lawsuit has been *filed*, but the legal system has not yet been activated because the defendant(s) involved in the lawsuit need to be *officially* notified that they are being sued.

A Civil Lawsuit: Step 4—The Involved Parties Are Notified (Notice/Service of Process)

Notifying a person that he or she is being sued is not as simple as just verbally telling them. Instead, the *Rules of Civil Procedure* requires that a defendant be *officially* notified that he or she is being sued. Official notification can only be performed through a mechanism known as service of process. But why go through the hassle of official notification? The main reason for requiring *official* notice of a lawsuit is to provide documented proof that a defendant has been officially notifed (served) of the lawsuit. The two most commonly used methods for official notification are posting by registered mail or receiving the notice from a process server.

 Legal Alert!

The Rules of Civil Procedure strictly forbid the plaintiff from directly handing the official notification to the defendant. The courts require that an intermediary (a person not involved in or that holds an interest in the lawsuit) to be responsible for "*officially*" notifying the defendant that they are being sued. The reason behind the strictness of this rule is to combat potential fraud by involving a third party in case questions arise as to whether a defendant was officially notified or not.

Registered Mail

The federal courts and most state courts allow service of process through registered mail (see Fig. 2-4). The post office delivers, by mail, a copy of the lawsuit to the defendant. Upon delivery, a person's signature is required on the signature card. The signature card is then returned to the plaintiff to prove that the lawsuit has been delivered and who accepted it. The plaintiff can then use the signature card as proof of service of process.

Process Server

In addition to registered mail, a professional process server can be hired to deliver the lawsuit to the defendant. The process server signs a form stating when, where, and to whom service of process was delivered. The verification form signed by the process server is the documented that proof a plaintiff needs to demonstrate that service of process has been completed.

Sidebar

There are two common misconceptions associated with service of process: 1) that you can refuse to accept a service of process; or 2) that you must physically touch the service of process in order to be officially notified. Where these myths got their origins is unclear, but they are often quoted as legal fact. In truth, you cannot avoid or refuse service of process.

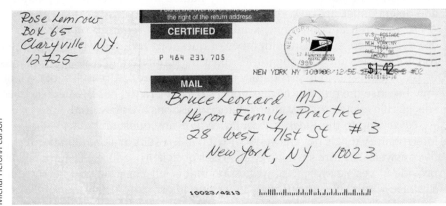

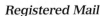

Fig. 2-4. Utilizing the post office's registered mail system is the most common way of notifying parties they are being sued.

Court Case

Collins v. Park

621 A.2d 996, 423 Pa. Super. 601 (1993)
Superior Court of Pennsylvania

FACTS: Ernest Collins filed a medical malpractice lawsuit against Dr. Guy Park stemming from a surgical procedure Dr. Park performed on him at Rolling Hill Hospital. A sheriff, attempting to make official notification through service of process, left the official notice with a receptionist at Rolling Hill Hospital. However, at the time the sheriff left the notice, Dr. Park was no longer working at the hospital. He did not maintain an office at the hospital nor did he admit patients to the hospital.

When the case reached the trial stage, a summons was issued for Dr. Park to appear at trial. At that time it was discovered that Dr. Park had been admitted to the hospital as a patient. The sheriff went to the hospital to serve the summons, leaving it with the ICU charge nurse.

ISSUE: Was the service of process effective, giving the court jurisdiction over Dr. Park?

RULE: Neither the receptionist nor the ICU charge nurse were authorized to receive the service of summons for Dr. Park. In addition, the sheriff did not effectively and officially notify Dr. Park that he was being sued. "The service of the summons attempted by the sheriff, therefore, was defective and did not confer upon the court jurisdiction to act against the person of Dr. Park."

EMPHASIS: There are legal requirements for service of process that must be satisfied. A party must be officially notified that they are involved in a lawsuit. That notification must comply with the legal requirements outlined in the law. In this case, leaving the service of process with the receptionist or the charge nurse did not satisfy the legal requirements for officially notifying someone that they were being sued.

Legal Alert!

If a party to a lawsuit is represented by an attorney, you have to be cautious about any contact that you have. Most of the time, the service of process will include statements such as *"any and all contact with [the party's name] must be made through the attorney or with the attorney's permission."*

interrogatories: a formal set of written questions provided to opposing parties in a lawsuit that help attorneys discover facts about the case

deposition: the taking of testimony of a witness, under oath, by an attorney before a trial

After official notice/service of process has been completed, the plaintiff takes the proof of official notification back to the court clerk's office. Once the court clerk has verified that all of the defendants have been officially notified, the court clerk will assign a judge and place the lawsuit on the court's docket.

A Civil Lawsuit: Step 5—A Pretrial Conference Occurs

Before a lawsuit is scheduled for trial, the parties will attend a pretrial conference. The purpose of the pretrial conference is to resolve any matters that need to be concluded before scheduling the trial. If a lawsuit has reached this point in the process, the parties are typically represented by an attorney.

Prior to appearing in court, attorneys need information that will assist them in developing their case. What tools are to be utilized and how they are to be handled is determined at the pretrial conference. The two most common investigative tools used in civil litigation are **interrogatories** and **depositions**.

Interrogatories

Interrogatories are written questions that are submitted to parties in the lawsuit. (The plaintiff attorney will submit written interrogatories to the defendant's attorney for the defendant to answer, and the defense attorney will submit written interrogatories to the plaintiff's attorney for the plaintiff to answer.) Only the parties that are actually named in the lawsuit, the plaintiff(s) and defendant(s), are given interrogatory questions to answer.

At the pretrial conference, a number of issues regarding interrogatories are determined, such as the number of questions to be allowed in the interrogatory, when the interrogatories must be submitted, and when they must be returned. Writing interrogatory questions requires a great deal of skill, not only because the number of questions is usually limited but because of a very special rule related to how interrogatory questions are answered.

According to the *Rules of Civil Procedure,* any question whatsoever on an interrogatory that is not answered or left blank results in an automatic affirmative answer. Or, more specifically, the rules of civil procedure will automatically provide a "yes" answer to any question that is left blank on an interrogatory. Because of this rule, an attorney, in writing interrogatory questions, wants to make sure that, if a question is left blank, that a yes answer will benefit their case. Answering interrogatory questions truthfully and honestly is not only crucial, but legally required. Any answer that is provided on an interrogatory questionnaire is subject to the penalty of **perjury**.

Depositions

Anyone who is a party to the lawsuit or is going to be called as a witness at trial can be deposed (the subject of a deposition). A deposition works very much like what you see in an actual trial. The exceptions are that no judge is present during a deposition, nor are other witnesses. The only people in the room during a deposition are the attorneys, the witness who is being deposed, and a stenographer. (Sometimes but not always the parties—the plaintiff and defendant—may be present.) The person who is giving the deposition testimony (the witness) is sworn in, and the attorneys start asking questions.

One of the key differences between a deposition and what occurs at trial is how objections to questions are handled. If an objection to a question is raised during a deposition, the objection is noted by the court stenographer and entered into the record. But, unlike a trial when the judge will tell you whether you have to answer the question or not, at a deposition the witness *must provide an answer*. Sometime after the deposition has occurred, the judge will review the deposition transcripts and rule on the objection and whether that particular line of questioning will be allowed at trial. Because the judge is not present during the deposition, the witness must provide an answer so that it is entered into the record. While this may initially seem unfair, there is a reason for the rule. If the judge were to rule that the witness had to answer the question, we would not have to go back and take another deposition, whereby the question would be answered. So the legal requirement that all questions be answered during a deposition is done so in the interest of judicial economy.

A Civil Lawsuit: Step 6—The Lawsuit Proceeds to Trial

After a lawsuit has been filed and all of the pretrial matters completed, the parties prepare for trial. For the small percentage of lawsuits that actually reach trial, the process starts with jury selection. The trial begins after the jury has been selected (see Fig. 2-5). The trial process involves:

- Opening Statements: Opening statements are made by the plaintiff attorney first and the defense attorney second. The purpose of an opening statement is to give the court a preview of the testimony that is going to be presented.
- Witness Testimony and Cross Examination: After opening statements have been made, the plaintiff attorney presents its case by calling witnesses to the stand to testify. Each witness is questioned by the plaintiff attorney first, followed by questions from the defense attorney. After the plaintiff has called all of its witnesses, the defense then calls its witnesses. Each defense witness is questioned by the defense attorney first, followed by questions from the plaintiff attorney.

perjury: intentionally lying under oath; a criminal offense for making a knowingly false statement under oath

 Concept Application

Interrogatories

Suppose that a plaintiff attorney (who is representing the patient in a negligence case) asks the following question on an interrogatory questionnaire:

Have you ever committed an act of negligence that you have not been sued for?

Because of the careful wording of the question, the answer that you provide can create problems, regardless of whether it is a yes or no answer.

NO: If you provide a no answer, are you admitting that you have committed a negligent act in the past, but that you just happened not to get caught? Or, are you stating that you have never committed any negligent act in the past before?

YES: If you provide a yes answer, or leave the space blank so that the court rules provide a yes answer for you, are you admitting that you have committed a negligent act in the past? If so, now you are on record for committing an act of negligence.

 The Ethics of Law

During a deposition related to a medical malpractice case, an attorney may ask any question regarding the patient's medical history. Because the patient brought the lawsuit alleging a medical mistake, *any* medical treatment that the patient has ever received in his or her lifetime may become relevant. This includes any psychiatric treatments, treatment for sexually transmitted diseases, and any and all medications taken, even extending to birth control, psychiatric medications, and medications for erectile dysfunction. While these questions may not be allowed at trial, they can be asked in a deposition, and because of the rules related to depositions they must be answered.

- Is that fair?
- Should an attorney be allowed to ask any question at all during a deposition?
- Do you think that requiring an answer at a deposition might deter some people from filing a lawsuit?

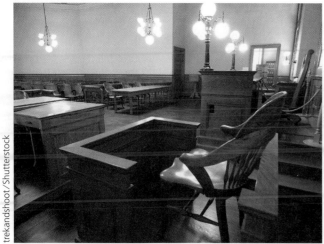

Fig. 2-5. The interior of a court of law. Of all the lawsuits that are filed, very few end up reaching the trial phase.

- Closing Arguments: After all witnesses have been called and all testimony and evidence has been presented, closing arguments are made. Closing arguments are used by the attorneys to sum up the case, and provide an overview of the testimony that has been provided.

- Jury Instructions/Deliberation: When closing arguments are completed, the judge will provide instructions to the members of the jury about how they should consider the testimony and evidence that has been provided for them The jurors will then retreat to the jury room, where they discuss the case (deliberate) and come up with a verdict.

Proofs

When a lawsuit reaches the trial stage, two different types of proofs are used, the burden of proof, which applies to a person, and the standard of proof, which applies to the evidence.

Burden of Proof In order for someone's lawsuit to be successful, they have to prove whatever claims or statements they are making. This legal requirement of proving claims is known as the burden of proof. The burden of proof identifies the *person* who is held legally responsible for providing the evidence and/or testimony needed to substantiate any claims or statements that are being made. For example, when a plaintiff files a lawsuit, he or she is claiming to have been harmed in some way. Since the plaintiff is making that claim, the plaintiff has the burden of proving that claim in court. It is important to identify who has the burden of proof because of the legal requirements associated with the burden of proof. Any person who has a burden of proof and does not fulfill that burden has not met the legal requirements necessary to substantiate his or her claim. If the party who has a burden of proving its claim does not meet that burden, the other party can move to have the case dismissed. To explain, suppose a patient files a negligence lawsuit against a healthcare worker. The patient, who is the plaintiff, has the burden of proving its claim of negligence. If the patient does not meet that burden, then the defendant healthcare worker, can ask the judge to dismiss the case.

But how does a person know whether he or she will have enough evidence to substantiate a claim? The answer is, by going back to the elements of the law that are contained in the definitional style writing of the law. A plaintiff who has enough evidence to support each of the elements of the law is likely to be successful in his or her lawsuit. However, without enough evidence to support even one aspect of his or her claim, the plaintiff has not met his or her burden of proving the claim.

Concept Connection
Witnesses and Expert Witness
A person who directly observed the event or incident that is focus of the lawsuit is called an eyewitness, which should not be confused with a witness at trial. Sometimes people are called to the stand to talk about relevant issues that pertain to the trial, even though they themselves did not observe the event under consideration. One example is an expert witness, which is commonly called to testify in medical malpractice cases.

Sidebar
The right to self incrimination does not apply to civil cases. The Fifth Amendment to the U.S. Constitution states: "… nor shall be compelled in any **criminal case** to be a witness against himself…." [emphasis added].

Concept Connection
Burden of Proof and Defenses
While the burden of proof typically belongs to the plaintiff, there are times when the burden of proof resides with the defendant instead. The most common occurrence of a defendant's burden of proof occurs when defenses are used.

Standard of Proof The standard of proof is different from the burden of proof. Instead of applying to a person, the standard of proof applies to the *evidence and testimony*. During jury deliberations, the jury will be asked to weigh the evidence and testimony that has been presented at trial. How much weight is given to the evidence and testimony is known as the standard of proof.

Three different standards of proof are used in court.

1. Balance of probabilities (also called *preponderance of the evidence*)
2. Clear and convincing evidence
3. Beyond a reasonable doubt

For civil litigation, the balance of probabilities (preponderance of the evidence (see Fig. 2-6)) is used to weigh the evidence and testimony at trial during jury deliberations. The balance of probabilities asks that you weigh the evidence to determine whether it is true or false, or believable or unbelievable. Or, if you are presented with conflicting testimony or evidence, which is more believable and/or reliable. Put another way, the jury is asked to *balance* whether something is *probably* true or *probably* not true. The other two standards of proof, clear and convincing evidence and beyond a reasonable doubt are only used in criminal cases and do not apply to civil litigation.

Appeals and the American Judicial System

Once a decision has been rendered by the jury and read in court, the decision is final and binding on all parties involved in the lawsuit. At this point, the only option available to counter

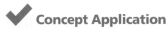

Concept Application

Proofs

In the trial of the century, O. J. Simpson was found *not guilty* of murder (in the criminal case), but found *guilty* of wrongful death (in the civil case). For the most part, both trials relied on the same evidence, the same testimony, and the same witnesses. So why did they end with different results? One of the reasons is that different standards of proof were used in the two cases. In the criminal case, the evidence was weighed using the "beyond a reasonable doubt" standard of proof. But in the civil trial, the evidence was weighed using the "balance of probabilities" standard of proof.

Balance of Probabilities Standard of Proof

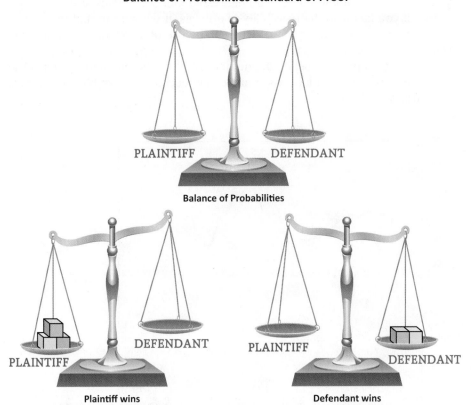

Fig. 2-6 Balance of Probabilities. In civil trial deliberations how the jury determines a verdict.

that decision is to file an appeal. An appeal is a legal procedure that is used to take a decision to a higher court for review.

When considering whether to file an appeal or not, the attorneys review every step that has occurred in the path of the lawsuit. In filing the appeal, the attorney must point to a specific legal error that occurred somewhere during the process of the lawsuit. When writing the appeal, the attorney must point out what the legal error was, why it was an error, and how it *adversely* affected the legal process. This distinction is an important one to make, because appeals can only be based on issues of law—meaning, you cannot appeal just because you disagree with the outcome or verdict.

Lawsuit Alternatives

There are alternatives to filing a lawsuit. At any point during the progression of a lawsuit, the parties can decide to settle their case, and not proceed on to the next step in litigation. In fact, the courts encourage the parties to discuss the possibility of reaching a settlement, in the hopes of avoiding trial. One of the main reasons for encouraging settlements is because of the outcome that occurs at trial: there is one winner and one loser. Having one person win and one person lose usually means that one party is happy with the result and the other party is unhappy. However, by reaching a settlement agreement both parties have the opportunity to walk away happy, or at least partially satisfied with the result. While settlement agreements are most common after a lawsuit is filed, there are alternatives that allow the parties to resolve their disputes without filing a lawsuit.

Alternative Dispute Resolution

Alternative Dispute Resolution (ADR) is a procedure that can be used instead of filing a lawsuit. ADR methods are being used with greater frequency in the United States. While the exact cause for this growth is unknown, one factor may be associated with time constraints. Most lawsuit take between two to five years to reach trial and come to a final resolution. Sometimes, it can be even longer if you factor in the possibility of appeals. If you add to that the cost of hiring an attorney and paying court fees, the use of alternatives to trial may seem like a more viable option.

Contrary to popular belief, the number of lawsuits that actually reach the trial phase in a court of law has dramatically decreased over recent decades. (see Graph 2-1).

Graph 2-1. Number of Tort Cases Resulting in Trial. This graph shows the number of tort cases filed in U.S. District Courts that actually reached trial. (Data compiled from the Administrative Office of the U.S. Courts, Annual Report of the Director, Table C-4 [1962–2002]).

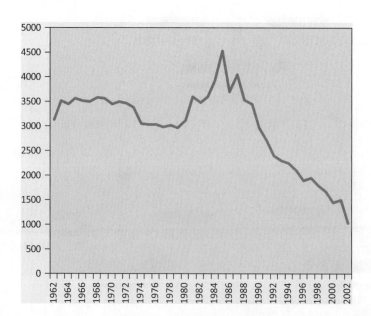

TABLE 2-3

Arbitration and Mediation Comparison

Arbitration	Mediation
May be optional, but is sometimes mandatory.	Always optional, never mandatory.
Is either binding or nonbinding.	Does not apply.
Utilizes a judge-like figure (an arbitrator).	Utilizes a referee (a mediator).
Operates like a court of law.	Operates like a business meeting.
Evidence and testimony is presented.	Evidence and testimony is presented.
Only used in civil cases. Not allowed for criminal cases.	Only used in civil cases. Not allowed for criminal cases.

Gunnar Pippel/Shutterstock

While lawsuits can take a lot of time to reach the trial phase, ADR methods can be completed within weeks or months, depending on the ADR method that is used. There are two types of alternative dispute resolution: **arbitration** and **mediation**. Table 2-3 provides a comparison.

Arbitration

Arbitration is very similar to what occurs at a trial. Instead of having a judge, there is an arbitrator—a neutral, unbiased person who acts like a judge. After listening to the evidence and testimony provided by both parties, the arbitrator renders a decision. In a court of law, the verdict is final, and both parties must adhere to the decision. But in arbitration, whether the parties adhere to the decision of the arbitrator, depends on the type of arbitration that the parties enter into. There are two types of arbitration, binding arbitration and nonbinding arbitration.

Binding Arbitration By entering into binding arbitration, the parties are agreeing to be bound to the decision of the arbitrator. That means, whatever decision the arbitrator reaches, each party is legally required to follow it. Because the parties entered into binding arbitration willingly, any lawsuit that is filed afterwards will likely be dismissed by the judge.

Nonbinding Arbitration Nonbinding arbitration means that neither side has to accept the decision of the arbitrator. Instead, they can either agree to accept the decision of the arbitration or reject it. If both parties agree to the arbitrator's decision, they will enter a settlement agreement. But, if both parties do not agree to the arbitrator's decision, they are free to file a civil lawsuit. Because the arbitration is *non*-binding, there is no restriction on filing a lawsuit.

So why use nonbinding arbitration if the parties can file a lawsuit? Nonbinding arbitration is usually used as a guide, to determine what an outcome *might be* if a case were to go to trial. It provides information, such as the strengths and/or weakness of a case, or what the opposing parties' trial strategy might be. In addition, arbitration can

arbitration: a process using a neutral, unbiased third party to make a final decision about a dispute

mediation: a process using a neutral party who gets the parties to work together to resolve their differences

 Beyond the Scope

There are rare exceptions when a judge might consider a lawsuit even though the parties have entered into a binding arbitration agreement. When this exception occurs is beyond the scope of this text.

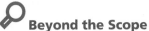 **Concept Connection**

Alternatives to Trial and Contracts

Both settlement agreements and binding arbitration are legal contracts. The formation of a contract is an essential component to arbitration agreements.

The Ethics of Law

Binding Arbitration

Another reason for the growth of alternative dispute resolution is that sometimes it may be a plaintiff's only option because they are legally precluded from filing a lawsuit. Most businesses have *mandatory*, or *binding*, arbitration clauses in the contracts that they use. For example, when you sign up for a credit card or apply for insurance, (both types of contracts) there is typically a clause in the contract stating that you agree to the use of binding arbitration and forego your right to file a lawsuit. To complicate matters, most companies that use binding arbitration clauses get to choose the arbitrator that will be used.

- Can you foresee any problems with the company selecting the arbitrator?
- Is this a fair process?
- Should a person be able to give up their right to file a lawsuit?

Legal Alert!

While settlement agreements in criminal cases (known as plea bargains) are commonplace; the courts strictly forbid the use of mediation or arbitration in criminal cases.

be completed in a short amount of time, so the parties do not have to wait for a judicial outcome.

Mediation

Mediation is another type of alternative dispute resolution. With mediation, the mediator works with the parties to reach a decision. Instead of listening to the parties and issuing a ruling, the mediator uses his or her skill to get the parties to work together in resolving their differences. The mediator usually starts by trying to find some common ground that both parties can agree to, and then work toward a resolution. If the mediator is successful in getting the parties to agree, a settlement agreement will be signed by the parties. If the mediator is unsuccessful, and the parties cannot agree, they are free to involve the courts to settle their differences. Because of how mediation works, mediation is not referred to as binding or nonbinding.

Make FALSE statements TRUE.

Rewrite the false statements below by replacing the bolded, italicized, and underlined word(s) to make it a true statement.

1. A ***civil law*** is any crime that is punishable by serving more than one year in jail or prison.

   _____

2. If a patient is suing a healthcare worker, the lawsuit will cite the patient as the ***plaintiff***.

   _____

3. Because of ***civil laws***, only certain lawsuits can be filed in only specific courts.

   _____

4. A person can ***file a lawsuit*** either through registered mail or a process server.

   _____

5. The only type of alternative dispute resolution that is binding or nonbinding is ***mediation***.

   _____

Circle Exercise

Circle the correct word from the choices given.

1. The focus of (**criminal laws, civil laws, arbitration**) is to maintain order between individuals.

2. Fortunately for us, (**apodictic, casuistry, definitional**) law writing makes identifying the legal elements of a law relatively easy.

3. To apply the law to the facts, we turn the elements into (**fill-in-the-blank, multiple choice, yes or no**) questions.

4. The only standard of proof that is used in civil cases is (**balance of probabilities, clear and convincing evidence, beyond a reasonable doubt**).

5. Only people who are a party to a lawsuit are involved in (**depositions, interrogatory, criminal laws**).

Matching

Match the numbered term to its lettered definition.

1. _____ arbitration

2. _____ civil laws

3. _____ defendant

4. _____ deposition

5. _____ interrogatories

6. _____ jurisdiction

7. _____ mediation

8. _____ perjury

9. _____ plaintiff

A. a formal set of written questions provided to opposing parties in a lawsuit that help attorneys discover facts about the case.

B. a law that covers the rights and remedies of individuals.

C. a process using a neutral party who gets the parties to work together to resolve their differences.

D. a process using a neutral, unbiased third party to make a final decision about a dispute.

E. intentionally lying under oath; a criminal offense for making a knowingly false statement under oath.

F. the authority provided to a court to preside (exercise authority) over specific legal matters.

G. the party who brings a civil claim of wrongdoing against another party; or, in criminal prosecutions, the state, district, or federal government.

H. the person accused of wrongdoing in a civil case; or the person charges with a crime in criminal prosecutions.

I. the taking of testimony of a witness, under oath, by an attorney before a trial.

Deliberations: Critical Thinking Questions

Question 1: Prosecutors have sole discretion on whether criminal charges are brought. While individual citizens can press charges against someone, that is not a guarantee that the prosecutor will agree and file criminal charges. Is that fair? Do you think that an individual citizen should be able to file criminal charges against another citizen?

Question 2: When performing a legal analysis, the law requires that all of the elements be satisfied in order for someone to break the law. Do you think that the law should be changed to only require one element to be satisfied in order to find someone guilty? Why or why not?

Question 3: People who are found to have broken a civil law can only be asked to pay a monetary fine. But what if they are unable to pay; what happens then? Does this allow a person who cannot pay the ability to break the law without suffering any consequences?

Question 4: If you and another person are involved in a legal dispute, and want to utilize alternative dispute resolution, which method would you choose? Do you think that mediation or arbitration is better? Explain your answer.

Question 5: The law of perjury applies to answering deposition questions, interrogatories, and testifying in court. But even though the law exists, do you think that everyone is always honest in those regards? Is there anything that the court can do to ensure that people's answers are truthful?

Closing Arguments: Case Analysis

Remember the scenario we used to analyze assault (pg 20)? We can use that same scenario to analyze battery as well. Mr. Jones, convalescing after hip surgery was trying to get out of bed. Ned the nursing assistant grabbed a pair of restraints and showing them to Mr. Jones said: "If you do not stay in bed I'm going to have to restrain you."

Under the common law: *Anyone who intentionally causes physical harm, which results in damages, is guilty of battery.*

Question 1: What are the two elements required for a person to be guilty of committing battery?

Question 2: Using the elements of the law of battery, turn each element into a yes or no question. Then, after reviewing the scenario determine whether the elements apply to Ned's actions.

Question 3: Is Ned likely or not likely to be found guilty of committing battery? Why or why not?

The Briefcase

This section repeats the objectives from the beginning of the chapter and provides a summary of the most important concepts for each objective. Use this section as a quick review and to check your understanding of the chapter's key points.

Objective 1: Describe the difference between criminal law and civil laws.
- Criminal laws:
  - actions that the legislature determines is a crime.
  - a punishment can include being sent to prison or jail.
  - charges can only be brought by a prosecutor
  - individuals cannot bring criminal charges against another individual.
- Civil laws
  - actions that the law will not allow when it occurs between individuals.
  - punishment is provided in the form of monetary award; there is no jail or prison.
  - civil lawsuits can be brought by any citizen.

Objective 2: Give an example of a civil law subcategory that can impact healthcare.
- See Table 2-2 on pg 19.

Objective 3: List the steps involved in a legal analysis.
- identifying the law's elements.
- applying the facts to the law.
- determining the outcome.

Objective 4: Identify who the parties are in a lawsuit.
- Plaintiff: the person who brings the lawsuit.
- Defendant: the person who is being sued in the lawsuit.

Objective 5: List the steps involved in a civil lawsuit.
- A wrong or injury occurs.
- The wrong or injury is discovered.
- The lawsuit is filed.
- The parties involved are notified.
- A pretrial conference occurs.
- The lawsuit proceeds to trial.

Objective 6: Provide an explanation of what jurisdiction gives a court of law.
- hear a case
- decide the issues
- make a decision
- enforce the application of law

Objective 7: Explain what interrogatories and depositions are and how they are used.
- Tools that are used by attorneys to find out information regarding their case.
- Interrogatories
  - Written questions that must be answered.
  - Leaving a question blank results in a yes answer.
  - Only parties to a lawsuit (plaintiff(s) and defendant(s)) answer interrogatories.
  - The law of perjury applies.
- Depositions
  - Testimony provided in person before the attorneys.
  - Anyone who may be called as a witness at trial can be deposed.
  - Objections can be raised, but the question must still be answered.

Objective 8: Describe the difference types of proof and when they are used.
- Burden of proof
  - Addresses question of law.
  - Can only be answered by a judge.
  - Determines which party (plaintiff or defendant) is required to prove their claim.
- Standard of proof
  - Addresses questions of fact.
  - Is answered by the jury.
  - Determines whether testimony or evidence is true/false or believable.
  - Three different types.
  - Balance of probabilities (used in civil trials)
  - Clear and convincing evidence (used in criminal trials)
  - Beyond a reasonable doubt (used in criminal trails)

Objective 9: Compare and contrast the different alternative dispute resolution methods.
- Settlement agreements.
- Arbitration
  - Binding arbitration
  - Nonbinding arbitration
- Mediation

Maximize Your Success with the Companion Website

The companion website to this textbook contains materials that can help you better understand the concepts presented in this chapter. Go to www.myhealthprofessionskit.com and click "Chapter 2.":

Web Links
- sample quizzes
- related web links
- learning games
- and more…

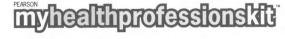

3

Working in the Healthcare Profession

The healthcare profession is unique. When patients seek treatment for their illnesses or injuries, they are often asked to expose some of the most personal and intimate parts of their bodies. They might be uncomfortable doing this in front of strangers. To complicate matters they may have their bodies touched, poked, and prodded, which can be humiliating and embarrassing, not to mention sometimes painful. In addition, patients might be asked to talk about things that are normally not discussed with strangers, such as moods, feelings, bodily functions, or sexual practices. Because of this personal involvement, healthcare professionals face situations not often seen in other professions. This chapter will explore what it takes to work in the healthcare environment and some of the laws that govern employment.

MEASURE YOUR PROGRESS: LEARNING OBJECTIVES

After studying this chapter, you will be able to:

- List the qualities needed to work in healthcare.

- Explain what defensive medicine is and how it relates to the practice of medicine.

- Define the importance that professional organizations have on the healthcare profession.

- Distinguish the difference between Medical Practice Acts and Medical Boards.

- Describe what the EEOC is and what areas of employment it governs.

- Define what the ADA is and how it protects employees.

- List the two areas covered by OSHA that have a direct impact on working in healthcare.

- Give an example of why a person might file a Workers' Compensation claim.

- List some of the reasons an employee may utilize FMLA.

KEY TERMS

certification

codes of ethics

credentialing

defensive medicine

licensure

medical practice acts

professional

reciprocity

standards of care

PROFESSIONAL HIGHLIGHT

Joan is the director for Community Health programs and services at the local community college. As part of her job, she counsels students on the different health programs that the school offers. To provide the information that students need to make a decision about which program to enter, Joan needs to have an understanding of the different types of credentials that are used in healthcare and the qualities that are required of healthcare professionals. This information will help students decide what type of healthcare professional they might want to become.

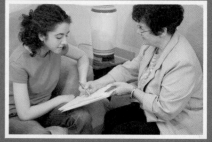

Lisa F Young/Shutterstock

Anyone who desires to work in the healthcare field has a variety of different professions to choose from. But even with all of the variety, there are basic characteristics that all healthcare professionals share. Regardless of which healthcare profession you choose to go into, they all require some form of academics and skill training. The different skills that each profession requires depends on the profession you have chosen to pursue. Besides academics, some healthcare professions need to fulfill additional requirements, such as obtaining a license or passing a certification exam. But before we get into the differences for each of the healthcare professions, we can start our discussion about the qualities that each of the healthcare professions share.

> The words *practice* and *professional* are used in healthcare, but how can a person practice at something and be a professional at the same time?

Qualities of a Successful Healthcare Practitioner

To be successful, all healthcare professionals need to be proficient in two vitally important skills: the technical skills associated with healthcare and the people skills that are needed when taking care of patients.

Technical Skills

Every profession requires the performance of particular technical skills. The healthcare profession that you choose to enter into will determine not only what technical skills you will be taught, but which technical skills you will be allowed to perform. Depending on the career you have chosen, these technical skills may include:

- administering medications,
- assessing patients and their conditions,
- identifying instruments,
- operating equipment,
- performing medical or surgical procedures, or
- taking and/or reading diagnostic images.

Technical skills are taught in a classroom setting, utilizing a combination of foundational knowledge and instructions. For example, in order to learn the technical skills that you need to take care of a patient with appendicitis, you first need an understanding of anatomy and physiology. Once that foundation has been learned, you then use that knowledge to learn the technical skills your profession requires. To continue our example: a radiology student will learn how to take images of the appendix; a surgical technologist student will learn what instruments a surgeon will need to operate on an appendix; and a nurse will learn the medications a patient with appendicitis might need to have administered.

People Skills

Most people who enter the healthcare profession already have the foundational people skills needed to work in healthcare (see Fig. 3-1). This usually comes from the caring nature of those who enter the healthcare field,

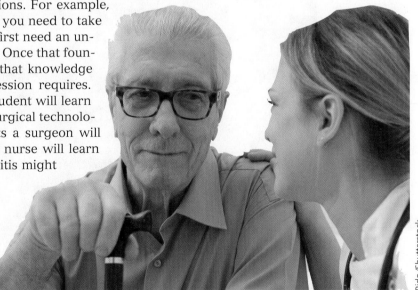

Fig. 3-1. Showing empathy is an essential skill in the healthcare profession.

Rido/Shutterstock

because most genuinely want to help people and assist those in need. People skills, sometimes referred to as *emotional intelligence*, include:

1. building the self-esteem of others
2. showing empathy for others
3. communicating effectively:
   a. by asking productive questions,
   b. demonstrating effective listening skills, and
   c. responding appropriately to emotional statements.

These three qualities are an essential component for the successful and compassionate practice of medicine.

The Practice of Medicine

Normally the public thinks that practicing medicine is limited to doctors, but it is really true of all healthcare professionals (see Fig. 3-2). The idea behind the *practice* of medicine is that medicine is not an exact science but instead something that is continually learned and fine-tuned. For example, the same treatments do not always work on all patients and not all diseases have the same outcome in all patients. Healthcare professionals will use the information that they learn from each patient to build a knowledge base that can only come with experience. The idea of *practicing* medicine, therefore, means that even though you have learned the foundations and technical skills that you need, you are still practicing to fine-tune those skills with every patient that you take care of.

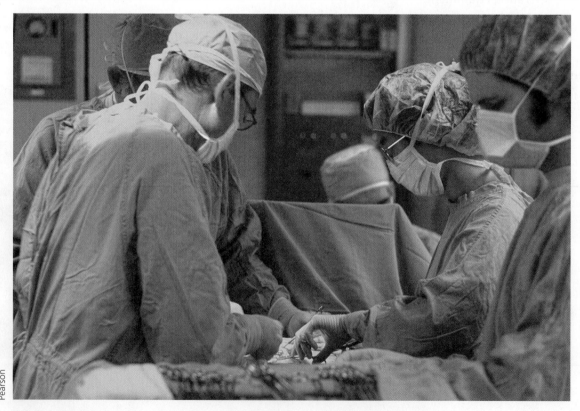

Pearson

Fig. 3-2. A surgical team practices its surgical skill on a patient in the operating room.

The main focus driving the practice of medicine in the past has been on the patient. We learn what one patient needs in order to determine what might help the next patient. But in today's litigious society, healthcare practitioners also need to focus on themselves when practicing medicine by including **defensive medicine** as part of their patient care.

The practice of defensive medicine is a direct result of the legal environment in which healthcare operates. It is no longer enough to perform the medical tests and treatments that a patient's condition requires. Instead, healthcare practitioners must also perform the medical tests and treatments that will protect the healthcare worker from lawsuits.

For example, if a patient were to slip and fall on the ice and complain of wrist pain and swelling, he or she will probably seek medical treatment. In the past, that medical treatment would consist of getting an X-ray and, depending on the result, possibly a cast, splint, or sling. But today, with the guise of defensive medicine, the patient will likely not only have an X-ray, but an electrocardiogram (EKG) or a head computed tomography (CT) scan, and possibly a complete blood count (CBC) as well. Why are these tests necessary in today's healthcare arena? What would an EKG, head CT, or blood work have to do with a wrist injury? The answers to these questions address a potential lawsuit, and not necessarily the patient's injury. Could the patient have hit their head when they fell? Could the cause of the fall have been from a stroke or a heart attack? While they have little to do with the actual injury to the wrist, these diagnostic procedures may be performed as a part of defensive medicine, to treat potential lawsuits instead of actual injuries.

Professions and Professional

Up to this point, we have talked about the technical skills and people skills that you need to practice medicine. The combination of these skills and how you use them distinguishes you as a **professional**.

The expertise, or how well crafted your technical and people skills are, will help you become a more experienced and seasoned professional. Even though you may just be starting your career, you still have special knowledge and expertise that makes you unique, because of the training, education, and experience that you have gained through your educational endeavors. Although you might not have a lot of experience at this point, you are still considered a professional.

Concept Connection
Practice and Malpractice/Negligence
The *practice* of medicine is one of the key differences between negligence and malpractice. Malpractice is often referred to as professional negligence.

---

defensive medicine: the type of medical practice used by healthcare workers to protect themselves against potential lawsuits

professional: a person who earns a living through the expertise of his or her work

---

Sidebar
Many healthcare practitioners are including lawsuits as a type of symptom that every patient has. Because the potential for lawsuits exist, including lawsuits as a symptom for every patient, reminds healthcare practitioners to consider when a lawsuit might occur so they can incorporate that symptom into their treatment plan.

Concept Connection
Defensive Medicine and Lawsuits
The defensive approach to the evaluation and treatment of patients is now commonplace in medicine. It directly addresses one of the first issues in the development of a lawsuit: a wrong or injury occurs. By preventing wrongs or injuries from occurring, utilizing defensive medicine, we can potentially stop a lawsuit from occurring in the first place.

Professional Organizations

When a student graduates from a school or program, his or her education is only beginning. Once a person graduates and starts working, he or she will continually learn additional and more advanced skills. To assist in that knowledge and growth, professional organizations exist to help further the profession. Professional organizations are associations of professional people who work to assist and advance the profession.

Professional organizations offer a variety of different resources, tools, services, and support for the professions they govern. But how do professional organizations get authority to govern a particular profession? The answer depends on the service the professional organization offers to the profession.

Many professional organizations focus on the educational aspect of their particular profession. They accomplish this goal by setting standards that an educational institution must follow if they want to offer a specific program. For example, the National League of Nursing (NLN), a professional organization for nurses, accredits colleges that offer nursing programs. The NLN receives authority to certify nursing programs by the U.S. Department of Education. But why is this relevant? One of the requirements that a person has to have when applying for licensure is to provide evidence that they have graduated from an accredited program. If the program is not accredited by the appropriate professional organization, the person will be unable to apply for licensure.

Another aspect of professional organizations, that specifically address some important health law considerations, is that professional organizations often write rules and standards for all members of the profession to follow. Those rules and standards are written in the form of **Standards of Care** and a **Code of Ethics**.

standards of care: written requirements that detail the responsibilities a professional will be held accountable for in the performance of his or her duties

code of ethics: written statements that detail the type of behavior a professional should strive toward when performing his or her professional duties

Standards of Care

All healthcare professions have at least one professional organization that publishes a standard of care. The organizations, in writing these standards of care, are detailing what minimal requirements they are going to hold a person practicing in that profession accountable to. Because these standards provide minimal requirements, they are most often written using generic and simple statements. For example, "The healthcare professional collects patient health data" is a standard of care typically found in most healthcare professionals' standard of care. By keeping things generic, a variety of different activities can be included in one standard (kind of similar to definitional law writing).

Codes of Ethics

Codes of ethics are similar to standards of care, but differ in that they describe the type of conduct a person practicing in that profession should have. As with standards of care, each profession has at least one professional organization that publishes a Code of Ethics.

⚙ Understanding Your Profession

To find some of the professional organizations that govern your chosen profession, check out the companion website at www.myhealthprofessionskit.com for links to your professional organization.

∅ Concept Connection
Standards of Care/Code of Ethics and Malpractice

Standards of Care and Codes of Ethics play an essential role in how malpractice is analyzed. Part of performing a legal analysis of malpractice, includes looking at the profession's Standard of Care and/or Code of Ethics.

Court Case

Corley v. State

749 So.2d 926 (La.App. Cir 2) (1999)
Louisiana Court of Appeals

FACTS: In 1978, Walter Corley was diagnosed with neurofibromatosis, a genetic disorder where nerve tissue grows tumors. In 1988, he started to develop low back pain, which he sought medical treatment for at E.A. Conway, a teaching hospital that is part of Louisiana State University. Throughout his many visits at E.A. Conway, Corley saw a total of four different doctors for his low back pain. Treatments concentrated on his back pain, with rare mention of his neurofibromatosis. Late in 1988 Corley developed shortness of breath and was diagnosed with bronchitis. A month later, with continued shortness of breath and marked weight loss, a very large mass was discovered in Corley's right chest. Mr. Corley passed away a few months later. Mr. Corley's wife and son filed a medical malpractice and wrongful death lawsuit against the hospital, the doctors, Louisiana State University, and the State of Louisiana.

ISSUE: At issue in this case was whether the doctors at E.A. Conway adhered to the standard of care for their profession. The plaintiff's expert, Dr. Schoendinger, noted "a physician who had a patient with neurofibromatosis should provide that patient with a general description of the disease process and possible symptoms, including the potential for malignant degeneration of neurofibromas." Failure to do so would, in Dr. Schoendinger's opinion, constitute a breach of the standard of care. The defendant's expert witnesses, most of whom were doctors and specialists employed by E.A. Conway, testified that the doctors followed the Standard of Care.

RULE: "Considering the above conflicting testimony, we cannot say that the trial court committed manifest error in finding that the physicians at E.A. Conway deviated from the applicable standard of care in their diagnosis and treatment of Walter Corley."

EMPHASIS: The importance of this case, for our present discussion, is to demonstrate how Standards of Care play an important role in medical malpractice cases. A professional's Standard of Care provides a baseline threshold that healthcare professionals will be held accountable for. The court stated in their opinion that "The physician will not be held to a standard of perfection nor evaluated with benefit of hindsight." And, "Physicians are obligated to rule out these imminent, serious and life-threatening causes first. Failure to eliminate these causes can subject a patient to a foreseeable risk of harm and would further constitute a breach of the applicable standard(s) of care."

Most professional organizations are national organizations. They publish national standards and codes that anyone in the country working in that particular profession must follow. In addition to these national standards and codes, there may be state level organizations, or even local organizations that might have additional standards and codes for a professional to follow.

State Medical Practice Acts and State Medical Boards

Under Article 4 of the U.S. Constitution, each state is free to operate independently, as a sovereign entity, as long as their actions and laws are not contrary to federal laws or interfere with another state's autonomy. One example is our current discussion concerning healthcare professions. If no federal law exists regarding healthcare, then each state is free to write their own laws describing how they want healthcare to function within their state.

At some point in your state's history, the state legislature wrote a **Medical Practice Act**.

While the requirements outlined in each state's Medical Practice Act will differ from state to state, all Medical Practice Acts have three things in common, they:

- create a medical board (or agency) that oversees healthcare delivery in the state, (see Fig. 3-3).

- write policies and procedures that dictate how healthcare is delivered in the state, and

- determine the scope of healthcare delivery and practice.

medical practice acts: laws that a state has passed to determine the requirements for healthcare and healthcare professionals

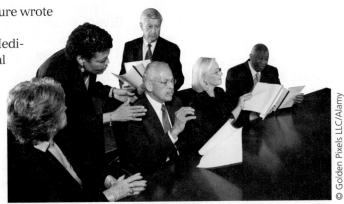

Fig. 3-3. Medical boards are made up of professionals, elected officials, and citizens.

© Golden Pixels LLC/Alamy

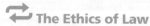
Understanding Your State

To find your state's medical board, check out the map of the United States on the companion website.

The Ethics of Law

Medical Boards

The rules and regulations written by the medical board of each state have the full force and effect of law, which the courts will uphold as law.

- But how can the medical board write laws, a power that is provided exclusively to the legislature?
- Should a nonlegislative body be able to write laws?
- Why would the courts uphold laws written by a nonlegislative body?

Create a Medical Board

The first part of your state's medical practice act will include language that creates a medical board. The medical practice act also defines the purpose and scope of the medical board and provides them with authority to write rules and regulations regarding the delivery of healthcare in the state. Part of those rules will determine:

- what the requirements are for entering the healthcare profession,
- what the requirements are for working as a healthcare professional, and
- how healthcare is delivered within the state.

Write Policies and Procedures

The medical board in each state is granted authority by the state's Medical Practice Act to write rules and regulations that govern healthcare within the state. The policies and procedures written by a state's medical board cover every aspect of healthcare. Of main importance for our current discussion about working in healthcare are the laws a state's medical board will write regarding the credentialing and scope of practice for healthcare professions within the state.

Determine the Scope of Practice Healthcare Delivery and Practice

One area of law that is not regulated at the federal level is the credentialing process and scope of practice for each of the different healthcare professions. Each state sets its own credentialing requirements because the **credentialing** of healthcare professionals is not regulated by the federal government.

credentialing: validation of an individual's background and qualifications, or fulfillment of the requirements established by the organization granting the verification

Credentialing: Certification and Licensure

While there are several different types of credentials, the two most commonly used in healthcare are certification and licensure (see Table 3-1).

Licensure The most commonly known type of credentialing process used in healthcare is **licensure**.

Obtaining a driver's license is an every day example of licensure. Each state has its own laws regarding the requirements a person must meet in order to obtain a driver's license. In most states, the applicant must pass a written exam and demonstrate proficiency by taking a hands-on driving test. Once a person has met the requirements, he or she is issued a driver's license. By issuing that license, the state is granting that person the authority to drive a motor vehicle on public roads.

licensure: a credentialing process where a person is granted the authority to perform particular tasks or skills, after demonstrating expertise

The process for obtaining a license in healthcare is relatively the same. Anyone who wants to obtain a healthcare license—such as a radiology technologist license, for example—has to meet the requirements established by the state for a radiology technologist license. The radiology technologist license, just like a driver's license, allows the professional to work as a radiology technologist within the state. But how do we know which healthcare professions require a license? That determination is made by the state.

All states in the United States require doctors and nurses to obtain a license. For other healthcare professions, the need for a license differs from state to state. For example, some states require massage therapists to be licensed, while some states do not. To determine what healthcare professions require licenses, consult your state's medical board. If a state requires licensure of a healthcare profession, then obtaining a license is mandatory in order to practice in that profession.

In addition to the requirements for obtaining a license, each state's medical practice act will include the procedures used for revoking or suspending a professional license. Just like a person's driver's license can be suspended, so too can a person's professional license. While statistics vary from state to state, the most common reasons for revocation of a professional license are:

- illegal activity (committing a misdemeanor or a felon, the most common having to do with the use of illegal drugs)
- not maintaining professional standards (staying up to date on continuing education)
- violating a profession's standards of care and codes of ethics

Certification Another type of credentialing used in healthcare is certification.

While the requirements for licensure are spelled out in a state's medical practice act and policies from the state medical board, the requirements for certification are determined by the person or institution issuing the certificate. Sometimes, the person or institution issuing the certificate has complete discretion over what the qualifying criteria is going to be. But for most certifications, like those used in healthcare, the criteria for obtaining a certificate can come from a variety of different sources. For example, most schools offer programs for certified medical assistants (CMA) or certified nursing assistants (CNA). The school, in offering those programs, will determine what the requirements are for issuing the certification. But, in doing so, it must adhere to requirements from other organizations, such as the Accrediting Bureau of Health Education Schools (ABHES) and the Commission on Accreditation of Allied Health Education Programs (CAAHEP) that accredit health educational programs.

Registration Some healthcare professionals are referred to as being registered, but registration is not a separate credentialing process. Instead, registration is a special designation that is used to differentiate members of the same profession. For example, both licensed practical nurses (LPNs) and Registered Nurses (RNs) are nurses, and each require a license. But there are some technical skills that a state will authorize RNs to perform but LPNs cannot. To differentiate which group of nurses has been authorized to perform those specific technical skills, the names of the nurses who are

certification: a credentialing process that confirms or guarantees that specific knowledge has been obtained or that a person has proven proficiency in a task or skill or demonstrated expertise in a particular area

Court Case

Poignon v. Ohio Board of Pharmacy

2004-Ohio-2709
Court of Appeals of Ohio Tenth Appellate District

FACTS: Daniel Poignon was a licensed pharmacist in the state of Ohio. During his employment for Rite Aid pharmacy, Poignon stole 1,888 units of drugs. Following his conviction of two felony counts of theft, the Ohio Board of Pharmacy suspended his license. While Poignon was given an opportunity to file an appeal, he missed the deadline. In accordance with Rule 4729-9-01(E) of the Ohio Administrative Code, the suspension/revocation of a license is permanent against both the license and licensee (the person who holds the license). Three years later, Poignon applied to the Ohio Board of Pharmacy for a pharmacist's license. The Board, in response to Poignon's application replied: "In short, your license was revoked, and that revocation is permanent as to you as well. Accordingly, we cannot process your application." Mr. Poignon filed suit asking the court to

force the board to process his application; or, in the alternative, providing him with an administrative hearing.

ISSUE: The issue before the court was whether Ohio's Board of Pharmacy had the right to *permanently* revoke a pharmacy license.

RULE: "[T]he board is not required to process relator's (plaintiff's) application or to hold a hearing on his application to be relicensed as a pharmacist in the state of Ohio inasmuch as the board has previously permanently revoked relator's (plaintiff's) pharmacy license."

EMPHASIS: The importance of this case is multifaceted. First and foremost, that illegal activity can result in revocation of a professional license. Second, and more related to our current discussion, that State Medical Boards have the authority to determine the criteria for licensure within the state. That determination includes not only the requirements for issuing a license, but when and how a license can be revoked or suspended.

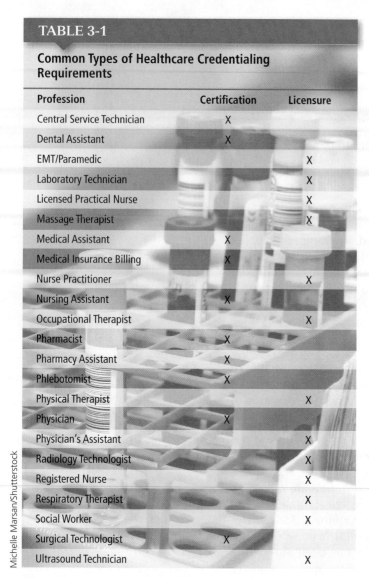

TABLE 3-1

Common Types of Healthcare Credentialing Requirements

Profession	Certification	Licensure
Central Service Technician	X	
Dental Assistant	X	
EMT/Paramedic		X
Laboratory Technician		X
Licensed Practical Nurse		X
Massage Therapist		X
Medical Assistant	X	
Medical Insurance Billing	X	
Nurse Practitioner		X
Nursing Assistant	X	
Occupational Therapist		X
Pharmacist	X	
Pharmacy Assistant	X	
Phlebotomist	X	
Physical Therapist		X
Physician	X	
Physician's Assistant		X
Radiology Technologist		X
Registered Nurse		X
Respiratory Therapist		X
Social Worker		X
Surgical Technologist	X	
Ultrasound Technician		X

Michelle Marsan/Shutterstock

reciprocity: the requirements established for the exchange of credentials from one state to another

authorized are placed on separate list (a registry), which classifies them as Registered Nurses.

Reciprocity Before we leave the topic of credentialing, we need to discuss a related topic, **reciprocity**.

Each individual state has the authority to set its own requirements for credentialing. But what if you obtain your credentials in one state, and then sometime later want to move to another state? Do you have to go through the entire educational and credentialing process all over again? Unfortunately the answer is, "It depends." Because each state sets its own requirements for entering the healthcare field, you will have to meet those requirements in order to practice medicine in that state. While the requirements for the different healthcare professions are pretty much standardized, there are some differences from state to state. Sometimes the state that you are moving to, after verifying your credentials, will simply issue you a license to practice. But, some states may require you to take additional classes or may require that you retake the licensure or certification exam. You need to contact that state's medical board and find out what its reciprocity policy is to find out the requirements.

Scope of Practice

Is anyone who enters the healthcare profession allowed to perform any medical procedure simply because he or she is a healthcare professional? The obvious answer is of course not. But with all of the different healthcare professions, how is a person suppose to know what each healthcare professional is allowed to do or not allowed to do? The answer to this question is determined by looking at that professional's scope of practice.

A profession's scope of practice sets the legal boundaries that each profession is authorized by law to perform. What those boundaries are is determined by the state Medical Board and Practice Acts. Instead of reinventing the wheel, most state medical boards determine

Court Case

Guanzon v. State Medical Board of Ohio

123 Ohio App.3d 489 (1997)
Court of Appeals of Ohio, County of Ohio, Tenth District, Franklin

FACTS: Dr. Noel A. Guanzon was a licensed physician in the state of West Virginia. On June 21, 1994, Guanzon applied for licensure in the state of Ohio. Prior to submitting his Ohio application, Guanzon was notified by the state of West Virginia that a patient had filed a complaint against him. He was ordered to appear before the West Virginia Board of Medicine's complaint committee. Instead of facing disciplinary action, Guanzon surrendered his West Virginia medical license. During the proceedings by West Virginia, his application for an Ohio licensure was approved. However, one year later, the Ohio Medical Board revoked Guanzon's license as well (presumably after being notified

by the state of West Virginia). Dr. Guanzon appealed the Ohio Medical Board's decision.

ISSUE: Did the Ohio medical board have a right to suspend a license based on actions by another state's medical board?

RULE: The court concluded that "Dr. Guanzon's conduct constitutes "fraud, misrepresentation, [and] deception in applying for or securing any license or certificate issued by the board..."

EMPHASIS: While the majority of this case focused on procedural rules, the emphasis for our current discussion relates to reciprocity. Each state sets their own requirements for licensure in their state. Part of applying for reciprocity will include listing any licenses that you have held in any state, and whether you have ever had your license suspended or revoked.

a profession's scope of practice by starting with the professional organization's Standards of Care. Since the baseline has already been established, states can use that as a foundation to write more stringent requirements if they so choose.

Working Outside Your Scope of Practice

When a state writes a professional scope of practice, it includes the technical skills that a professional is allowed to perform independently. But what about technical skills that are not included in your scope of practice? Can a healthcare professional perform technical skills as long as someone who is authorized to perform that skill supervises them? The short answer is no; absolutely not, never under any circumstances. Now for the long answer.

State medical boards write healthcare credentialing and scope of practice laws to protect the public. A person who seeks medical care, does not always have the time to verify whether a person is licensed or what their scope of practice is. Because patients blindly put their trust in healthcare provider's hands, the law wants to make sure that trust is not violated by allowing nonauthorized healthcare professional to provide medical care that they are not licensed to provide. At some time in your career, a person you are working with may ask you to do something that is outside of your scope of practice. Just because someone asks you to do something, (even if they are higher up than you) does not mean that you can. The person asking may not know what you are authorized and are not authorized to do.

The law requires that as a professional you know what your scope of practice is. The law puts the emphasis on you knowing your boundaries, instead of others. Think of it this way, we cannot expect every healthcare professional to know all of the rules, regulations, scope of practice, and limitations of each and every healthcare profession. Instead, the law requires that each person know what their scope of practice is and not step outside of it. Because; under the law, *you* are legally required to know what your scope of practice is, if you step outside of your scope of practice, you run the risk not only of losing your credentials but exposing yourself to a potential lawsuit.

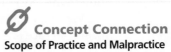

Concept Connection

Scope of Practice and Malpractice

A person who works outside of their scope of practice alters how malpractice is analyzed. If a person steps outside of his or her scope of practice, we do not use the standards of care of the person's profession, but instead use the standards of care of the profession that person stepped into to determine if malpractice has occurred.

Court Case

O'Sullivan v. Mallon

390 A.2d 149, 160 N.J.Super. 416
New Jersey Superior Court, Law Division (1978)

FACTS: The plaintiff was employed by the defendants as an x-ray technician. During her employment, the plaintiff states that she was ordered to perform catheterizations, which she refused to do. The plaintiff claims that she informed her employer that she did not have the proper training or education to perform such a procedure, and that catheterizations could only be performed by licensed nurses and doctors. The x-ray technician was discharged from her employment and filed a lawsuit against her employer.

ISSUE: At issue in the case was whether an employee has the right to discharge an employee who refuses to perform an illegal act.

RULE: "[E]mployment at will may not be terminated by an employer in retaliation for an employee's refusal to perform an illegal act. This rule is especially cogent where the subject matter is the administration of medical treatment, an area in which the public has a foremost interest and which is extensively regulated by various state agencies."

EMPHASIS: While this is an employment case, it demonstrates the importance of working within your scope of practice and knowing what your limitations are. After the x-ray technician's discharge, "the New Jersey Board of Medical Examiners concluded that such an act performed by her would be in violation of the Medical Practice Act. . . .the State Board of Nursing issued a cease and desist order to these defendants forbidding the performance of catheterizations by persons not licensed as nurses." The main issue of this case, for our present discussion, is that you cannot *just follow orders*. Only a state medical board has the authority to determine what your scope of practice is.

> I know that I'm probably going to have to work over-time at some point. Are there specific laws that relate to employment that I need to know about?

Employment Law

One of the specialty areas of law is employment law, which covers issues related to employment and the employer/employee relationship. While there are no specific employment laws that cover only healthcare issues, there are many different employment laws that apply to anyone working in the United States. Employment laws can be broken down into three areas:

- applying for a job
- working on the job, and
- losing a job.

Eployment Laws: Applying for a Job

Anyone who applies for a job has the legal right to be considered for that position based on the merits or their ability to perform the job's requirements. There are several laws, governmental agencies, and federal programs that ensure that legal right is maintained.

Equal Employment Opportunity Commission (EEOC)

Hiring decisions should be based on a person's ability to perform the job that they are applying for. Unfortunately though, discrimination in hiring practices occurs. In 1964, with the passage of the Civil Rights Act, the federal government created the EEOC to fight discrimination in the workplace. The EEOC is charged with enforcing the federal laws that prohibit discrimination in the workplace, which included both the public and the private sector.

While the initial concept for creating the EEOC was to fight discrimination based on race and gender, the list has since been expanded to include:

- age
- disability
- national origin
- pregnancy
- race
- religion
- sex

While the EEOC investigates complaints concerning workplace discrimination, it readily admits that most forms of discrimination in hiring practices are not easily identifiable. For example, suppose a position opens that an applicant named Mohammed has applied for. Because of the name, a person

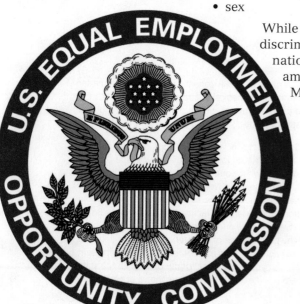

⇄ The Ethics of Law

Sexual Orientation and Employment

Did you notice that sexual orientation is not included on the list of protection provided for by the EEOC? While some states have included sexual orientation as a protected class, there are other states where a company can legally refuse to hire or fire an employee based on their sexual orientation.

- Should sexual orientation be included under the EEOC?
- What reasons can you think of that might explain why sexual orientation is not included as a protected class?

who is prejudiced against such individuals would most likely not consider him for the position. Because the applicant was not contacted for an interview, he is likely unaware that it was due to discrimination.

Affirmative Action

In the late 1950s and early 1960s, the civil rights movement was at the forefront of our national concerns. Even after passage of the Thirteenth, Fourteenth, and Fifteenth Amendments to the U.S. Constitution and the 1866 Civil Rights Act, minorities were still facing severe discrimination in the workplace.

The words affirmative action were first used in President John F. Kennedy's Executive Order 10925, which required federal contractors to take "affirmative action" to ensure that applicants for a job were not discriminated against based on race, creed, color, or national origin. (President Lyndon Johnson later expanded those rights to include gender.) Part of the reason for implementing affirmative action was to redress the overt wrongs that had been committed against minorities in hiring practices throughout the United States, by creating diversity in the workplace.

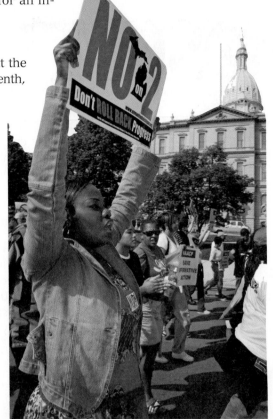

Americans With Disabilities Act (ADA)

There are many facets to the Americans with Disabilities Act (ADA). For our current discussion, the ADA prohibits discrimination in employment for people with disabilities. Any qualified candidate must be considered for a job, without consideration of his or her disability. As with affirmative action, if a person is unable to perform his or her job duties, an employer is not required to hire that person just because he or she has a disability. For example, suppose a healthcare provider has had his or her dominant arm amputated and wears a prosthesis. If the person applies for a job but is unable to perform the duties required of that position, the ADA would not require the hospital to hire him or her.

Employment Laws: Working on the Job

All of the laws that we have discussed so far cover discrimination. And, while the focus has been applying for a job, affirmative action, the EEOC, and the ADA are still in place after a person has obtained a job. A person cannot be discriminated against in promotion practices or decisions related to layoffs or termination.

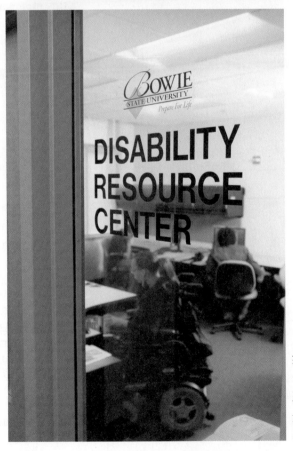

> ⇄ **The Ethics of Law**
>
> **Affirmative Action**
>
> Affirmative action is not without its critics; even from those who affirmative action was designed to protect. Some argue that if everyone is truly equal, then there is no need for affirmative action laws. By having affirmative action laws, some critics believe, the government is indicating that minorities are in fact different, because they are in need of special protection to make them equal. What do you think?

Most of the laws that apply to working on the job focus on maintaining a safe work environment.

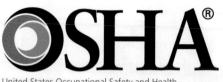

United States Occupational Safety and Health Administration.

Occupational Safety and Health Administration (OSHA)

In 1971, the Occupational Safety and Health Act established the Occupational and Health Administration (OSHA), an agency of the federal government overseen by the U.S. Department of Labor. OSHA was designed to protect workers from job-related deaths, injuries, and illness.

OSHA ensures that employers are providing a safe work environment for their employees and that the laws related to workplace safety are enforced. Compliance comes in the form of investigations or through OSHA's complaint bureau. While the number and type of OSHA's regulatory areas are numerous, there are two areas overseen by OSHA that specifically relate to employees working in the healthcare environment; bloodborne pathogens and Material Safety Data Sheets (MSDS).

Bloodborne Pathogens A bloodborne pathogen is any disease that can be contracted if you come in contact with another person's blood or body fluids. OSHA publishes the Bloodborne Pathogen Standard (29 CFR 1910.1030, 29 USC 655(b)), which details the policies healthcare institutions must follow relating to bloodborne pathogens. Among other things, the policy outlines:

- what bloodborne pathogens are,
- universal precautions,
- how exposures are handled, and
- disposing of medical waste.

Material Safety Data Sheets (MSDS) Another area that is covered by OSHA, in conjunction with the U.S. Food and Drug Administration, relates to the hazardous materials you may encounter as an employee. Many employees, even those that work outside of healthcare, encounter potentially dangerous substances, chemicals, or materials that could cause harm. In the healthcare arena, you may encounter caustic items, such as cleaning solutions or radioactive materials. If, through your employment, you could be exposed to any of the caustic materials identified by OSHA, an MSDS is placed in a file at your workstation that you can readily access. These data sheets include information on:

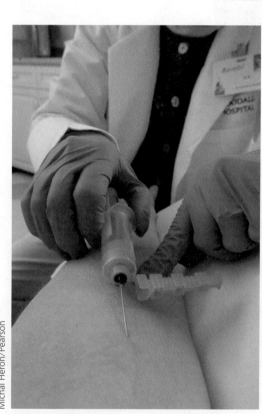

- what the substance is
- what the chemical makeup of the substance is
- how it can be harmful
- how to properly handle and store the substance
- what the risks are for exposure
- what to do if you are exposed

Workers' Compensation

If you are injured or become sick while working on the job, you may be entitled to Workers' Compensation. The idea behind Workers' Compensation is that if you are hurt because of your job, your job should pay for you being hurt. Workers' Compensation is provided for all employees, regardless of who they work for or where they work. Every state, and the federal government, requires employers to provide Workers' Compensation for all of their employee's.

Michal Heron/Pearson

One of the most common misconceptions related to Workers' Compensation is when an injury or illness is covered under Workers' Compensation. When evaluating a Workers' Compensation claim, two questions are used to determine whether Workers' Compensation benefits will be provided. "Did the employee's injury/illness *arise out of* the work that they were asked to perform?" Or, "Did the employee receive the injury/illness *in the course of* their employment?"

For approved injuries and illnesses under Workers' Compensation, there are two types of benefits, medical expenses and wages.

Because employers are required by law to carry Workers' Compensation, concessions are made regarding the type and amount of benefits that are paid under Workers' Compensation. If an employee misses work because of a compensable injury or illness, the employee may be entitled to receive wages. Because of the amount of fraud that has occurred with Workers' Compensation, all states limit the amount Workers' Compensation of wages that are paid under Workers' Compensation. While the actual amounts vary for state to state, the normal is 75 percent of the employee's regular income—up to a maximum of $1,500 a month. The rationale used to support this limitation is that Workers' Compensation should not be an avenue for people to make money and every effort should be made to return a person to his or her job as quickly as possible.

In addition, the amount of money a healthcare provider is paid for providing medical services to injured workers is also reduced; typically by 25 percent. For example, if a doctor's office would normally bill an insurance company $50 for a routine office visit, that same visit under Workers' Compensation would only be reimbursed $37.50. Because Workers' Compensation laws set the amount of money a healthcare provider is allowed to charge, that is the only amount they can receive. Meaning, the doctor's office cannot bill the patient to make up the difference. Part of the rationale provided for reduced fees is to provide only reasonable and necessary treatments and to cut down on malingering.

One common question regarding Workers' Compensation is whether an employer can require an employee to show up for work and perform duties other than what they normally perform? Yes, an employer can require a person to return to work as long as the employer accommodates the medical restrictions that the doctor provides for the patient. While an employee has the right to refuse that work assignment, if they do, they are giving up their right to receive Workers' Compensation wages. The main rationale for this argument is to encourage employees to get well and back to work instead of lingering in the Workers' Compensation system.

Sidebar

Some ambulance and fire companies are using iPhones, PDAs, and Blackberrys to assist them with hazardous material emergencies. MSDS forms can be downloaded onto these electronic devices and used by first responders, should they be called to treat an employee who has been exposed to a hazardous substance at work.

Sidebar

Most of the time people think of Workers' Compensation as covering injuries or accidents on the job. But illness may also be covered if it is related to one's job duties, keeping in mind the "arise out of" and "in the course of" questions. For example, mesothelioma is a type of cancer that results from exposure to asbestos, and might be work-related for employees who were exposed to asbestos as part of their employment.

Sidebar

One employer went as far as they could to make accommodations for an employee's return to work. The employee's doctor had restricted the employee to sitting at a desk for no more than an hour at a time, to be followed by at least two hours of bed rest. To accommodate the employee, the employer closed off some offices at the end of the hallway and had a hospital bed delivered for the employee to sleep in. Because the employee made these accommodations, the employee either had to accept that work assignment or forfeit Workers' Compensation wages.

Concept Connection

Workers' Compensation and Vicarious Liability

One of the legal theories for requiring employers to provide Workers' Compensation is the theory of vicarious liability, a concept that is found in many different aspects of the law.

Family Medical Leave Act (FMLA)

Prior to passing the Family Medical Leave Act (FMLA), some employees lost their jobs when they had extended absences due to medical problems. Initially, the problem arose when women were taking time off from work after childbirth, only to find that their job was no longer available upon their return. In 1993 Congress passed the FMLA to protect those jobs.

While the initial intent of FMLA was to protect women, men soon cried foul and sued under reverse discrimination, because they too should be allowed to take time off from work to care for their newborn child. Congress agreed, and expanded the FMLA rules. Currently, an employee can utilize FMLA:

1. for the birth and care of the newborn child of the employee;
2. for placement of a child in their home by adoption or through foster care;
3. to care for an immediate family member (spouse, child, or parent) with a serious health condition; or
4. to take medical leave when an employee themselves has a serious health condition.

Under FMLA an employee can take up to 12 weeks of unpaid leave within one year without risk of losing his or her position.

Fair Labor Standards Act (FLSA)

The Department of Labor, which oversees the FMLA, governs another area of employment law. The Fair Labor Standards Act (FLSA) set up requirements related to the minimum wage and how overtime is compensated. While the FLSA is specific about *how* overtime is paid, it does not regulate the number of hours a person can work.

Unfortunately mandatory overtime has become commonplace in healthcare today. This is due, in part, to healthcare staffing shortages and the increased number of patients needing care. In order to compensate, some healthcare institutions have to resort to mandatory overtime in order to cover staffing shortages and patient care needs.

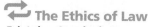
The Ethics of Law

Fair Labor Standards Act

While mandatory overtime is an unpopular subject amongst healthcare workers, most healthcare institutions use mandatory overtime to provide adequate staffing ratios and to maintain a level of care that the patient population requires.

- How affective do you think a person is when they are working overtime?
- If a mistake is made while a person is working mandatory overtime, who do you think should be at fault, the healthcare worker or the employer?

Employment Laws: Losing a Job

While no one wants to lose his or her job, it is an unfortunate occurrence in the business world. Whether a person is laid off or terminated, there are specific laws that cover an employee if this unfortunate event happens.

Every company's policy and procedures manual must outline the process that is used for terminating an employee. Usually that process involves receiving a verbal warning first, a written warning second, and then termination. Because businesses are required to have such a policy, they are also legally required to follow that policy. But, as we have noted with the law, there are exceptions.

There are certain situations where an employer can automatically terminate an employee without having to go through the termination process outlined in their policy and procedure manual. Some examples include showing up to work intoxicated, being verbally or physically abusive to fellow employees, or failing to follow safety protocols that endanger the workplace or employees.

Just Cause

An employee cannot fire an employee for any reason. Instead, an employee can only be terminated for just cause. Or, put another way, the *cause* for termination must be *justified*. The just cause requirement ensures that employers are terminating employees for reasons that are related to their job performance. Meaning, the termination cannot be arbitrary or discriminatory but based on a valid reason. Typically, to satisfy the just cause requirement, employers will utilize language in employee's job descriptions to justify the termination, should it become necessary.

Unions

Many companies and organizations, healthcare included, are unionized. Unionized employers and employees are bound by the labor agreements that they have entered into. If a labor agreement exists, employees and employers are required to follow that agreement. Labor agreements usually provide more stringent requirements than what employment laws require.

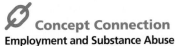 **Concept Connection**

Employment and Substance Abuse

Substance abuse, whether from legal or illegal substances, is a problem that can affect any business. Reporting impaired employees is a concept directly connected to employment laws and part of an employee's professional responsibilities.

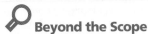 **Beyond the Scope**

Unions bring to employment law some very complicated exceptions and special rules. The intricate complexities involving unions and employment law are beyond the scope of this text. The reader is encouraged to consult outside resources if they desire more information related to unions and the workplace.

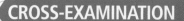

Make FALSE statements TRUE.

Rewrite the false statements below by replacing the bolded, italicized, and underlined word(s) to make it a true statement.

1. <u>***State medical boards***</u> issue standards of care that healthcare professionals must follow.

   _____

2. Part of the reason for implementing <u>***Workers' Compensation***</u> was to redress the overt wrongs that had been committed against minorities in hiring practices throughout the United States, by creating diversity in the workplace.

   _____

3. <u>***The EEOC***</u> creates policies on bloodborne pathogens and material safety data sheets.

   _____

4. "Arising out of" or "in the course of" are questions used to address whether <u>***FMLA***</u> applies or not.

   _____

5. Under the <u>***Fair Labor Standards Act***</u>, a person can take up to 12 weeks of unpaid leave without risk of losing his or her job.

   _____

Circle Exercise

Circle the correct word from the choices given.

1. (**People Skills, Practice of Medicine, Technical Skills**) is sometimes referred to as emotional intelligence.

2. A person who holds a license and wants to move to another state must check the other state's (**autonomy, professional organization, reciprocity**) agreement.

3. The (**affirmative action, EEOC, FLSA**) is charged with enforcing the federal laws that prohibit discrimination.

4. One of the requirements of (**EEOC, FLSA, OSHA**) is that employers provided documentation that their employees have been trained in bloodborne pathogens.

5. Employees having "ready access" relates to (**affirmative action, material safety data sheets, Workers' Compensation**).

Matching

Match the numbered law to its lettered area of coveage.

1. _____ ADA
2. _____ affirmative action
3. _____ Bloodborne Pathogens
4. _____ EEOC
5. _____ employment at will
6. _____ FLSA
7. _____ FMLA
8. _____ MSDS
9. _____ Workers' Compensation

A. discrimination against race, creed, color, or national origin
B. discrimination in the workplace
C. employee termination
D. employees with disabilities
E. exposure to infectious diseases
F. job-related injuries
G. unpaid leave job security
H. wages and overtime compensation
I. working with hazardous material

Matching

Match the numbered term to its lettered definition.

1. _____ certification
2. _____ code of ethics
3. _____ credentialing
4. _____ defensive medicine
5. _____ licensure
6. _____ medical practice acts
7. _____ professional
8. _____ reciprocity
9. _____ standards of care

A. a credentialing process that confirms or guarantees that specific knowledge has been obtained or that a person has proven proficiency in a task or skill, or demonstrated expertise in a particular area.

B. a credentialing process where a person is granted the authority to perform particular tasks or skills after demonstrating expertise.

C. a person who earns a living through the expertise of his or her work.

D. laws that a state has passed to determine the requirements for healthcare and healthcare professionals.

E. the requirements established for the exchange of credentials from one state to another.

F. the type of medical practice used by healthcare workers to protect themselves against potential lawsuits.

G. validation of an individual's background and qualifications, or fulfillment of the requirements established by the organization granting the verification.

H. written requirements that detail the responsibilities a professional will be held accountable for in the performance of his or her duties.

I. written statements that detail the type of behavior a professional should strive toward when performing his or her professional duties.

Deliberations: Critical Thinking Questions

Question 1: As we have seen, not all healthcare professions require a license. Some states are considering requiring licensure for all healthcare professions. What are your thoughts? Do you think that all healthcare professionals should be required to obtain a license of some kind? Explain your answer.

Question 2: Can a person perform the tasks that are governed by a license without obtaining one? A person can get behind the wheel of a vehicle and drive on the public roads without obtaining a driver's license. Does the same holds true for a healthcare license? Can a person practice medicine or perform medical tasks and procedures without actually holding a license? What mechanism do you think might be in place to stop or identify this type of practice? How is the public protected from unlawful practice by an unlicensed person?

Question 3: The practice of defensive medicine is commonplace in healthcare today. But, because some of the tests and procedures that we order for patients, in the name of defensive medicine, do not directly address the medical issues for which patients are seeking care, some insurance companies are discussing the possibility of denying payments for defensive

medicine procedures. Do you think that it is fair? Should insurance companies pay for defensive medicine, or is that something that the healthcare institution should absorb?

Question 4: Mary is a massage therapist working in a state that does not license massage therapist. Even though licensure for massage therapist is not mandatory, to add credibility to her business Mary would like to undergo voluntary licensure. However, when she contacts the state, she finds out that there is no such thing as voluntary licensure. Why would a state not offer voluntary licensure?

Question 5: A doctor has decided to buy lunch for his office staff. The receptionist has been asked by the doctor to run across the street and pick up their lunch, because the restaurant does not provide delivery. On her way to pick up the lunch, in the office parking lot, the receptionist trips on a pot hole and twists her ankle. Would this injury be covered under Workers' Compensation? Explain why or why not. Regardless of which answer you chose, identify some arguments that a person might have regarding the decision opposite of what yours was.

Closing Arguments: Case Analysis

Abby is working on the surgical floor of the local hospital as a certified nursing assistant. Part of her job duties requires that she give bed baths to patients who are bedridden. One of the patients that she has to bathe is Mr. Arthur, who is recovering from a traffic accident. Because Abby has been working there for a long time, the nurses trust her. Nancy, a nurse on the floor, knows that Abby is getting ready to give Mr. Arthur a bath. Because Mr. Arthur needs a suppository, Nancy asks Abby to administer it to the patient while she is giving him his bath. Pretend that you are Abby, knowing that as a certified nursing assistant you are not allowed to administer medications. But, you understand that this is a simple thing, and having given suppositories to your children before know that it is not a big deal.

Question 1: What should you do?
As Abby is giving Mr. Arthur his bath, he suffers from a seizure, causing his intravenous lines to disconnect, which scratches Abby

on the arm. Unfortunately, Mr. Arthur is HIV positive, which greatly concerns Abby. Abby contacts employee health and is seen by the doctor and preventive measures are taken. The next day, Abby reports to work, but her supervisor is worried about the possibility of infection and wonders if Abby should take time off from work until the results come back.

Question 2: Should healthcare workers who become infected with HIV be allowed to continue working with patients? Does it matter whether a person was infected on the job or not?

Question 3: What are the potential ramifications of allowing an HIV-infected healthcare worker to continue to work with patients? What are the potential ramifications of not allowing an HIV-infected healthcare worker to continue to work with patients?

The Briefcase

This section repeats the objectives from the beginning of the chapter and provides a summary of the most important concepts for each objective. Use this section as a quick review and to check your understanding of the chapter key points.

Objective 1: List the qualities needed to work in healthcare.
- technical skills
- people skills
- professionalism

Objective 2: Explain what defensive medicine is and how it relates to the practice of medicine.
- It helps protect healthcare workers against a lawsuit.
- It helps prevent a wrong or injury from occurring.

Objective 3: Define the importance that professional organizations have on the healthcare professions.
- Govern the healthcare profession
- Support and control the healthcare profession
- Publish requirements for the profession, including:
  - Standards of care
  - Codes of ethics

Objective 4: Distinguish the difference between medical practice acts and medical boards.
- Medical Practice Acts
  - create a medical board that oversees healthcare delivery in the state
- Medical Boards
  - oversee licensure
  - formulate policies and procedures that dictate how healthcare is delivered in the state
  - determine the scope of practice for healthcare professionals.

Objective 5: Describe what the EEOC is and what areas of employment it governs.
- discrimination in the workplace
- affirmative action

Objective 6: Define what the ADA is and how it protects employees.
- It protects employees with disabilities
- It helps employers by defining what accommodations need to be made for a disabled employee

Objective 7: List the two areas covered by OSHA that have a direct impact on working in healthcare.
- bloodborne pathogens
- material safety data sheets

Objective 8: Give an example of why a person might file a Workers' Compensation claim.
- For injuries or illnesses that are employment related
- To pay for medical expenses
- To pay for lost wages
- Two rules are used to determine if an injury/illness is compensable
  - arising out of
  - in the course of

Objective 9: List some of the reasons an employee may utilize FMLA.
- to take care of ill family members
- to care for newly arrived family members, by birth or adoption
- to take time off for a serious illness

Maximize Your Success with the Companion Website

The companion website to this textbook contains materials that can help you better understand the concepts presented in this chapter. Go to www.myhealthprofessionskit.com to access:

- sample quizzes
- related web links
- learning games
- and more…

PEARSON
myhealthprofessionskit™

Medical Records, Insurance, and Contracts

Communication consists of five language skills: reading, listening, analyzing, writing, and speaking. When working in the healthcare field you will utilize all five of these language skills. While each language skill is important in healthcare, this chapter will concentrate on the language skill of writing, specifically, the three most common forms of writing you will face as a healthcare professional: medical records, insurance, and contracts.

MEASURE YOUR PROGRESS: LEARNING OBJECTIVES

After studying this chapter, you will be able to:

- List the five different purposes that medical records serve.

- Provide examples of what type of court cases medical records can be used for.

- Briefly describe the two perspectives related to charting in a medical record.

- Identify what a *subpoena duces tecum* is and when it is used.

- Compare and contrast the ownership of medical records.

- Using the key terms *premiums* and *actuarial tables*, briefly define how insurance works.

- Provide an example of how international classification of disease (ICD) codes and current procedure technology (CPT) codes affect upcoding.

- Compare and contrast *respondeat superior* with vicarious liability.

- Explain how the reasonable person standard is applied to implied contracts.

KEY TERMS

actuarial tables

contract

insurance

legal document

reasonable person standard

respondeat superior

subpoena duces tecum

upcoding

vicarious liability

PROFESSIONAL HIGHLIGHT

Mary is a medical records technician at a large healthcare institution. She is not only responsible for ensuring that all documentation is included in the medical records but also works closely with medical coding and billing and insurance companies. In order to ensure that the hospital is in compliance with all of the regulatory agencies and insurance company requirements, Mary has to have a thorough understanding of the laws related to medical records, documentation, insurance, and contracts.

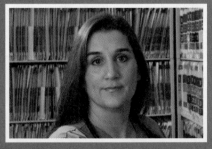

Condor 36/Shutterstock

What to write in a patient's medical records is not an easy question to answer. A lot depends on the circumstances, the patient, what care you are providing, and what role you are performing. While there is no simple formula to tell you exactly what to document, there are some guiding principles that will help you figure out what to write. But before we get into a discussion about what to write in a patient's medical records, we should review the purposes that medical records serve. Understanding what purpose medical records serve will help you determine what you need to document and why.

> How do I figure out what to write in a patient's medical record?

Medical Records

While the most common purpose for medical records is the documentation of patient care, medical records serve many other purposes as well. Medical records can be used to:

- manage healthcare
- track healthcare
- provide clinical data
- meet regulatory requirements
- document healthcare

Managing Healthcare

Managing a patient's healthcare needs can be difficult and time-consuming. But instead of the patient having to repeat his or her medical history whenever care is received, we can accomplish the same goal by looking at the patient's medical records. By reviewing a patient's medical records, we can ascertain: what diseases a patient has had in the past, medications they have taken, if they have any allergies, or what surgeries have been performed. In addition to what care has been provided in the past, we can also find out what response the patient had to those treatments, to help us plan future medical care. For example, if a patient had a lot of post-operative pain on a previous surgery, the physician might investigate different approaches to pain management or consider prescribing a different type of pain medication.

Tracking Care

Whenever a patient has an encounter with a healthcare provider, that encounter is documented in the medical record. This allows healthcare providers to track:

- why a patient sought medical care (signs and symptoms, injury, follow-up),
- where a patient received medical care (such as doctor's office, hospital, or outpatient clinic),
- what medical care was provided,
- when a patient received medical care (often, routinely, rarely), or
- how the patient responded to the medical care that was provided.

For example, a patient may have cut his finger while opening a can, but cannot remember when he received his last tetanus shot. By looking at the patient's medical record, the healthcare provider can track down when the last tetanus shot was given to determine whether another tetanus shot is needed. This concept applies to other areas as well, such as determining when routine diagnostic tests, such as a mammography or prostate exams, need to be scheduled.

Providing Clinical Data

The data provided in a patient's medical records can be a wonderful resource of information for research and statistical purposes. The data of several patients can be reviewed to determine useful information to clinicians and practitioners alike. For example, public health officials might want to look at several patients' medical records that have been diagnosed with an infectious disease. If public health officials find common similarities, they can take appropriate action, such issuing a boil water order or looking at one particular restaurant where people ate.

Concept Application

Medical Records—Providing Clinical Data

When the human immunodeficiency virus (HIV) first surfaced in the early 1980s, experts in epidemiology at the Centers for Disease Control and Prevention (CDC) used the valuable information contained in patients' medical records to trace the route of infection, allowing them to better understand the disease and how it was spread. This information gave healthcare providers the tools they needed to identify other patients that might be infected.

Meeting Regulatory Requirements

All of the regulatory agencies that govern healthcare require patient care to be documented. One of the largest and most significant governmental agencies, the Joint Commission on Accreditation of Healthcare Organizations (JCAHO), accredits and certifies healthcare organizations. As part of the accreditation process, inspectors from JCAHO will evaluate the patient's medical records to ensure that the institution is meeting required performance standards. Without accreditation and certification by JCAHO, a healthcare institution cannot bill Medicare and Medicaid for services. Most insurance companies follow suit, requiring JCAHO certification in order to receive payment as well.

Documenting Health Care: What to Write?

When students first start learning about documenting in a patient's medical record, there are some common questions, such as: What do you write, how much do you write, and can you write too much or too little? Unfortunately there is no simple answer to these basic questions because it all depends on the type of care that has been provided. Some care, such as providing medication, only requires initialing a box, writing a couple of words, or maybe writing one sentence. Other, more complex medical care, such as a surgical procedure, usually requires a few pages of documentation. But even though there is no simple formula to tell you what to write, there are two approaches to documenting that will help you determine what to write and if you have written enough (see Fig. 4-1).

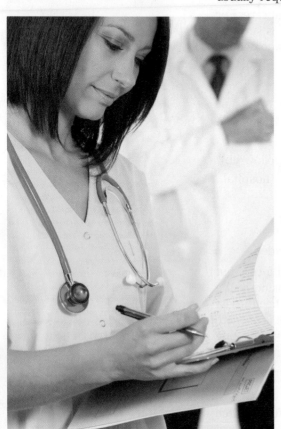

Fig. 4-1 Medical documentation is an essential part of working in the healthcare environment. Knowing what to document is just as important as the medical care that you provide.

auremar/Shutterstock

Medical Approach to Documenting

In the medical perspective approach to documenting, you write down any pertinent information related to the care you have provided to the patient. But that begs the question, what is pertinent? As we previously discussed, medical records serve many different purposes. Because of the different purposes medical records serve, a number of different people could possibly look at a patient's medical records. Any time that a person looks at a patient's medical record, he or she is looking for specific information. That information is dependant on the purpose that the medical record serves.

When a person looks at information that has been entered into a patient's medical records, you typically will not be around to answer questions. Or, even if you are, you may not remember what care you provided to the patient, especially if it was three years ago. When documenting in a patient's medical record, you want to be able to provide the information that a person might be looking for. This takes us back to the what, where, when, why, and how purposes that medical records serve. If your documentation can answer those questions, then you will be providing the information that a person needs. After you have finished documenting on a patient's chart, go back through and review what you have written.

Court Case

Caruso v. Pine Manor Nursing Center

538 N.E.2d 722, 182 Ill. App, 3d 879 (1989)
Appellate Court of Illinois, First District, Fifth Division

FACTS: After several hospitalizations for Parkinson's disease, dementia, organic brain syndrome, nephritis, periodontal disease, renal insufficiency, urinary tract infections, and a kidney infection; Phillip Caruso was admitted to Pine Manor Nursing Center. During his initial examination, a doctor found him to be in stable condition, with good skin turgor (evidence of adequate hydration). As part of his nursing care, Phillip received three meals a day, three snacks a day, and medications four times a day; all of which included water or other liquids. In addition, when he was repositioned or changed during the night, Phillip was offered something to drink. Seven days after Phillip was admitted to Pine Manor, he developed tremors, weakness, and confusion and was taken to the Emergency Room. The ER doctor noted that Phillip had poor skin turgor (evidence of *inadequate* hydration) and admitted him to the hospital where a nephrologist diagnosed him with renal insufficiency with superimposed

dehydration. The family, on behalf of Phillip, filed a medical malpractice lawsuit against Pine Manor. In response to the lawsuit, Pine Manor admitted that they did not document Phillip's intake and output, something that, because of Phillip's medical history, they were required to document.

ISSUE: While this case focused on procedural issues that occurred at trial, one important issue, for our present discussion, was the lack of documentation.

RULE: "[T]he evidence presented showed a proximate cause of Phillip's dehydration as a result of his stay at Pine Manor; it was not unreasonable for the jury to conclude that Phillip did suffer dehydration and that Pine Manor's treatment of him caused his dehydration."

EMPHASIS: Without the documentation of Phillip's intake and output, Pine Manor had no proof of what medical treatment was provided nor what the response to that treatment was. This case demonstrates the importance of documenting in a patient's medical record and the varying reasons documenting is performed.

Legal Approach to Documenting

While the main purpose for documenting in a patient's records is for medical reasons, there are additional considerations to think about. Medical records are **legal documents**, which brings into the discussion about documenting some unique legal rules and requirements.

Almost anything that contains a writing can be considered a legal document. The importance of what makes a document a "legal" document, is whether the writing can be attributed to the author. If a writing can be attributed to the author, then it is considered a legal document. The receipts that you receive at a store, the instructions included in the latest electronic gadget you purchased, and even the notes that you take during class are all legal documents, because they can be attributed to the author. The main importance, for our purposes, is when medical records are used as legal documents (see Table 4-1).

Because medical records are legal documents, there is a possibility that what you write might be used in a legal proceeding. Or, because you were the author of a document, you might be called as a witness if that document is used at trial. These possibilities underline one of the main reasons you document using a legal approach.

If a healthcare provider is on the witness stand and is asked by an attorney what care he or she provided to a patient three years ago, it is doubtful that the healthcare provider would be able to remember. If you were asked on the witness stand what care you provided to Mr. Jones three years ago, would you be able to remember off the top of your head?

From a legal perspective, then, healthcare workers should write enough so that by rereading their records they can refresh their memory about the care that they provided. Looking at the medical records, you will be able to testify as to the what, where, when, why, and how questions that might be asked of you. The answers to these questions will probably have legal significance in a medically related lawsuit. If there is not enough information in the medical record to answer an attorney's question, then they will only have your testimony to rely on.

 Beyond the Scope

In addition to what you write in a patient's medical record, there are several different formats that outline how you write. Some of these formats include the SOAP (Subjective, Objective, Assessment, Plan) method; the DAR (Data, Action, Response) method; and charting by exception.

legal document: any writing that provides information or ideas that can be attributed to the author

Table 4-1

How Medical Records can be Used In Different Legal Settings.

Type of Law	Medical Documentation Used
Administrative Law	A person who becomes disabled will have to apply for benefits. Part of the application for disability will include medical documentation substantiating the disability and the medical treatment that has been received.
Bankruptcy, Debtor, and Credit Law	One of the leading causes of bankruptcy in the United States is medical expenses. If a person is filing for bankruptcy, they will be asked to demonstrate the expenses that they have. They will be required to show proof of expenses, such as billing statements, to substantiate their bankruptcy proceedings.
Criminal Law	The use of medical records is commonplace in criminal law. Autopsy reports are used in murder or manslaughter cases; psychiatric records are used for insanity defense; treatment records are used as evidence in criminal assaults, battery, rape prosecutions, and abuse cases.
Employment/Labor Law	A person filing a Workers' Compensation claim will have to provide medical documentation to support their claim. The medical records will be used to demonstrate that the injury a person sustained was related to their employment.
Family Law	There are many aspects of family law that use medical records. Divorcing parents may introduce medical records during custody disputes to demonstrate injuries a child has received or the lack of medical care the other parent may not have provided.
Tort Law	All torts, to be successful, must demonstrate some kind of injury. If that injury is a medical injury, the plaintiff will have to provide documentation detailing the injury that they have received and the medical treatment they have sought.
Wills, Estates, and Trust Law	Medical records are commonly used in competency issues related to wills and estates. In addition, living wills and medical power-of-attorney documents (which are part of the medical record) are also included in estate planning and wills.

Andy Dean Photography/Shutterstock

> **"If it is wasn't written down, it wasn't done!"**
>
> teacept/Shutterstock

Beyond the Scope

Each healthcare institution has specific rules regarding how to correct mistakes in documentation. Because of the varied rules, how to correct mistakes is beyond the scope of this text. For more information regarding correcting mistakes, consult the healthcare institution where you are working.

What Is Not Written

Just as important as what *is* written in a patient's medical records is what is *not* written. There is a legal principle related to documenting that states: "*If it wasn't written down, it wasn't done.*" Based on that principle, even though care may have actually been provided, if that care is not documented in the medical record, then, according to the law, that care *was not* provided. While you may very well have provided the care, but forgot to document it, under the law if the care is not documented, then it was not *legally* provided.

Along with the legal requirements for documenting medical care, there are laws related to how corrections in a medical record are handled. For example, if a mistake has been made in a hand-written chart, a single line is drawn through the mistake. Obliterations, white-out, and the blacking out of entries is not allowed. With the increasing use of electronic medical records, the issues related to how corrections are made are becoming more and more obsolete, as computer software automatically makes corrections according to legal standards.

Subpoena Duces Tecum

If documents are required for use in court or other legal proceedings, they are obtained by an attorney or judge issuing a *subpoena duces tecum*.

Any legal document can be requested through a *subpoena duces tecum*. In healthcare, the most commonly requested document is the patient's medical records. But why would an attorney go through the hassle of issuing a

subpoena duces tecum: "bring with you under penalty of punishment"; a requirement that documents be delivered to a court or brought with you to court

Court Case

Keene v. Brigham and Women's Hospital, Inc.

439 Mass. 223, 786 N.E.2d 824 (2003)
Massachusetts Supreme Judicial Court

FACTS: Dylan Keene was born on May 15, 1986 at 1:07 AM. A few hours after his birth, he developed respiratory problems and was transferred from the regular care nursery to the neonatal intensive care unit (NICU). At 6:25 AM, blood tests were performed, including a blood cultures, and the patient was sent back to the regular care nursery. The NICU discharge note stated to watch for signs of sepsis (infection) and to withhold antibiotics pending the results of the blood tests. On May 16, 1986 at 2:30 AM, Dylan started having seizures. Antibiotics were ordered and administered. Tests performed afterwards determined that Dylan had contracted neonatal sepsis and meningitis. Whether from the infection or the seizure, Dylan suffered severe brain damage. He has little or no voluntary control over any part of his body, suffers from repeated seizures, and requires numerous medications and treatments.

At issue in this case are the events that occurred between 6:25 AM (May 15) and 2:30 AM (May 16). However, what actually occurred during that timeframe is only speculative, because the medical records for that time-period have been lost.

ISSUE: This case raises several different and important issues. However, for our present purposes, one issue is whether the defendant hospital could demonstrate to the court what care had been provided to Dylan?

RULE: The court ruled that ". . . a party who has negligently or intentionally lost or destroyed evidence known to be relevant for an upcoming legal proceeding should be held accountable for any unfair prejudice that results."

EMPHASIS: The court in this case looked at the medical records as evidence. The court reasoned that: 1) Documenting in a patient's medical record is done, in part, for legal purposes. 2) Medical records are created, in part, for use in legal proceedings. 3) Because medical records are often used as evidence, an institution has the responsibility to maintain those records as evidence even though an actual lawsuit has not been filed.

subpoena? Why not just send a letter to the institution and ask for a copy of a patient's medical records? The main reason attorneys use *subpoena duces tecums* is because it is a legal request that you are obligated to comply with. Failure to comply can result in court fines and penalties. Another reason attorneys use *subpoena duces tecums* is because of a special distinction associated with medical record ownership.

Medical Record Ownership

While it is the healthcare provider's responsibility to document medical care, the care that they are documenting is information about a specific patient. Who owns the medical records, the patient or the healthcare institution? Medical records are dually owned by both the patient and the healthcare institution.

Medical Record Ownership: Healthcare Institution

All healthcare providers are required to create and maintain medical records. This requirement comes from regulatory agencies, insurance companies, and licensing authorities, to name a few. When you combine this requirement with the multifaceted purpose that medical records serve, it is easy to see why healthcare institutions are reluctant to part with medical records.

Because healthcare facilities create the medical records, they have the right of ownership to the record itself. Or, more specifically, they own the pieces of paper that constitute a person's medical record. But while healthcare institutions own the paper, the information that is on that paper belongs to the patient.

Medical Record Ownership: Patients

Patients request copies of their medical records for varying reasons. One of the most common is for consultations with other healthcare providers. Because the healthcare institution owns the documents, a patient is not entitled to the documents themselves. But the patient is entitled to the information

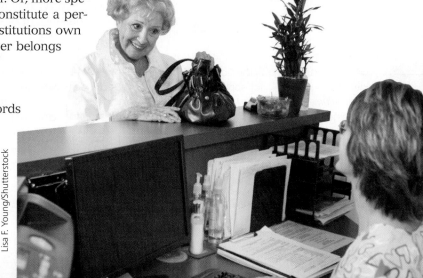

Lisa F. Young/Shutterstock

that is on the documents. With the growing use of electronic health records, this premise may be a little clearer. If a healthcare institution uses electronic health records, a patient would be entitled to a printout of the record, but not the electronic discs and computers that contain the records.

Medical Record Ownership: Doctrine of Professional Discretion

While patient requests for medical records are usually freely granted, there is one noted exception. If a patient requests a copy of their medical records, the doctor(s) must first approve that request before the chart is copied. The Doctrine of Professional Discretion allows a physician to decide whether to release a patient's medical records or not. The doctor can decide to release the entire records, only part of it, or none at all to the patient. This exception is contrary to the general rule that the patient owns the information and is entitled to that information because, sometimes, having the information can be detrimental to patient safety and well-being.

Hypochondriacs Hypochondriacs are patients who have a preoccupation with disease and illness, often misunderstanding bodily sensations. They often fear that they have a devastating medical problem. Providing hypochondriacs with access to their medical records can augment misconceptions about disease. For example, a hypochondriac may visit a doctor complaining of dizziness. The physician might make a notation that because of the dizziness, he needs to rule out the possibility of a stroke. Even though a stroke might have been ruled out, if a hypochondriac patient sees that notation, he or she may be convinced that he or she had a stroke and will not only return to the doctor but mention it as part of his or her past medical history. If a doctor believes that giving a hypochondriac patient access to medical records will be devastating to either his or her physical or mental health, the doctor can withhold access under the doctrine of professional discretion.

Psychological/Psychiatric Records While doctors can utilize the doctrine of professional discretion for hypochondriac patients, the most common application of the doctrine is for a patient's psychiatric record. Information contained in the psychiatric record could be devastating if read by the patient. For example, a physician may note in a patient's chart that because of their depression, the healthcare team should place the patient on a suicide watch and take suicide precautions. A psychiatric patient may not have considered suicide, but upon reading it in his or her records, either entertains the idea or worse, makes an attempt. By withholding the medical records, or at least that portion of it, the physician is protecting the mental health of the patient making the request.

Storage and Retention of Medical Records

All healthcare institutions are required to maintain and store medical records. Keeping medical records indefinitely presents problems for healthcare institutions because of the amount of space that is required and the inevitable cost of

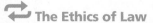

Legal Alert! The Doctrine of Professional Discretion does not apply to a *subpoena duces tecum*, as the request is court ordered and not something a doctor can override. The Doctrine of Professional Discretion only applies to individual requests for copies of medical records.

The Ethics of Law

Doctrine of Professional Discretion

Under the Doctrine of Professional Discretion, a doctor does not have to give a reason for denying a patient's request for their medical records. Is that fair?

- Should a doctor be required to provide a reason for the denial?
- Since no reason for the denial is required, what is to stop a doctor who committed an act of negligence from hiding behind the Doctrine of Professional Discretion?
- Are there any ways around this exception to the rule?

storage. While advances in electronic forms of documentation have minimized these problems, electronic records still need to be maintained (see Fig. 4-2).

There are specific rules and guidelines related to the maintenance and retention of medical records. Remember the legal principle *"If it wasn't written down, it wasn't done!"* This demonstrates why records need to be stored for a specific period of time. If we cannot provide proof of care, because of missing records, then that care was not performed.

The rule of thumb for maintaining medical records is 20 years after the last treatment was provided. Where this number comes from is significant, because it is directly tied to a law known as the Statute of Limitations.

Insurance companies are businesses. They have an obligation to pay money on the policies they have written. But how insurance companies make money has come under sharp criticism in the past few decades.

Insurance

With the growing cost of healthcare in the United States, very few people are able to pay for their own healthcare. Most people in the United States rely on healthcare **insurance** benefits provided through their employer.

Insurance policies can be written for almost anything and can cover almost any loss. How insurance coverage, insurance policies, and insurance companies work is complex. To better understand some of these complexities, we can examine a type of insurance that most are familiar with: car insurance.

When you apply for car insurance, you fill out an application that asks questions related to your driving record, the type of car you drive, how old you are, where you live, and other demographic information. A person at the insurance company, known as an underwriter, evaluates this information to determine what their *risk of loss* is, or what their chances are of having to pay money on your behalf. Statistically, a younger driver is more likely to be involved in an accident than a middle-aged driver is. Additionally, people living in large cities are more likely to be involved in accidents than people living in rural areas are. Based on the amount of financial risk involved, underwriters calculate what they are going to charge for that risk; that amount is referred to as a premium. Any change in the information, such as your age or location, will alter their risk of loss and change the premium you pay. Another example that can affect the insurance company's risk of loss and therefore your premium is the deductible amount. If you agree to a large deductible, the amount of money the insurance company might have to pay out will be decreased, which

> **insurance:** the transfer of an obligation from one party to another, usually in exchange for a fee

> I know that healthcare is dependent on insurance companies, but how do insurance companies work?

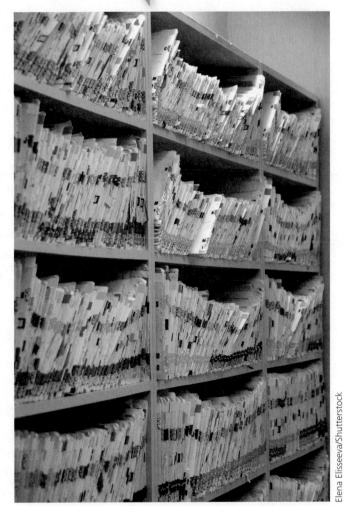

Fig. 4-2 Healthcare institutions are required to maintain patient medical records.

Elena Elisseeva/Shutterstock

⌀ Concept Connection
Record Retention and Statute of Limitations
The 20-year rule of thumb for maintaining medical records is based on the Statute of Limitations. The Statute of Limitations is a legal defense that determines how long a person has to bring a lawsuit.

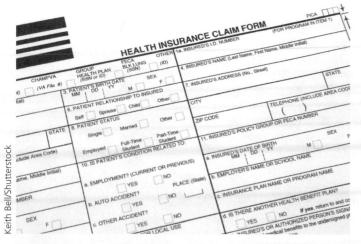

Fig. 4-3. Insurance claim form.

actuarial tables: a comprehensive list of statistical data; used most often by insurance companies to determine illness, disease, and accident projections

will also decrease your premium. If you do not want to have a deductible, the amount of money the insurance company might have to pay out will increase, which will also increase your premium.

Health insurance works the same way. When you apply for insurance, you provide information about yourself, your health habits, and any diseases or injuries that you have had. All of this information is used to determine what the health insurance company's risk of loss might be. This helps the company to determine the premium you will pay. If you are a smoker, the chances of you developing disease is much greater, which will increase the insurance company's risk of loss, creating a larger premium. Just as insurance companies know that statistically a young driver is more at risk for an accident, they also know statistically what a person's risk for disease or injury is. The statistical information used by underwriters is found on **actuarial tables**.

Statisticians have been gathering information about illness and injuries for centuries. Some of that information is provided by governmental agencies, other from the insurance claim forms (see Fig. 4-3). All of this information is plugged into tables where sophisticated mathematical formulas calculate a risk of loss. For example, if an underwriter is evaluating a policy for a 23-year-old, nonsmoker with a family history of heart disease, the underwriter can look up the actuarial table and ascertain what the statistical chances are of that person developing diabetes. That statistic, along with many others, is used to determine what an insurance company's risk of loss might be.

Now that we have an understanding about how insurance companies work, the only remaining question is how insurance companies make money. The premiums that you pay to an insurance company are partially invested. These investments help the insurance company generate income and a profit. And while insurance companies are free to invest how they see fit, they cannot invest all of the money that they have.

When a person becomes sick or injured, the insurance company is required to remove money from its general account and place it in a special account called a reserve account. The money placed in these special accounts is *reserved* for that purpose only, to pay for the illness or injury. The money in a reserve account cannot be used for investments or business expenses. Ideally, insurance companies would like to limit the amount of money they are required to place in reserve accounts, so they can keep that money in their general account and use it for investment purposes.

Managed Care

In the 1970s and 1980s, insurance companies grew concerned about the skyrocketing cost of healthcare. To help combat rising costs, they developed a concept referred to as managed care. Prior to the implementation of managed care, hospitals provided care and insurance companies paid the bill. But insurance companies voiced concern over whether they were paying for something that was not really necessary. For example, in the not too distant past, it was common to admit a person to the hospital overnight so he or she could have laboratory work performed or X-rays taken the next morning. After the tests were completed, the patient would recoup in a hospital room until he or she was comfortable enough to be discharged home.

⇄ The Ethics of Law

The Ethics of Law: Insurance—A Right or a Privilege?

A right is something that everyone is entitled to equally. For example, freedom of speech and freedom of religion is a right provided to every citizen under the U.S. Constitution. Access to healthcare and insurance is not a legal right that everyone is entitled to. But should it be?

- Should healthcare be a right that everyone is entitled to equally?
- Or should healthcare be a privilege that only a few should be entitled to?

With cost of healthcare skyrocketing, insurance companies become more active in managing the care that patients received. But technically, that statement is incorrect. Under managed care, health insurance companies are not dictating what healthcare a person can or cannot receive. Instead, they are stating what care they will, and will not, pay for. The patient, the doctor, and the institution still get to decide what treatment a patient receives. But that treatment may not be paid for by the insurance company. With the implementation of managed care, healthcare providers were asked to take part in the fiscal responsibility of healthcare. The way that this responsibility was accomplished was by insurance companies' changing the payment structure.

Suppose you need to have your house painted, and solicit estimates from different companies. One company gave you a great hourly rate, but a competitor is going to charge you a flat fee to get the job done. While you can probably foresee some of the inherent problems each option has, essentially what managed care accomplished was changing payment from an hourly rate to a flat rate payment system.

ICDs, and CPTs Codes

In 1983, Medicare released a new, flat rate reimbursement structure based on the International Classification of Diseases (ICD). Each disease, illness, or injury is assigned a number, which is located in a special codebook. To understand further, look at the following example.

A patient who is admitted to the hospital for appendicitis is assigned an ICD-9 code of 540.xx. (The number 9 after ICD indicates that it is the ninth version, which is currently in use today; and, the "xx" after the number 540 indicates the requirement for a fourth and fifth digit for accurate coding.) When the bill is submitted, the insurance company will look up the ICD code to determine the dollar amount they will pay to the hospital. To use an arbitrary figure for discussion purposes, assume that an ICD code of 540.xx is allotted $5,000. Once the insurance company receives the bill with the ICD code of 540.xx, they will issue a check to the hospital for $5,000. But how do ICD codes save money?

When a hospital takes care of a patient, they have to utilize all of the resources that the patient's medical condition requires. If those resources cost the hospital $6,000 (and they are only going to be reimbursed $5,000), then the hospital will lose money. But, if the hospital can economize, and find a way provide care by only spending $4,000, then the hospital will be able to make a profit of $1,000.

Patients who are admitted to the hospital are assigned ICD codes. Outpatient procedures, such as the visits to a doctor's office or the treatments received at an outpatient clinic, use Current Procedure Terminology (CPT) codes. Just like ICD codes, each CPT code is assigned a number and a reimbursement amount.

Upcoding

Even though ICD and CPT codes are now the norm in healthcare, they are not without problems. One highly illegal and unethical practice that has resulted from this payment structure is the occurrence of **upcoding**.

Some hospitals and doctors' offices were unhappy with the small reimbursements that they are provided with ICD and CPT codes. In order to receive a larger reimbursement, they would assign a completely different ICD or CPT code number. For example, a routine office visit, where a patient spends 15 minutes with the doctor, is assigned a CPT code of 99211, which will be reimbursed at a rate of, say, $50. But, in order to get more money from the insurance company, the doctor would upcode using a CPT code of 99212 instead, which might allow for a $75 reimbursement. However, a CPT code of 99212 requires that the physician spend 30 minutes with the patient. If the doctor has not spent that much time with the patient, billing for that service is paramount to fraud.

upcoding: using an incorrect ICD or CPT code to gain a larger insurance payment

Court Case

United States of America v. Robert W. Stokes, D.O.

United States District Court, Western District of Michigan, Southern Division (2007)

FACTS: Dr. Stokes, a dermatologist practicing in Grand Rapids Michigan, was convicted of fraud resulting from upcoded bills he submitted to Blue Cross/Blue Shield, Aetna, and Medicare. In addition to upcoding, it was alleged that Dr. Stokes re-used medical equipment that was not properly sterilized and performed surgical procedures to remove tissue from patients that were not cancerous (in order to receive payment for his services); improperly billing insurance companies for equipment he had re-used and for procedures that he did not perform.

ISSUE: Does the billing of procedures not performed, and the upcoding of procedures constitute a crime?

RULE: Dr. Stokes was convicted of three counts of insurance fraud and sentenced to 10 years in prison and ordered to pay a $1.3 million fine. In addition, the state of Michigan revoked Dr. Stokes license to practice medicine.

EMPHASIS: As healthcare providers, we are only allowed to charge for the services that we provide. Although reimbursement may not provide the amount a person would like to receive for their services, performing illegal and unlawful actions is not the way to address those concerns. (This particular case cites the criminal proceedings against Dr. Stokes. In addition to this criminal case, Dr. Stokes faced multiple civil lawsuits.)

The practice of upcoding was commonplace when ICD and CPT codes were first utilized. But insurance companies and Medicare quickly clamped down on the problem, severely increasing the fines and penalties associated with upcoding. In order to substantiate the codes that are being applied, it is common for copies of patients' medical records to be sent with the bills to the insurance company. The documentation must coincide and substantiate the charge, or code, that is being billed.

> What about malpractice insurance? How does that work? Is it only for doctors or should all healthcare professionals carry it?

Before we leave the topic of insurance, we should take a look another type of insurance that affects healthcare workers, that of malpractice insurance. Malpractice insurance, like car insurance and medical insurance, is based on the potential risk of loss. However, the risk of loss with malpractice insurance is the cost of defending a healthcare worker in court and paying a judgment.

Any healthcare provider can obtain malpractice insurance. By far, doctors pay the highest premiums for malpractice insurance, with some specialty physicians paying $150,000 a year. Nurses, respiratory therapists, and radiology technologists can obtain malpractice insurance policies as well. But the amounts those professions pay for their premium is much smaller; about $150 per year, on average.

All states in the United States require that licensed healthcare professionals be covered by malpractice insurance. A healthcare institution that hires healthcare professionals must provide malpractice insurance for all of its employees. But why would the law require the healthcare institution to carry malpractice insurance instead of the individual healthcare practitioner?

Employment Provided Malpractice Insurance

If a patient is injured because of a medical mistake, he or she deserves to be compensated. Most individuals could not afford to pay the thousands or millions of dollars that a medical mistake might cost. Two legal theories exist that support the requirement that healthcare employers provide malpractice insurance for their employees: *respondeat superior* and vicarious liability.

Respondeat Superior

An employer has a lot of control over its employees. It decides what the qualifications are for a position, the amount and type of training that employees will receive, and the policies and procedures that an employee is required to follow. Because of the control an employer has over its employees, it is also responsible for the actions of its employees. This responsibility is quantified in the legal doctrine know as *respondeat superior*.

Because of the amount of control an employer has over the employee, employers are held legally responsible for the actions of their employees. Even though an employer may not have done anything wrong, if an employee makes a mistake on the job, it is the employer that is held legally responsible. But why would an employer be held legally responsible for something, if it did nothing wrong? The answer is through a legal concept called **vicarious liability**.

Vicarious liability is liability without fault. That means that even though a person may not have done anything wrong (they are not at fault), he or she is still held legally responsible for any damages that are caused. To better understand the concept, consider the following example:

Suppose a child breaks a window while playing baseball. The person whose window was broken needs to get it repaired. But should they absorb the cost of repair simply because a child will be unable to pay for it? Under the law, the child's parents will be held legally responsible for fixing the window, even though the parents did nothing wrong. This same premise, in the larger scheme of things, demonstrates how an employer can be held vicariously liable for the actions of its employees.

> **respondeat superior:** "let the master answer," a concept where the employer is responsible for the actions of its employees

> **vicarious liability:** liability without fault; a person is held legally responsible for the actions of others even though they themselves did nothing wrong

Court Case

Hoffman v. Moore Regional Hospital Inc.

114 N.C.App. 248, 441 S.E.2d 567 (1994)
Court of Appeals of North Carolina

FACTS: Ruth Hoffman underwent a radiological procedure that was performed at Moore Regional Hospital. The radiologist, Dr. Lina, performed a renal angioplasty, during which Mrs. Hoffman suffered complications and had to be transferred to another healthcare facility. Her condition continued to deteriorate and she passed away on January, 9, 1990.

Dr. Lina was not an employee of Moore Regional Hospital, but worked for Pinehurst Radiology Group. This group performed most, if not all, of the radiology services for Moore Regional Hospital. A lawsuit was filed by Mrs. Hoffman's family against Moore Regional Hospital, claiming that as *respondeat superior*, Moore General Hospital was vicariously liable for Dr. Lina's actions. Moore General Hospital contends that they are not responsible for Dr. Lina's actions because they are not his employer, but instead Dr. Lina is an independent contractor.

ISSUE: The issue before the court was "whether the alleged employer has the right to supervise and control the details of the work performed by the alleged employee."

RULE: "We conclude that no genuine issue of material fact exists as to whether Dr. Lina was an employee of the Hospital. As a matter of law, he was not."

EMPHASIS: A main part of the law of *respondeat superior* is the ability to control the actions of their employees. In this case, the court found that Dr. Lina was not an employee of the hospital, and therefore the hospital did not have the necessary control over her actions to satisfy the *respondeat superior* required. The case against Moore General Hospital was dismissed, but the case against Dr. Lina was allowed to continue.

Contract law is a unique and very specialized category of law. There are numerous requirements and conditions that need to be in place to form a contract and laws that dictate how a contract is carried out. While you may not initially think that contract law applies to healthcare, you will deal with contracts every day that you provide patient care. In addition, there are unique characteristics to contract law, some of which have a direct impact on patient care that you need to be aware of.

> **Why do I need to know about contract law if I am going to be working in healthcare?**

Contracts

Because healthcare professionals deal in contracts every day, it is important that we discuss some of the basics of contracts, what they are, how they are formed, and how they are used. To start our discussion, we need to identify what a **contract** is.

In order for a court to recognize an agreement, specific requirements need to be satisfied. Those requirements are outlined in the common law definition of a contract, which is *an offer that has been accepted with due consideration.*

> **contract:** an agreement between parties that the law will recognize

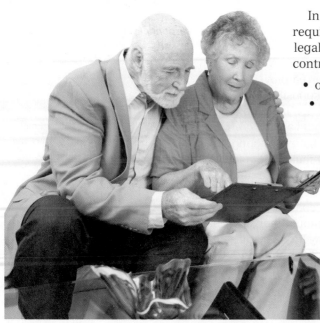

In order for a contract to exist, it must have the legal requirements, or elements, that the law requires. Using the legal definition of a contract, the elements required to form a contract are:

- offer
- acceptance
- consideration

Offer

All contracts begin with an offer. An offer is thought of as the desire to enter into an agreement. You probably are not aware of it, but you encounter offers every single day. Advertisements, such as the commercials you see on television or in the newspaper, are offers to enter into a contract. While we typically think of contracts being only in written form, verbal offers can form the basis for creating a contract. In addition, the mere existence of certain circumstances can be considered an offer as well. For example, a healthcare institution that has an emergency room is offering emergency services to the community.

Acceptance

Acceptance is, generally, the taking of the offer, and like an offer it can come in several forms. Acceptance does not require a verbal response, such as "I accept your offer," but can come in the form of action. If you respond to an advertisement by walking into a store and giving them money for the item advertised, you are accepting their offer. To use a healthcare example, a person who comes to an emergency room is accepting the offer of healthcare services.

Consideration

The consideration element required to form a contract is much more complex than what can be analyzed here. Essentially, what the consideration requirement is asking is whether the parties have thought about what they are giving up when entering into the contract. For example, if you walk into a store to purchase an advertised product, have you thought about how handing over your money might impact your finances? Even though complex, for our purposes, consideration is an important concept because it has a direct impact on healthcare; not everyone has the ability to provide consideration, but contracts still need to be formed.

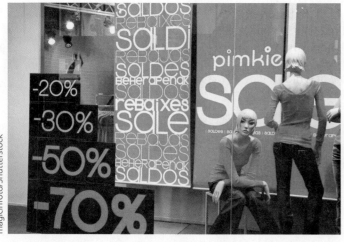

Contractual Capacity

Contractual capacity is not an element used to determine whether a contract is formed. It is used to address the element of consideration. If a person lacks the mental capacity to enter into a contract, then the consideration element of a contract cannot be satisfied.

In the healthcare arena, we have patients who are under the influence of drugs (both illegal and prescription), or who do not have the mental capacity to form the requisite consideration (such as a child or the mentally impaired). Even though a person may not have the contractual capacity required to form a contract, we still need to form a contract in order to provide healthcare services. In certain situations, the law will allow the formation of a contract by those who lack contractual capacity.

Implied Contracts

Each time a patient seeks healthcare, he or she has to provide consent in order to receive treatment. Normally, when a patient arrives at a healthcare institution he or she is asked to sign a Consent for Treatment form. However, there are times when medical conditions exist where patients are unable to provide actual consent. For example, what if an unconscious patient is brought into the emergency room following an accident? Obviously, we cannot wait for an unconscious person to wake up and give consent before we start treating that person. In situations like this, the law will determine that an implied consent exists so that healthcare can provide the treatment a person needs. This implied consent addresses the consideration element that might be lacking to form a contract from those who do not have the ability to do so.

The essence behind an implied contract is that if the person were able to do so, they would have agreed to treatment, and therefore entered into a contract for healthcare services. By coming to the hospital, or being taken to the hospital, it is *implied* that the person wishes to be treated and thereby gives their consent to treatment—even if they are medically unable to do so. As a healthcare professional you need to understand the situations in which a court would determine that an implied contract was formed.

Suppose a child fell off a swing set at the school playground and is brought into the emergency room. All attempts have been made to reach the parents, but no one has been able to make contact with either, in order to get consent for treatment. Under implied contracts, the emergency room staff can provide basic medical care, such as respiratory support, treat wounds, and administer some medications. But what if the child requires a blood transfusion? Can we give a blood transfusion to a child under the implied contract theory? How is someone in healthcare supposed to know or understand what the limits are? Within the law, there is a legal standard that is used in situations such as these called the **reasonable person standard**.

The reasonable person standard is used to answer a variety of different legal questions and can be used in a variety of different contexts. The reasonable person standard asks the question:

What would a reasonable and prudent person do in the same, or similar, circumstances?

Returning to our example concerning the child who needs a blood transfusion, the court would ask: "What would a reasonable and prudent parent (person) do if their child was in need of a blood transfusion (the same, or similar, circumstance)?" Do you think that a reasonable and prudent parent would offer consent to a blood transfusion in this situation? If the answer is yes, then we can consider giving the blood transfusion under implied consent. But if the answer is no, then we will not be allowed to give a blood transfusion under implied consent.

Making tough decisions such as this one, is further evidence of why all healthcare professionals need to know about health law and medical ethics. Have you thought about whether the child's family belongs to a particular religious group, such as Jehovah's Witnesses, which do not receive blood transfusions for religious reasons?

reasonable person standard: a legal standard used to determine whether the actions of a party are warranted

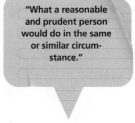

"What a reasonable and prudent person would do in the same or similar circumstance."

teacept/Shutterstock

The Statute of Frauds

At the beginning of this section, we looked at the definition of a contract: an agreement between the parties that the court would recognize. As we noted, the definition does not require that agreement to be in writing, as the courts may recognize oral contracts as well. But even though the definition of a contract does not require a writing, there are times when the law does. The Statute of Frauds is a law that indicates when a contract must be in writing in order for the courts to recognize that contract. The Statute of Frauds requires written contracts for:

- Executor/administrator agreements (such as wills and trusts)
- Anything that cannot be completed within a one-year time-frame (such as employment contracts for over a one-year period)
- Interests in land (such as the purchase of a home)
- The sale of any item priced at $7,500 or more (such as a vehicle or piece of equipment)

While you may not be exposed to the Statute of Frauds requirements as an entry-level healthcare practitioner, it does have implications on your personal life, so you should be aware that it exists and what situations it covers.

Make FALSE statements TRUE.

Rewrite the false statements below by replacing the bolded, italicized, and underlined word(s) to make it a true statement.

1. There are two perspectives related to what to write in a patient's medical record, the ***licensure*** perspective and the ***patient*** perspective.

   _____

2. According to the legal principle, "If it wasn't written down, it ***likely may still have been performed***."

   _____

3. When writing an insurance policy, an underwriter will use ***premiums*** to determine a person's ***actuarial table***.

   _____

4. ***Diagnostic Related Groups*** are used for coding outpatient procedures to insurance companies.

   _____

5. ***Respondeat superior*** helps explain why an employer is responsible for the actions of an employee even if the employer did nothing wrong.

   _____

Circle Exercise

Circle the correct word from the choices given.

1. A (**diagnostic related group, doctrine of professional discretion, subpoena duces tecum**) is a special request used to obtain a copy of patient's medical record.

2. A (**current procedure terminology, doctrine of professional discretion, subpoena duces tecum**) allows a physician to rule against a patient's request for medical records.

3. (**Acceptance, Contractual Capacity, Offer**) is sometimes used to address the element of consideration.

4. Insurance companies developed (**premiums, managed care, upcoding**) to help combat the rising costs of healthcare.

5. The (**Malpractice Insurance Policy, Premiums, Statute of Frauds**) will determine when a contract is required to be in writing in order to be enforced by the courts.

Matching

Match the numbered term to its lettered definition.

1. _____ actuarial tables

2. _____ contract

3. _____ insurance

4. _____ legal document

5. _____ reasonable person standard

6. _____ *respondeat superior*

7. _____ subpoena duces tecum

8. _____ upcoding

9. _____ vicarious liability

A. a comprehensive list of statistical data; used most often by insurance companies to determine illness, disease, and accident projections.

B. a legal standard used to determine whether the actions of a party are warranted.

C. an agreement between parties that the law will recognize.

D. any writing that provides information or ideas that can be attributed to the author.

E. "bring with you under penalty of punishment"; a requirement that documents be delivered to a court or brought with you to court.

F. "let the master answer," a concept where the employer is responsible for the actions of its employees.

G. liability without fault; a person is held legally responsible for the actions of others even though they themselves did nothing wrong.

H. the transfer of an obligation from one party to another, usually in exchange for a fee.

I. using an incorrect ICD or CPT code to gain a larger insurance payment.

Deliberations: Critical Thinking Questions

Question 1: The legal principle "If it wasn't written down, it wasn't done" demonstrates the importance of documenting care. But does the opposite hold true? Just because care is documented, does that mean that care was actually provided? Is there a way to tell whether care was provided or not, even though it was not documented?

Question 2: You are caring for a patient recovering from a heart attack. A common medication provided to heart attack patients is nitroglycerin, which can cause headaches. The doctor has provided the following order for pain medication: two tablets of 325mg aspirin every four hours as needed for headaches.

During the night the patient puts his call light on requesting something for his headache. You give him the aspirin that the doctor orders. Twenty minutes later you check on the patient and find that he is fast asleep.

Using that example, write what you would document in the patient's medical record.

Question 3: The survival of any healthcare institution relies heavily on the reimbursement that they receive from insurance companies. Operating as a business requires that healthcare institutions operate within a budget and perform cost/benefit analysis on the products that they offer. Should a hospital focus on patient care requirements or approach healthcare from a business decision perspective? Is there a way for them to do both?

Question 4: A pedestrian was hit by a car and brought into the emergency room unconscious. There was no identification on the patient to indicate who he is or who his family is. Besides his head injury, he has also suffered severe trauma to his left lower leg. The surgeon is recommending amputation as the best course of treatment for his leg injury; waiting too long could result in severe blood loss, infection, gangrene, and even death. However, because the patient is unconscious, he is unable to provide consent. And because there is no identification on the patient, no way to know if he has family to contact. A decision needs to be made now. How would you decide? What factors would you use to make that determination?

Question 5: A doctor is unhappy with the reimbursement amounts being provided by an insurance company. Although he does not increase the amount of time he spends with each patient, he has the patients wait in the examination room for additional time. That timeframe can then be used to charge a higher amount under the CPT classification. As a medical assistant working in the doctor's office, you become aware of what the doctor is doing. What should you do?

Closing Arguments: Case Analysis

Danny is a registered nurse working on a busy orthopedic floor at the local hospital. He has had a particularly busy day, with several of his patients either being discharged home or sent to surgery.

Because of this, he has not had time to document his care as it happened, but has jotted down notes. He is now at the end of his shift and sits down to complete his documentation.

Danny is documenting the care that he provided to Mr. Jones. After he has written a few sentences, the unit clerk gives Danny some lab work that just came back on Mrs. Smith. After reviewing the lab work, Danny returns to his documentation but mistakenly writes some notes about Mrs. Smith's lab work in Mr. Jones's chart.

Question 1: How would you suggest Danny correct this mistake?

Question 2: A few weeks later, Mr. Jones requests a copy of his medical records so that he can send them to a specialist for a

second opinion. A person working in the medical records department has received the request and obtained the doctor's approval to provide Mr. Jones with a copy. But, while she is copying the medical record for Mr. Jones she notices that there is documentation about Mrs. Smith in the chart. What suggestions do you have about how to resolve this issue?

Question 3: Because the office copied the patient's medical records, they submit a bill to her insurance company as a simple office visit. The insurance company denies the payment. Should the doctor's office absorb this cost or bill the patient? Explain your answer.

The Briefcase

This section repeats the objectives from the beginning of the chapter and provides a summary of the most important concepts for each objective. Use this section as a quick review and to check your understanding of the chapter key points.

Objective 1: List the five different purposes that medical records serve.
- Manage Healthcare
- Tracking Healthcare
- Provide Clinical Data
- Meet Regulatory Requirements
- Document Healthcare

Objective 2: Provide examples of what type of court cases medical records can be used for.
- See Table 4-1 on pg. 60.

Objective 3: Briefly describe the two perspective related to charting in a medical record.
- Medical perspective demonstrates what care has been provided, taking into account all actions surrounding the care and the affect of that care.
- Legal perspective provides enough information so that you will be able to accurately recall it at a later time.

Objective 4: Identify what a subpoena duces tecum is and when it is used.
- medical records
- to bring with you under penalty of punishment
- malpractice cases

Objective 5: Compare and contrast the ownership of medical records.
- Institutions own the paper
- Patients own the information
- Doctrine of Professional Discretion

Objective 6: Using the key terms premium and actuarial tables, briefly define how insurance works.
- Premiums are monthly fees paid by the insured.
- Actuarial tables are used by underwriters to determine risk of loss.

Objective 7: Provide an example of how ICD codes and CPT codes affect upcoding.
- ICD codes are for inpatients
- CPT codes are used for outpatient procedures
- Using a different code to receive more money from the insurance company

Objective 8: Compare and contrast *respondeat superior* and vicarious liability.
- respondeat superior gives the employer responsibility over the actions of the employee
- vicarious liability creates liability even though someone did nothing wrong.

Objective 9: Explain how the reasonable person standard is applied to implied contracts.
- Implied contracts are formed when it is implied that a person would want a contract, but is unable to do so.
- A reasonable person in the same situation would want to form a contract.

Maximize Your Success with the Companion Website

The companion website to this textbook contains materials that can help you better understand the concepts presented in this chapter. Go to www.myhealthprofessionskit.com to access:

- sample quizzes
- related web links
- learning games
- and more…

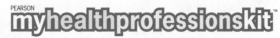
PEARSON
myhealthprofessionskit™

5 Privacy and Confidentiality

When we take care of patients, we sometimes have to ask them very private things (feelings, moods, sexual practices, etc.). This environment of trust is essential to healthcare, because patients need to feel comfortable about giving private information; especially for those things that might affect their health. For example, drug interactions are a major concern for any patient. If a patient is taking illegal drugs, as healthcare providers we need to know that information to avoid any drug interactions.

Because we are asking patients to provide us with private information based on medical need, the patient needs to be assured that we will only use that information for medical purposes. And, in providing that private information, that we do not disclose it to anyone who is not directly involved in providing medical care to that patient. In this chapter, we will discuss the laws of privacy and confidentiality associated with healthcare.

MEASURE YOUR PROGRESS: LEARNING OBJECTIVES

After studying this chapter, you will be able to:

- Describe what common laws exist that relate to privacy and confidentiality.

- List the two different laws that are incorporated into HIPAA

- Identify who HIPAA applies to, and how that determination is made.

- Analyze what information HIPAA refers to as protected health information (PHI).

- Explain how HIPAA makes sure that private information stays private.

- Determine who private information can be disclosed to and why.

- Provide examples of how information is disclosed under HIPAA.

- Detail the steps involved for Office of Civil Rights (OCR) reviews for HIPAA complaints or infractions.

- Define the different penalties a person can receive for violating HIPAA.

KEY TERMS

accountability

compliance

covered entity

de-identify

liable

limited data set

portability

privacy

slander

PROFESSIONAL HIGHLIGHT

Hisoka is the compliance officer at the local hospital. As the compliance officer, he is responsible for ensuring that the institution is complying with the state and federal laws that relate to healthcare. Over the past few years, a large part of Hisoka's job has focused on the new privacy laws that relate to healthcare, such as HIPAA. Without a thorough understanding of the law and how healthcare works, Hisoka would not be able to ensure that the institution and its employees were maintaining compliance with the law.

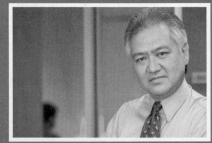

When the Health Insurance Portability and Accountability Act (HIPAA) was first introduced, it sent shock waves through the healthcare community. Much of the concern had to do with the drastic changes that HIPAA was going to require of healthcare institutions. Part of this concern came from the fact that Congress, for the first time, was legislating an area of healthcare that they had not legislated before, that of **privacy**.

Privacy and confidentiality are not new concepts to either healthcare or the law. Healthcare and the law have always taken the issue of privacy and confidentiality seriously. But prior to HIPAA, only a few laws existed to address issues of privacy and confidentiality.

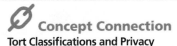

I've heard so much about HIPAA over the past few years. What's the big deal and why is it so important to healthcare?

Privacy Common Laws

Normally when you think about how the law addresses the harms a person receives, it is common to think of physical harm; such as broken bones, wounds, or pain and suffering. But, with privacy laws, the injury is not physical; instead the harm is to the person's personality or reputation.

privacy: something that belongs to or is intended only for an individual or particular group

Defamation

One of the oldest existing laws related to privacy is the tort of defamation, also known as defamation of character. The common law definition of defamation is:

an intentional false or defamatory statement about another person that results in damages.

The legal elements required to establish the tort of defamation are:

1. intentional
2. false or defamatory statement
3. of another person
4. causing damage

Although the tort of defamation is uncommon in healthcare, when it does occur it provides a good example of how a person's reputation can be harmed.

As a healthcare professional, your patients and friends will commonly ask about other healthcare professionals; such as,

⊘ Concept Connection
Tort Classifications and Privacy
Torts are categorized according to the harms a person receives. There are many different tort classifications; harms to personality is one of them.

⇄ The Ethics of Law

The key to defamation in the healthcare setting is whether you are making the statement as a healthcare professional or as an individual. As an individual, you are entitled to your personal opinions and can share those personal opinions with family and close friends. If your parents were to ask you about a specific doctor, you can respond to them with your personal opinion, because you are being asked as their child. But, if a patient asks you that same question, because you are being asked as a healthcare professional, you have to give a professional response.

- What if a patient asked you about Dr. Smith, who is someone you did not care for?
- How would you respond, as a professional, to the patient's question, "Is he a good doctor?"

 Sidebar

One way to think about defamation is by looking at the word components; the prefix *de-* (taking away) and the word root *fame*. By committing defamation, you are *taking away* their *fame;* what makes a person famous or the reputation that they have.

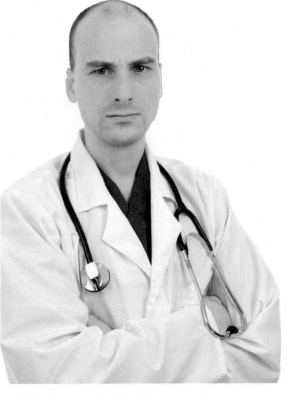

spaxiax/Shutterstock

"Is Dr. Smith a good doctor?" While you may have strong opinions about Dr. Smith, what if you responded to the patient by saying, "I would not let him treat my dog!" Is that statement going to cause harm to Dr. Smith's reputation? Note: the law of defamation does not require that the statement be false. Instead, the statement can be false *OR* defamatory.

There are two subcategories to the tort of defamation, libel and slander. Prior to the electronic revolution, slander was much more common than libel was. But today, with social media such as MySpace, Facebook, and Twitter, libel is becoming more common.

libel: the communication of a false or defamatory statement that is written or seen

slander: the communication of a false or defamatory statement that is spoken or heard

Invasion of Privacy

The common law definition of the tort invasion of privacy is:

the intentional prying or intruding into another person's privacy that causes damage.

The legal elements required to establish the tort of invasion of privacy are:

1. intentional
2. prying or intruding into
3. another person's privacy
4. causing damage

The tort invasion of privacy requires someone to take affirmative steps, by *"prying or intruding"* into a person's privacy. But what about the opposite of that; someone that has private information and releases it to another person? Since there was no *prying or intruding*, the tort of invasion of privacy would not apply. Neither would the common law tort of defamation, because there was no false or defamatory statement.

With all of the changes that were occurring in society and technology, Congress grew concerned about whether the common laws related to privacy would be sufficient to cover breaches in privacy or confidentiality. One of the main concerns was how patient information was going to be kept private, in today's electronic age. To ensure that patient information was kept private, Congress enacted HIPAA, the Health Insurance Portability and Accountability Act.

Health Insurance Portability and Accountability Act (HIPAA)

The initial catalyst for creating HIPAA grew out of concerns over Internet safety and technological security. At that same time that HIPAA was being considered, another bill was working its way through Congress concerning

Court Case

Pachowitz v. LeDoux

265 Wis.2d 631, 666 N.W.2d 88 (2003)
Wisconsin Court of Appeals

FACTS: Katherina LeDoux worked as an EMT for Tess Corners Volunteer Fire Department. On April 21, 2000 she responded to the home of Julie Pachowitz for a possible overdose. Upon arrival, Pachowitz was found to be unresponsive and had poor vital signs. Because Pachowitz worked as an employee at West Allis Memorial Hospital, her husband requested that the patient be taken to Waukesha Memorial Hospital instead, "to avoid disclosure of her need for emergency medical care to her fellow employees."

After taking the patient to the hospital, EMT LeDoux telephoned a fellow worker and friend of Pachowitz named Slocomb. LeDoux testifies that she made the phone call "because she was concerned about Pachowitz and thought Slocomb could possibly be of assistance . . ." Pachowitz filed a defamation and invasion of privacy lawsuit against LeDoux and the volunteer Fire Department. The jury found in favor of Pachowitz.

ISSUE: At issue in this case, was whether LeDoux breached Pachowitz's privacy because of the telephone call that she made.

RULE: The court ruled that disclosure of private information depends on the giving and receiving of the information.

EMPHASIS: While the defamation portion of the lawsuit was dropped, the invasion of privacy portion continued to trial. The importance of this case demonstrates that, even though LeDoux may have acted out of genuine concern, healthcare professionals are still required to keep patient information private.

health insurance. Because both bills had to do with healthcare, the two bills were combined. There are two different components to HIPAA:

1. laws that regulate health *Insurance Portability*, and
2. laws that regulate health *Accountability*.

Health Accountability

When you talk to people about HIPAA, most think about the health **accountability** section that covers privacy and confidentiality.

The health accountability section of HIPAA requires that healthcare professionals keep certain information confidential and private. Or, put another way, requires that healthcare professionals be held *accountable* for the private information that they have. But what information is HIPAA referring to and how does the law ensure accountability?

While the initial catalyst for creating HIPAA had to do with the electronic exchange of private information, the statute grew to cover *all forms* of communication; verbal, written, electronic, or otherwise. To understand exactly what HIPAA is and how it works, we can examine the legislation from three different angles:

- who HIPAA applies to,
- what HIPPA regulates, and
- how HIPAA is enforced.

Covered Entities

The first issue to address is to determine whom does HIPAA apply to. HIPAA only regulates specific organizations and the organization's employees. HIPAA is not a blanket confidentiality policy that affects all businesses and citizens. HIPAA only applies to what the legislation defines as a **covered entity**.

The definition of a covered entity under HIPAA includes:

- any healthcare provider,
- any health insurance company, or
- any health-related company that gives or receives patient information.

Any organization that provides patient care is a covered entity, that includes hospitals, doctor's offices, home health agencies, and outpatient clinics. Health-related business, such as durable medical equipment companies, transcription services, or billing companies are also covered entities under HIPAA, because they receive health information as part of doing business. Health insurance companies are also covered entities under HIPAA, but other types of insurance, such as automobile insurance or life insurance, are not covered entities. (see Fig. 5-1)

Because of some common confusions about HIPAA, the law makes the distinction in determining what a covered entity is and is not. Just because a business or individual has health information does not mean that HIPAA automatically applies to them. For example, elementary schools have health information regarding the vaccinations that their students have received. Even though schools have health information, they are not covered entities under HIPAA. (However, just because they are not covered entities under HIPAA does not mean that other privacy and confidentiality laws do not apply either. They still are subject to the laws of invasion of privacy, defamation, libel, and slander.)

accountability: being held responsible; being required to answer to a situation

covered entity: an institution or group that is the subject of a regulation or law

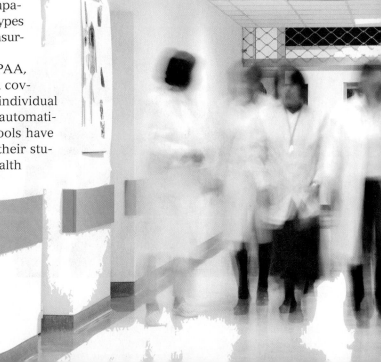

Fig. 5-1. Only institutions that meet the definition of a covered entity are subject to the laws and requirements of HIPAA.

© Vilevi/Dreamstime.com

Now that a covered entity has been identified, we can move forward in our discussion to determine what HIPPA regulates and how they regulate it. To ensure that patient information is kept private and confidential, the health accountability section of HIPAA contains two rules, the Privacy Rule and the Security Rule.

The Privacy Rule

One area of concern prompting the passage of HIPAA was how the business of healthcare exchanged information; especially in the electronic age. The Privacy Rule of HIPAA specifically addresses those concerns. The purpose of HIPPA's Privacy Rule, as stated in the statute, is:

"to assure that individuals' health information is properly protected while allowing the flow of health information needed to provide and promote high quality health care and to protect the public's health and well being."

HIPAA's Privacy Rule tells us:

1. what patient information is private,
2. to whom discloser is allowed, and
3. if disclosure is allowed, how is information disclosed.

What Information Is Private

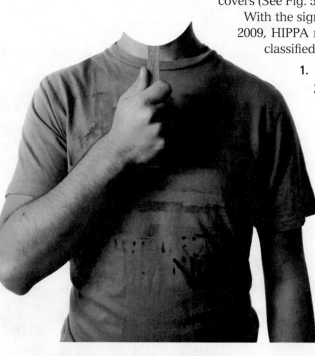

In order to understand what we are actually dealing with when complying with HIPAA, we have to know what type of information HIPAA is referring to when they say "private patient information." HIPAA defines private patient information as Protected Health Information (PHI). What kind of information do we use to identify a particular individual? If you were told about a man, living in New York City, would you be able to readily identify who that specific person is? But what about an unmarried Caucasian male, born on April 1, 1976, who resides at 123 Avenue A in New York City, New York? Does that information readily point to one particular individual? Any information that is unique to an individual or can pinpoint a specific individual is the type of information that HIPAA covers (See Fig. 5-2).

With the signing of the American Recovery and Reinvestment Act of 2009, HIPPA now identifies 11 different types of information that are classified as PHI:

1. Names
2. Geographic information (addresses)
3. All dates that directly relate to an individual, such as a date of birth or dates that services were provided
4. Telephone numbers, including fax numbers and cell phone numbers
5. E-mail addresses
6. Social Security numbers
7. Account numbers, which includes medical record numbers or health plan (insurance) numbers
8. Certificate or license numbers
9. Web site addresses, URL's or http addresses
10. Biometric identifiers, including fingerprints and voice prints
11. Photographic and comparable images

After reviewing this list, you might be saying to yourself that most of it is not health information at all but personal information. Do not be confused by the word "health" in Protected *Health* Information. Most of the information identified as PHI is not really information about a person's health at all. But remember, in order for HIPAA to apply, the organization must be a covered entity. Therefore, the word *health* is used in the designation, not to identify what health information is but to identify the setting in which that information is used, that of health care.

Who You Can Disclose To

One of the initial concerns raised by HIPAA was whether the implementation was going to impact patient care. With the strict standards regarding privacy, some thought that HIPAA was going to limit healthcare workers from talking to each other. The application of HIPAA's Privacy Rule allows for the exchange of PHI so that information can be used and shared:

- to coordinate treatment and care,
- to ensure that healthcare workers provide good care,
- with family, friends, relatives, or others designated by the patient (unless the patient objects),
- to pay health providers,
- to protect the public health, and
- to make required reporting to governmental agencies.

To Coordinate Treatment and Care In order to identify that we are providing the correct treatment to the correct patient, certain PHI needs to be disclosed to other healthcare workers that are providing care. How would a healthcare worker be able to provide patient care, without disclosing some type of PHI? HIPAA allows for the disclosure of PHI to a healthcare worker who is providing care to the patient or involved in coordinating patient care. What HIPAA does not allow is disclosure of PHI to a healthcare worker just because they are a healthcare worker.

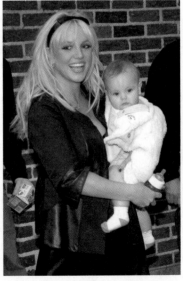

Fig. 5-2. A patient signs in on an electronic sign-in sheet. To protect patient information, many healthcare institutions have switched to electronic sign-in sheets.

Glenda M. Powers/Shutterstock

✔ Concept Application

Britney Spears and HIPAA

In September 2005, pop star Britney Spears gave birth at UCLA Medical Center. During her hospitalization, several hospital employees who were not directly involved in Spears' care accessed her medical records. When the hospital discovered this breach of confidentiality and privacy, they reprimanded the employees and instituted mandatory HIPAA training.

Three years later, in January 2008, Spears had a much publicized emotional breakdown, and was again admitted to UCLA Medical Center. Because of the press coverage related to the breakdown, combined with the past infraction, the hospital took a proactive stance. It sent out notices, e-mails, and announcements to all hospital employees reminding them of the past violations and the importance of HIPAA. Despite this warning, 19 employees who were not involved in Spears' care accessed her medical records. The hospital terminated 13 employees and suspended the 6 others. UCLA Medical Center immediately notified governmental officials about the HIPAA infraction and worked with them to develop a contingency plan so that something like this would not happen again. Because of their proactive measures, and how the hospital handled the infractions, no HIPAA fines were levied against UCLA Medical Center.

© Everett Collection Inc/Alamy

Court Case

Jose N. Proenza Sanfiel, R.N. v. Department of Health

749 So.2d 525 (1999)
Florida Court of Appeals

FACTS: Jose Proenza Sanfiel, a psychiatric Registered Nurse, claims that he purchased a computer for $20 at a thrift shop that had been previously owned by Charter Behavioral Health System, a psychiatric hospital in Orlando Florida. (This claim is disputed by Charter, stating that they never sold or donated any computer equipment.) When Proenza Sanfiel got the computer home, he discovered that it contained patient records, including names, admission dates, types of addiction(s), treatments, and psychiatric disorders.

At this same time, Charter was being investigated for defrauding the government. Proenza Sanfiel contacted law enforcement agencies, believing that a crime had been committed by leaving the information on the computer before donating it. But, law enforcement officials did not file charges against Charter because it was outside their jurisdiction. Next, Proenza Sanfiel contacted local news agencies and allowed them to see the information that was stored on the computer. Even though Proenza Sanfiel requested that the patient information be blurred out, when the story aired patient information was not obscured. To supplement the story, a few journalists tried to interview some of the patients on the computer list.

Upon learning about the story, Florida's state medical board issued an emergency suspension of Proenza Sanfiel nursing license. They asked that Proenza Sanfiel turn over the computer's hard drive; which he refused to do. Charter asked Proenza Sanfiel to turn over the computer as well, but instead of doing so voluntarily, he offered to sell the computer to Charter for $20,000.

Testifying, Proenza Sanfiel admitted that he made the disclosure. He also admitted that he knew that as a psychiatric nurse that he could be disciplined for disclosing confidential patient information. But, he argued that his action of releasing the information to the media was done so as a private citizen, not as a healthcare provider.

ISSUE: While this particular case focused on the authority of the medical board to suspend Proenza Sanfiel's nursing license, the reason for the suspension centered on his unprofessional conduct by releasing private patient information.

RULE: "It is reasonable to characterize Proenza Sanfiel's actions as unprofessional conduct even though Proenza Sanfiel was acting in a 'private' capacity."

EMPHASIS: The importance of this case is multi-faceted. First, it demonstrates that actions you take as a private citizen can have professional repercussion. Second, that medical information can only be released if a person has a medical need for that information. And third, the law regards confidentiality and privacy as very important.

The privacy rule of HIPAA applies to the giving and receiving of information. If you have a medical reason for obtaining a patient's private information, HIPAA's Privacy Rule allows you to do so. But if you do not have a medical reason for obtaining a patient's PHI, then you are not allowed to obtain a patient's PHI. The same holds true for whom you can give information to. If you have patient PHI, you can only provide information to those people who are authorized to have that information. Meaning, you can only give what PHI you have to a person who has a medical reason for obtaining that PHI.

To Ensure That Healthcare Workers Provide Good Care There are times that healthcare workers need a patient's private information, even though they are not directly involved in the patient's medical care. HIPAA allows this exception, if the purpose is to ensure that healthcare workers provide good care.

In 2005, the Patient Safety and Quality Improvement Act (PSQIA) was passed. This act provided a mechanism for healthcare institutions to gather information about patient care to improve the quality of care they are providing. For example, pharmacists at a local hospital may notice that they are not dispensing as much pain medication as they have in the past. They ask that the quality improvement department develop a report to identify the exact reason for the decrease in pain medication so that they can identify if a problem exists that they need to address. Specialists in the quality improvement department will comb through patient medical records to gather the information that they need to formulate that report. While these quality specialists are not directly involved in patient care, they are allowed access to patient information to improve the quality of care that is being provided.

Concept Connection

HIPAA and Medical Research

Medical research is another avenue where medical information will be obtained by personnel who are not providing direct medical care to patients. Because the goal of medical research is to improve the quality of medical care, HIPAA allows certain patient information to be obtained by research personnel.

Family, Friends, Relatives Family, friends, and relatives provide a vital support structure for patients. To provide that support, they will sometimes need to have private patient information. HIPAA does not preclude healthcare workers from providing information to family, friends, and relatives, but there are limitations.

First, we can only release information to the people that the patient authorizes us to release information to. When a patient is admitted to the hospital, or sees a doctor for the first time, they will be asked to fill out a questionnaire. One of the questions will ask whom healthcare information can be released to. While patients will typically list family members, they can designate anyone that they like.

Second, we need to be careful about the information that we release. Although a patient may authorize disclosure, that does not mean that we can give out any and all private information. Unfortunately, there are no specific guidelines to determine what information should or should not be disclosed to authorized family members. Instead, the only rule that we can follow is common sense.

Protecting The Public There are times when patient information needs to be released to law enforcement or other governmental agencies. For example, notifying child protective services about suspected child abuse is a legal requirement that all healthcare practitioners must adhere to. Because the legal requirement for mandatory reporting is found in laws other than HIPAA, they supersede HIPAA's requirements.

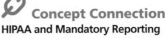

Concept Connection

HIPAA and Mandatory Reporting

Even though the law of HIPAA ensures patient privacy, there are times when other laws require healthcare professionals to release information. Mandatory reporting laws are a part of a healthcare practitioners professional responsibilities.

Paying Health Providers One of the first uses of the Internet in the healthcare setting was the electronic submission of information to insurance companies for payment of services. In order for insurance companies to be able to pay healthcare providers, they need to know what patient they are paying for and what services have been provided. HIPAA allows the disclosure of PHI to health insurance companies for the payment of services.

How Information Is Disclosed

Even though HIPAA allows disclosure of information, that does not mean that any and all information can be disclosed to any authorized individuals or businesses. Instead, HIPAA requires that when we release private information, we release only the *minimal amount* of PHI that is necessary for the person receiving it. To accomplish this goal, the Privacy Rule of HIPAA requires that we **de-identify** patient documents that contain PHI.

de-identify: the process of removing any information from documents, or restricting electronic access to information, that a person is not authorized to receive

To de-indentify a document, you start by making a copy of the medical record or report that is being requested. The document is then reviewed and any PHI that is not required by the recipient is blacked out on the copy. Or, if using electronic forms of records, individuals are not provided access to particular fields or pages of information. But wait a minute! Previously, we stated that altering medical records was not allowed. So why is HIPAA now telling us that we have to?

The answer is that what you are blacking out, to de-indentify, is not the original record but a copy. You never want to black out the original medical record.

Sidebar

Copies of medical records provided to an attorney under a *subpoena duces tecum* are not de-identified. Since the subpoena is court ordered, you do not have to de-identify the documents. In addition, because the patient is working with the attorney in filing the lawsuit, he or she is providing authorization for the information to be disclosed.

Once a document has been de-identified, it is referred to as a **limited data set**.

Even though identifying information has been removed from a document, that does not mean that the information provided is open to the public. A person or organization that receives a limited data set as a covered entity is still obligated to institute the safeguards required of HIPAA to protect that information.

limited data set: a document that has had some, or all, of the patient's private information removed

Court Case

In Re Application of the Milton S. Hershey Medical Center of the Pennsylvania State University. Appeal of John Doe, M.D. in Re Application of the Harrisburg Hospital. Appeal of John Doe M.D.

595 A.2d 1290, 407 Pa. Super. 565 (1991)
Superior Court of Pennsylvania

FACTS: A resident physician, referred to as Dr. John Doe (a pseudonym) was working at both Hershey Medical Center and Harrisburg Hospital. During an invasive, internal surgical procedure, the attending physician accidently cut Dr. Doe on his finger. (Whether there was a transfer of Dr. Doe's blood to the patient is unknown, court records only state "apparently there was not.") Dr. Doe voluntary took an HIV test, which came back positive, which were confirmed by later tests. Upon learning about his HIV status, Dr. Doe took a voluntary leave of absence.

Hershey Medical Center and Harrisburg Hospital identified 447 patients that had received care from Dr. Doe. The hospitals filed a joint petition, citing "compelling need" to release information about Dr. Doe and his medical condition to the patients he had provided care to.

The trial court order that the hospital could release Dr. Doe's name only to physicians, so they could identify which patients to notify. Patients could only be told that a resident physician involved in their care had tested HIV positive. Dr. Doe, through his attorney, appealed the decision of the trial court allowing the limited release of his information.

ISSUE: The issue, on appeal, was whether the trial court had the authority to allow the hospital to disclose information about Dr. Doe and his medical condition.

RULE: "After weighing the competing interests in this case, we find that the scales tip in favor of the public health, regardless of the small potential for transmittal of the fatal virus." The appellate court ruled that the trial court did not abuse its discretion.

EMPHASIS: This case involves very important issues that must be handled delicately. While the over-riding principle of the law is to keep patient information private, there are limited exceptions. But, as this case demonstrates, those exceptions cannot be taken lightly.

Incidental Disclosure

Even though HIPAA has several rules regarding patient privacy, sometimes disclosure cannot be prevented. HIPAA does not require that healthcare institutions implement every conceivable safeguard to protect patient privacy. Nor does HIPAA require covered entities to guarantee protection of patient information from any and all possible disclosures. For example, if a patient has a cardiac arrest, and the nursing assistant yells out into the corridor, "The patient is coding!" and that statement is overheard by a visitor, that would be considered an incidental disclosure that cannot be helped; nor is it something that HIPAA is trying to prevent. Instead, HIPPA requires that healthcare institutions implement reasonable safeguards. What safeguards are used will depend on the institution, the type of medical care that they provide, and the situation. Sometimes, the only way to evaluate whether safeguards are appropriate or need to be changed is after an incidental disclosure occurs.

HIPAA Violations

When Congress drafted HIPAA, they granted the U.S. Department of Health and Human Services (HHS) with administrative authority to oversee HIPAA and provide the necessary tools for its implementation. To help HHS to accomplish those goals, HHS joined forces with two additional governmental agencies; the OCR and the U.S. Department of Justice (DOJ) to ensure that individuals and covered entities are in **compliance** with HIPAA's requirements.

Because a person's privacy is an essential component of a person's civil rights, HHS grants the OCR the authority to investigate HIPAA complaints. Although complaints can be filed at any time, OCR recommends that a complaint be filed within 180 days of the occurrence.

Step 1: Filing a Complaint A patient who believes that his or her privacy has been violated is encouraged to file a complaint with the covered entity first. While not a legal requirement, allowing the institution to address the issue first gives it a chance to investigate what happened and to take any corrective action that may be necessary. That corrective action may include changes to policies and procedures or counseling the employee(s) that committed the infraction.

compliance: the adherence to a policy or rule

If patients do not want to file a complaint with the covered entity, or they feel that the covered entity has not addressed their concerns adequately, they can file a complaint directly with OCR.

Step 2: Informal Review If OCR receives a complaint, an informal review process is initiated. One of the first things that OCR will determine is whether the disclosure was an incidental disclosure or a breach of confidentiality. To make this determination, it will ask the covered entity to submit a report about the situation, detailing what occurred, what policies and procedures it has in place, and any corrective action that was taken. If OCR is satisfied with the report, it will close its investigation.

Step 3: Formal Review If the infraction is serious enough, or the healthcare institution's report is deemed inadequate, OCR will initiate a formal review. A formal review typically involves personnel from OCR making a site visit to the covered entity. Key personnel will be interviewed and questioned, and the healthcare institution and policies inspected. Once the formal review is complete, OCR will determine what corrective action, if any, is going to be required of the covered entity, and if it is going to be subjected to any penalties.

HIPAA Penalties OCR can impose a $100, per violation, penalty against an institution that has committed a HIPPA infraction. (There is a $25,000 per calendar year cap.) The violations that are imposed by OCR only apply to institutions; not to individuals. Under the doctrine of *respondeat superior*, since an institution is responsible for the actions of the employees, they are liable for those actions. So even though an employee may cause the violation, they are not subject to the civil fines that are levied by OCR.

> **⊘ Concept Connection**
> **HIPAA Fines and *Respondeat Superior***
> Employees are responsible for the actions of their employees, under the doctrine of *respondeat superior*; a type of vicarious liability.

While civil monetary fines are the most common type of penalty, it is not the only type allowed. At the beginning of this chapter we mentioned that when HIPAA was first introduced, it sent shockwaves throughout the healthcare community. The major reason for this concern was not because of the Privacy Rule, but because HIPAA includes criminal punishment for certain types of violations and infractions.

An individual who violates HIPAA's Privacy Rule by "knowingly obtaining or disclosing identifiable health information" can receive:

> **⊘ Concept Connection**
> **HIPAA and Criminal Law**
> When writing a law, the legislature makes the determination whether that law falls into the civil category or criminal category. If the punishment for breaking a particular law includes the possibility of a jail or prison sentence, it is classified as a criminal law.

- up to $50,000 in fines *and* sentenced up to 1 year imprisonment
- up to $100,000 in fines *and* sentenced up to 5 years' imprisonment (if done under false pretenses)
- up to $250,000 in fines *and* sentenced up to 10 years' imprisonment (if intent to sell, transfer, or use for commercial advantage, personal gain, or malicious harm)

Because OCR does not have the authority to levy criminal punishment, HHS gave the DOJ authority to prosecute the criminal component of HIPAA violations. Did you notice in the beginning of this paragraph, that only *individuals* are subject to criminal punishment for HIPAA violations? Healthcare institutions are not subject to criminal penalties, only individuals. While this may not seem fair, it does have practical application; you cannot place an institution in prison.

Before leaving the topic of HIPAA violations, it is important to make a legal distinction. Only HHS, OCR, and the DOJ can bring a cause of action (lawsuit) under HIPAA. HIPAA is not a law that private individuals can use to sue other citizens or institutions for. Meaning, if a patient believes that their privacy has been breached, he or she cannot bring a HIPAA lawsuit against a healthcare

Court Case

United States v. Richard Gibson

No. CR04-0374 RSM (2004)
United States District Court, Western District of Washington

FACTS: Richard Gibson was a phlebotomist working for Seattle Cancer Care Alliance in Seattle Washington. Without medical necessity or authorization, Gibson accessed patient information, which he fraudulently used to obtain credit cards. When it was discovered what Gibson had done, he was arrested for violating HIPAA. After his arrest, Gibson entered a plea agreement with prosecutors, agreeing to sixteen months in jail and paying restitution to the credit card companies.

ISSUE: Can an individual be subjected to criminal punishment for violating a person's privacy?

RULE: Even though the majority of HIPAA's violations is related to civil law, drafters of the legislation took the issue of patient privacy seriously enough to include individual punishment by placing a would-be violator in prison or jail. Because the legislature is granted the sole discretion of creating the law, they also have sole discretion to determine what the punishment will be.

EMPHASIS: HIPAA was enacted by Congress and first took effect in 1996. For several years after HIPAA went into effect, no one had been criminally prosecuted. It left some to wonder whether or not HIPAA had any intention of utilizing the criminal component of HIPAA. But, that all changed when Gibson was arrested. Gibson is the first person to have served jail time for violating the criminal section of HIPAA.

worker or healthcare institution. However, that does not mean that the patient is precluded from filing a lawsuit. While individuals cannot file a HIPAA lawsuit, they can, under tort law, file an invasion of privacy lawsuit against a healthcare worker or institution.

Security Rule

The last part of the Health Information portion of HIPAA is known as the Security Rule. The Security Rule requires:

"appropriate administrative, physical and technical safeguards to ensure the confidentiality, integrity, and security of electronic protected health information."

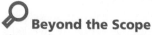 **Beyond the Scope**

The specific requirements of the Security Rule included in HIPAA are beyond the scope of this text. If you need more information regarding the Security Rule, you are encouraged to view the Health and Human Services website and consult other outside resources.

For example, if a healthcare organization is using electronic medical records, the Security Rule requires that firewalls be installed and passwords incorporated to limit access to certain types of information.

Like the Privacy Rule, the Security Rule is not meant to be a hindrance to the delivery of healthcare. Instead, the purpose of the Security Rule is to "protect the privacy of individual's health information while allowing covered entities to adopt new technologies to improve the quality and efficiency of patient care."

Health Care Portability

At the beginning of this chapter, we mentioned that there were two aspects to HIPAA: the Health Accountability Section and the Health Insurance Portability Section. The second part of HIPAA, the Health Insurance **Portability** section has not received the attention that the Health Accountability section has.

At the same time that HIPAA was being introduced in the legislature, another bill was being considered relating to employees and their healthcare insurance. Prior to HIPAA, when an employee changed jobs, their new insurance company could deny coverage based on any preexisting medical conditions they had. If an employee who developed diabetes under an old employer's insurance changed jobs, the insurance offered by the new employer could deny coverage of diabetes as a pre-existing condition. Such situations have caused many employees either to stay at their current job or pay those expenses out of pocket. The portability section of HIPAA no longer allows insurance companies to deny coverage of pre-existing conditions.

portability: the ability of something to be moved or transported from one place to another

Make FALSE statements TRUE.

Rewrite the false statement below by replacing the bolded, italicized, and underlined word(s) to make it a true statement.

1. The damages that the tort of defamation requires is the harm to a person's ***individuality***.

   _____

2. The initial catalyst for creating HIPAA grew out of concerns over ***slander and libel***.

   _____

3. The health accountability section of HIPAA contains two different rules, the Privacy Rule and the ***Confidentiality*** Rule.

   _____

4. HIPAA defines private patient information as ***de-identifying***.

   _____

5. The PSQIA address the ***friends and family*** exception to information disclosure.

   _____

Circle Exercise

Circle the correct word from the choices given.

1. There are two subcategories to the tort of (**defamation, invasion of privacy, HIPAA**) libel and slander.

2. The health accountability section, the HI in HIPAA, deals with (**insurance, information, individuality**).

3. Under HIPAA's criminal section, the maximum jail time a person can receive is (**5, 10, 15**) years.

4. The portability section of HIPAA refers to (**insurance, information, individuality**).

5. Any health provider, health insurance company, or health-related company is described by HIPAA as a (**covered entity, limited data set, Privacy Rule**).

Matching

Match the numbered term to its lettered definition.

1. _____ accountability
2. _____ compliance
3. _____ covered entity
4. _____ de-identify
5. _____ libel
6. _____ limited data set
7. _____ portability
8. _____ privacy
9. _____ slander

A. a document that has had some, or all, of the patient's private information removed.

B. an institution or group that is the subject of a regulation or law.

C. being held responsible; being required to answer to a situation.

D. something that belongs to or is intended only for an individual or particular group.

E. the ability of something to be moved or transported from one place to another.

F. the adherence to a policy or rule.

G. the communication of a false or defamatory statement that is spoken or heard.

H. the communication of a false or defamatory statement that is written or seen.

I. the process of removing any information from documents, or restricting electronic access to information, that a person is not authorized to receive.

Deliberations: Critical Thinking Questions

Question 1: You are working as a medical assistant in Dr. Jones's office, who is a general practitioner. Dr. Jones went to medical school with Dr. Smith, who is a cardiologist in town, and someone he commonly refers patients to. Your mother went to see Dr. Smith last year and did not like his bedside manner. Because of this, she decided not to see Dr. Smith but another cardiologist instead.

One day at work, Dr. Jones refers a patient to Dr. Smith; this new patient asks you, "Is Dr. Smith a good doctor?" If you were to tell the patient your personal opinion, how do you think this might impact the relationship that Dr. Jones and Dr. Smith currently have? Are there any other ramifications that you can think of?

Question 2: An elementary school hires a school nurse to maintain health records, such as immunizations, on the students enrolled at the school. In addition, the nurse provides medical support for students who are sick and injured. Is the school a covered entity under HIPAA? What about the school nurse? Even though an institution might not be a covered entity, does that mean the healthcare professionals that they hire are not subjected to privacy laws?

Question 3: A patient who is separated from her husband, but is not yet divorced, has been admitted to the hospital following a car accident. On her admission form, she specifically stated that she does not want information released to her husband. During the night the patient's condition changed and she required emergency surgery. She is currently on life support recovering in the ICU. In the morning, the patient's husband calls the hospital inquiring about his wife. Because he is the father of the children, he wants to know what is going on so that he can make child-care arrangements. What do you do?

Question 4: You are working as a medical assistant in an oncologist's office. Just before noon, your spouse stops by the office to take you out to lunch. Sitting in the waiting room is your church pastor. Is seeing patients in the waiting room a violation of HIPAA? During lunch, your spouse asks you questions about why your pastor was there. What kind of information can you tell your spouse?

Question 5: The doctor's office where you work has had a particularly busy month. In order to catch up on some paperwork, the doctor allows you to take your laptop computer home. While stopping to pick your children up from daycare, someone breaks into your car and steals your laptop, which contains patient files and private information. Have you committed a HIPAA violation? What safeguards should be taken so that information does not fall into the wrong hands?

Closing Arguments: Case Analysis

Hillary's son Chad developed a fever during the night that did not respond to over-the-counter medications and cool bathes. Hillary calls their pediatrician, who directs her to take Chad to the emergency room.

Question 1: When Hillary arrives at the ER she is triaged by a nurse. The questions that the triage nurse is asking, and the answers that Hillary is providing, can be overheard by other patients in the waiting room. Is this a HIPAA violation? What suggestions do you have about how the ER can minimize patient privacy?

Question 2: After Hillary waits for 30 minutes, a staff member calls her back into the emergency room. This particular night, the ER is extremely busy. The only place that is available is an open room that has six gurneys separated by curtains. As she enters the room, she can see other patients waiting, and is able to see, through openings in the curtains, that medical staff are performing medical procedures. Is anything that Hillary has experienced so far a HIPAA violation? Do you have any suggestions for the hospital?

Question 3: The next day, Hillary's neighbor comes over, who works at the hospital. She states that she saw you in the ER, but could not stop and say hi. She asks you what is going on and if everything is OK? You are upset that your neighbor not only saw you last night, but that she asked about your medical condition. Hillary is concerned that her neighbor has breached her privacy and thinks she has committed a HIPAA violation. Hillary calls the hospital and wants to file a complaint. As the department manager, how would you handle this complaint?

The Briefcase

This section repeats the objectives from the beginning of the chapter and provides a summary of the important concepts for each objective. Use this section as a quick review and to check your understanding of the chapter's key points.

Objective 1: Describe what common laws exist that relate to privacy and confidentiality.

- Defamation
  - Libel
  - Slander
- Invasion of Privacy

Objective 2: List the two different laws that are incorporated into HIPAA.

- Health Insurance Portability
- Health Accountability

Objective 3: Identify who HIPAA applies to, and how that determination is made.

- Covered Entities
  - any healthcare provider
  - any health insurance company
  - any health-related company that gives or receives patient information

Objective 4: Analyze what information HIPAA refers to as Protected Health Information (PHI).

- Private Health Information
- Information that can be used to identify a unique individual

Objective 5: Explain how HIPAA makes sure that private information stays private.

- The Privacy Rule
- The Security Rule

Objective 6: Determine who private information can be disclosed to and why.

- Healthcare Professionals
  - to coordinate treatment and care
  - to ensure that healthcare workers provide good care
- Family, Friends, Relatives
- Pay health providers
- Public Health
- Governmental Agencies

Objective 7: Provide examples of how information is disclosed under HIPAA.

- de-identifying
- limited data set

Objective 8: Detail the steps involved for Office of Civil Rights (OCR) reviews for HIPAA complaints or infractions.

- Filing a Complaint
- Informal Review
- Formal Review

Objective 9: Define the different penalties a person can receive for violating HIPAA.

- Civil Fines (OCR)
  - $100 per violation
  - $25,000 cap per calendar year
- Criminal Punishment (DOJ)
  - up to $50,000 in fines *and* up to 1 year in prison
  - up to $100,000 in fines *and* up to 5 years in prison (false pretenses)
  - up to $250,000 in fines *and* up to 10 years in prison (sell, transfer, or use for commercial advantage, personal gain, or malicious harm).

Maximize Your Success with the Companion Website

The Companion Website to this textbook contains materials that can help you better understand the concepts presented in this chapter. Go to www.myhealthprofessionskit.com to access:

- Web Links
- Games
- and more …

PEARSON
myhealthprofessionskit™

6

Negligence, Malpractice, and Other Torts

As a healthcare professional, you are provided with special education and training. Part of that education and training includes being proficient in the technical skills that are required of your profession. Because the law is granting you the authority to perform those skills, you are going to be held accountable for performing those skills. In this chapter, we will discuss the tort of negligence and the other torts commonly encountered by a healthcare professional in the performance of their duties.

MEASURE YOUR PROGRESS: LEARNING OBJECTIVES

After studying this chapter, you will be able to:

- Identify the two different classifications of torts.

- List the four different categories of harm.

- Categorize the different torts according to their harm category.

- Given the common law definition of a tort, list a tort's elements.

- Describe the different types and categories of damages allowed by the courts.

- Explain the concept of mitigation and damages.

- Compare and contrast negligence and malpractice.

- Differentiate between misfeasance, malfeasance, and nonfeasance.

- List the different defenses that are available to a defendant.

KEY TERMS

chattels

damages

malfeasance

misfeasance

mitigate

negligence

nonfeasance

res ipsa loquitur

torts

PROFESSIONAL HIGHLIGHT

Maria works in the Risk Management department of her local hospital. The Risk Management department is responsible for evaluating, minimizing, and preventing any legal risk that the institution might have. Maria investigates patient complaints and reviews incident reports to determine if any torts have been committed. In addition, if a lawsuit has been filed against the hospital, Maria works with the hospital attorney to evaluate the claim, and perform other pre-trail matters. All of the information that Maria obtains during the performance of her duties also helps her to develop continuing education and training for hospital staff. In order for Maria to minimize the legal risk for the hospital, she needs to have a thorough understanding of how healthcare operates and tort law.

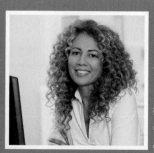

Goodluz/Shutterstock

The word *tort* comes from the *Latin* word *tortus*, which means twisted, and from the French word *tort*, which means calamity, injury, mischief, or wrong. Tort law is a category of law that addresses the harms individuals can inflict on others. Coming up with a definitive definition of what torts are can be difficult. In part, the difficulty comes from the many exceptions that exist, and the exceptions to the exceptions within the law. To add to that complexity, the law of torts has grown over the years because there are many new and different ways in which a person can harm another. For our purposes, we will concentrate on the basics of tort law and review the most common torts that you will encounter as a healthcare professional.

> **What are torts and what do they have to do with healthcare?**

Torts

The most common type of civil law that you will encounter as a healthcare professional is **tort** law.

The practice of tort law has become one of the largest areas of legal practice in the United States. Because the field of tort law is so large, most attorneys who handle torts limit their practice to only one type of tort, such as negligence, or concentrate on a specific subcategory of torts, such as personal injuries.

There are two different ways to classify torts, either by action or type.

1. Torts can be categorized by the *action* that causes the harm.
2. Torts can be categorized by the *type* of harm that is received.

torts: the area of civil law that addresses the harms a person receives, except for harms arising out of contracts

Torts Classified by Action

In the world of law and the legal community, torts are classified based on the action that causes the harm. The law makes a distinction between actions that are intentional and those that are unintentional.

Classifying torts by their action can be problematic, and typically causes confusion. The main problem with classifying torts by action has to do with understanding the difference between intentional and unintentional actions. A person who commits a tort does not typically set out with the intent of causing harm. For example, if a driver causes a car accident, the intentional action the law looks at is the act of driving, not that the driver intended to cause an accident. Because of this confusion, it is usually easier when first studying torts to classify them according to the type of harm that is received.

Fig. 6-1. If an accident occurs, the person who causes the accident is known as the tortfeasor.

Torts Classified by Harm

When classifying torts according to harm, we concentrate on how a person is injured. (see Table 6-1 for the legal elements of different torts classified by harm; Table 6-2 compares Classification by Harm with Classification by Action) The person who causes the harm is known as a tortfeasor (see Fig. 6-1). Tortfeasors can cause::

- harm to a person's body,
- harm to a person's personality, or
- harm to a person's property.

There is also another category of harm called strict harm. The requirements for strict harm have unique variations in the law that we will discuss at the end of this section.

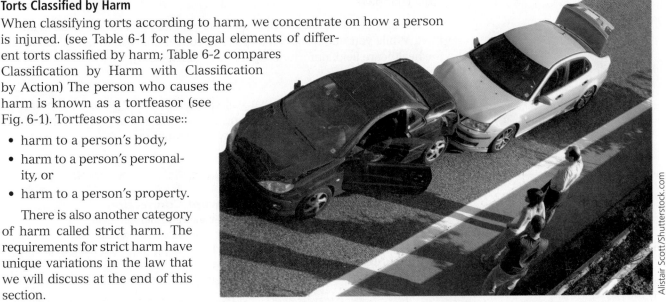

Alistair Scott/Shutterstock.com

Harm to Property

Harms to a person's property are uncommon in the healthcare environment, but they can occur. The torts that cause harm to a person's property include:

- Trespass to Land
- Trespass to Chattels
- Conversion

Trespass to Land The common law definition of the tort trespass to land is:

the intentional intrusion or invasion of another person's property (land) causing damage.

From a healthcare perspective, trespass to land rarely occurs. One of the only times that it might happen is when home healthcare providers enter onto someone's property other than the patient they are providing care for. To add to the rarity, the mere entrance onto the property is not enough to satisfy the requirement for this tort. Instead, the entrance onto another person's property must cause damage of some kind, which is why this tort is unlikely in the healthcare arena.

Trespass to Chattels Before we get into a discussion about the remaining harms to property, an important legal distinction needs to be made. Under the law, land (including homes and buildings) is referred to as *real property* or simply as *property*; belongings (personal property) are referred to as **chattels**.

chattels: a person's belongings, other than land

The common law definition of the tort trespass to chattels is:

the intentional interference with another person's chattels (personal property).

The key to the commission of this tort is the *interference* element. Patients bring personal belongings with them to the hospital and doctor's office all the time. Inevitably, some of those items may get lost when patients are transferred to different departments within the hospital or different rooms within an office. If we misplace a patient's personal items, we may be trespassing on their chattels.

Conversion The common law definition of the tort conversion is:

the intentional taking of another person's chattel (personal property) and making it your own.

The tort of conversion is similar to its criminal counterpart, the crime of theft. While you might think that theft or conversion would not occur within the healthcare field, unfortunately it does—albeit rarely.

Harms to Personality

There are two different torts that can cause harm to a person's personality; defamation (which includes libel, slander) and invasion of privacy. These torts address harms to a person's personality or reputation.

 Sidebar

The three most common objects that come up missing in the healthcare arena are glasses, dentures, and hearing aids. Whether they get wrapped up in the linen, mistakenly thrown out with the garbage, or not placed with a patient's belongings interferes with patients' personal property and can lead to trespass to chattels.

 Concept Connection

Civil Lawsuit and False Imprisonment

The torts of defamation, libel, slander, and invasion of privacy are dealt with in sections discussing confidentiality. Confidentiality laws, like HIPAA, are an important concept to healthcare professionals.

Harm to The Body

Because of the different ways that a person's body can be harmed, the torts that cause harm to the body are much more common in the healthcare environment than the other tort categories. The four most common harm to body torts that you will encounter as a healthcare professional are:

- assault
- battery
- false imprisonment
- negligence

False Imprisonment The common law definition of false imprisonment is:

the intentional confinement of a person who is aware of their confinement.

The legal elements required to establish the tort of false imprisonment are:

1. Intentional
2. Confinement
3. Of a person
4. Aware of confinement

One area of confusion related to the tort of false imprisonment is that some think that it only applies if a person is placed in jail or prison. The word *prison* comes from the French word *prisoun*, which means "physically confined." When talking about imprisonment, therefore, we are talking about physically confining a person, or restricting their movements; which can occur almost anywhere—not just in a prison (see Fig. 6-2).

Did you notice that the elements of invasion of privacy do not require a time frame? Because there is no minimum time requirement, any amount of time that a person is confined will satisfy that element of the tort. In addition, there is the element of awareness of confinement that

> ### ⊘ Concept Connection
> **Torts and Legal Elements**
> In order to understand how a legal analysis is performed, the torts of assault and battery are typically discussed, because they contain similar elements. To better understand the torts of assault and battery, perform a legal analysis.

Fig. 6-2. The most common occurrence of false imprisonment in healthcare is associated with the use of restraints.

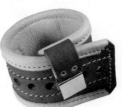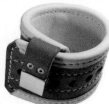

dcwcreations/Shutterstock

✔ Concept Application
False Imprisonment

The use of restraints has become a hot topic in healthcare. To use restraints correctly in a healthcare setting, they are applied only to protect the safety and welfare of the patient. For example, patients who are under the effects of anesthesia may need to be restrained so that they do not unknowingly pull out important tubes or intravenous lines.

In the past however, restraints were commonly used for staff convenience rather than patient safety. For example, restraining elderly patients in order to stop them from wandering in the hallways was commonplace. Because restraints were overused and misused in the healthcare arena in the past, regulatory agencies that govern healthcare have clamped down on how and when restraints are used.

Beyond the Scope

There are specific requirements regarding when restraints can be used in the healthcare setting. What those requirements are, are beyond the scope of this text. For more information, the reader is directed to their institution's policies and procedures and other resources.

TABLE 6-1

Torts and their Elements

Assault	Invasion of Privacy
• Intentional Threatening • With Physical Harm	• Intentional • Prying or Intruding Into • Another Person's Privacy • Causing Damage
Battery	**Negligence**
• Physical Harm of Another • Causing Damage	• Duty • Breach • Damages • Causation
Conversion	**Trespass to Chattels**
• Intentional Taking of • Another Person's Chattels (Personal Property) • Making it Your Own	• Intentional • Interference with • Another Person's Chattels (Personal Property)
Defamation	**Trespass to Land**
• Intentional • False or Defamatory Statement • Of Another Person • Causing Damage (Includes the torts of Libel and Slander)	• Intentional • Intrusion or Invasion • Of Another's Property (Land) • Causing damage
False Imprisonment	
• Intentional • Confinement • Of a Person • Aware of Confinement	

Alex Staroseltsev/Shutterstock

is important to note. A person who is not aware of having been confined has not been falsely imprisoned. While this is not usually an area of concern for the public, it has a common application in healthcare. We often take care of patients who, because of either a medical condition (dementia, unconsciousness) or medical treatments (sedation, anesthesia), may not be aware of a confinement if it were to happen to them. But, that does not mean that we can restrict a person's movements, just because they are not aware.

Negligence The common law definition of the tort of negligence is:

a breach of duty that causes damages.

The elements required to establish the tort of negligence are:

1. Duty
2. Breach
3. Damages
4. Causation

An in-depth explanation and analysis of the tort of negligence will follow in the next section of this chapter.

Strict Harm

All of the torts that we have discussed thus far have very specific elements that need to be satisfied. But the torts associated with strict harm are different. Strict harm torts relate to a special type of liability within the law; vicarious liability, or liability without fault. The two most common strict harm torts you may encounter in your healthcare career are product liability torts and strict liability.

Product Liability Product liability lawsuits focus on products and the manufacturing process. Because healthcare professionals are not involved in the manufacturing of products, they will not be sued for product liability. But it is common for healthcare professionals to be called as witnesses in product liability trials, so we should be aware of what they are.

A products liability lawsuit focuses on one of three different aspects, a:

• design defect,

• manufacturing defect, or

• failure to warn.

Product liability lawsuits will allege that a product was faulty in either the design (the initial concept, or blueprints of how the product was conceived); manufacturing (how the product was put together, such as on the assembly line); or a failure to warn (not informing a person how a product can cause harm, such as the side effects of medications). One of the most famous examples of a failure to warn product liability lawsuit is the McDonald's hot coffee case. While not a specific healthcare example, it does provide insight on product liability and will give you some interesting information that you may not be aware of.

Court Case

Liebeck v. McDonald's Restaurants

No. D-202 CV-93-02419, 1995 WL 360309
Bernalillo County, N.M. Dist Ct. (Aug. 18, 1994)

FACTS: Stella Liebeck ordered food and coffee at a McDonald's drive-thru window. After receiving her order, Liebeck put the coffee cup between her knees and took off the cap to add cream and sugar. The coffee spilled into her lap and soaked into the pair of sweatpants she was wearing. The heat from the coffee (estimated to be 180°F) caused third-degree burns to her inner thighs, perineum, buttocks, genitals, and groin. Because of the injuries she sustained, and their location, she required not only wound debridement but skin grafting surgeries as well.

ISSUE: The issue before the court was whether McDonald's had *failed to warn* about the dangers related to extremely hot coffee. The court struggled with the concept that coffee is supposed to be hot. But in this particular case, the temperature of the coffee exceeded industry standards (which an expert witness testified was 140°F).

During the trial, the plaintiff was able to demonstrate that McDonald's had repeatedly ignored warnings that the temperature of its coffee exceeded industry standards and could cause severe burns. Therefore, the issue was not whether coffee is supposed to be served hot, but whether McDonald's coffee was so hot that it could cause severe injuries, and by ignoring those warnings were they liable?

RULE: The jury awarded Liebeck $200,000 in compensatory damages (which was later reduced to $160,000) and $2.7 million in punitive damages (later reduced to $480,000). During the appeals process, Liebeck and McDonald's entered into a settlement agreement which contained a nondisclosure clause. Therefore, the final amount paid to Liebeck is unknown.

EMPHASIS: Even though the case was highlighted in the news, many do not know the specific facts of the case and why it was an important concept in the law. Yes, coffee is supposed to be hot, but it is not supposed to be so hot that it causes third-degree burns.

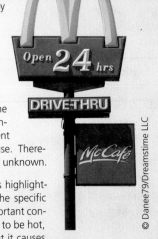

© Danee79/Dreamstime LLC

Strict Liability There are certain items that the law considers to be so inherently dangerous that, regardless of the precautions taken, the person who owns them or uses them, is held legally responsible for any harms that they cause, regardless of whether they did anything wrong or not.

In the healthcare arena, there are some materials that we use that can cause harm, such as radiation, chemotherapeutic agents, and others that have medical benefits. Having the materials is the only requirement for a strict liability claim, in that by mere possession the owner is responsible. The hospital can do everything in its power to safeguard those items, but if a person is harmed because of the materials, a strict liability claim could be brought. (Note: there is a legal difference between a harm and a side effect or complication. Side effects and complications are medically acceptable consequences and do not fall under the strict harm requirements.)

Like product liability torts, healthcare workers are not sued for strict liability because they do not own the materials. Instead, because the hospital is the owner of the materials, healthcare workers can be called to testify in strict liability cases at trial.

Johnny Habell/Shutterstock

 Concept Application

Strict Liability

Anyone that owns an animal is responsible for any damages that animal causes despite any safeguards they have taken. For example, the owner of a dog can tether a dog to a lead, build a fence around the property, and put a bite guard on the dog. But if the dog escapes, gets out of his bite guard, and injures someone, an owner will still be held legally responsible for the injuries because he or she owns the dog. (Strict liability only applies when the person has not done anything wrong. A dog owner who does not put his or her dog on a leash and allows the dog to run wild would be considered negligent, and strict liability would not apply.)

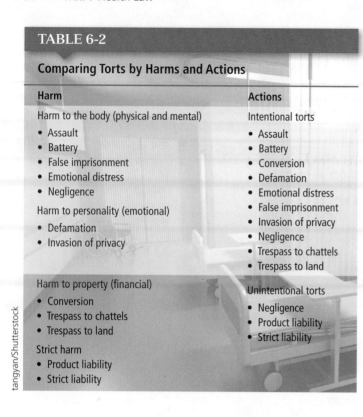

TABLE 6-2

Comparing Torts by Harms and Actions

Harm	Actions
Harm to the body (physical and mental)	Intentional torts
• Assault	• Assault
• Battery	• Battery
• False imprisonment	• Conversion
• Emotional distress	• Defamation
• Negligence	• Emotional distress
	• False imprisonment
Harm to personality (emotional)	• Invasion of privacy
• Defamation	• Negligence
• Invasion of privacy	• Trespass to chattels
	• Trespass to land
Harm to property (financial)	Unintentional torts
• Conversion	• Negligence
• Trespass to chattels	• Product liability
• Trespass to land	• Strict liability
Strict harm	
• Product liability	
• Strict liability	

damages: a quantified amount of money used to demonstrate a loss or injury to a person or property

Fig. 6-3. If the commission of a tort results in a broken arm, the fracture is an example of the physical damage a person has suffered.

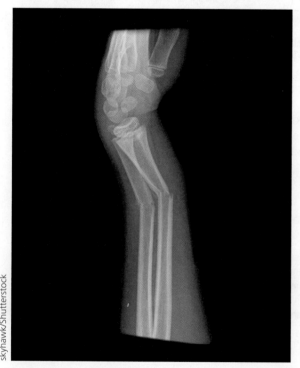

Damages

All of the torts that we have discussed require that the person bringing the lawsuit suffer some type of harm. In order to be successful in any of these tort actions, a person needs to provide evidence of the harm that they have received. In the law, the harms that a person suffers are referred to as damages.

When a civil lawsuit is filed, the plaintiff is required to quantify what the harm is and how he or she arrived at the amount of damages the defendant is being asked to pay. When listing these damages, the plaintiff has to classify those damages according to their type and category.

Type of Damages

The types of damages a person suffers are based on *how* a person is injured. There are three main types of damages:

• physical damages
• mental/emotional damages
• financial damages

Physical Damages

Physical damages are the most common type of damages sought in medical lawsuits. Physical damages relate to the physical injuries that a person sustained (see Fig. 6-3). For example, if a person's arm is broken because of the commission of a tort, the fracture is an example of the physical damages that a person has sustained. In addition, the amount of pain and suffering that a person goes through is also considered physical damage. The problem, however, is quantifying what pain and suffering is worth. This is something that the courts struggle with all the time.

Mental/Emotional Damages

Mental and emotional damages are different than pain and suffering. If a person is asking for mental and emotional damages, the damages have to relate to some psychological harm that the person suffered because of the tort. Lawsuits cannot be brought on principle alone, because hurt feelings are not enough to substantiate mental or emotional damages. Instead, the harm or injury must be severe enough to cause someone to seek medical treatment, such as from a psychologist or psychiatrist.

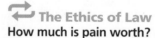 **The Ethics of Law**

How much is pain worth?

Quantifying pain and suffering is difficult, because pain is subjective.

• How much money is pain and suffering worth? Is there a way to put a value on it?

• Suppose you were sitting on a jury and were asked to come up with a dollar amount for a person who broke their arm. What formula would you use, or how would you arrive at a dollar amount?

Financial Damages

The last type of damage is financial harm. Financial harm relates to an amount of money that has been lost as a result of the tort. A person can be financially damaged through lost wages (including lost earning capacity), damaged property that needs to be fixed, or bills that need to be paid, such as medical expenses.

Categories of Damages

Once the plaintiff has identified the *type* of damages that they are asking for, they next have to categorize those damages. There are three different categories of damages:

- compensatory damages
- consequential damages
- punitive damages

Compensatory Damages

A plaintiff who is asking for compensatory damages is asking to be *compensated* for a loss. As the name implies, compensatory damages are not based on an arbitrary figure that a plaintiff would *like* to receive. Instead, compensatory damages are provided to reimburse an amount of money that the plaintiff has already paid or will be required to pay.

Plaintiffs who ask for compensatory damages as part of a lawsuit must include a calculation of how they arrived at the amount that they are asking for. Medical bills, estimates to fix damaged property, or receipts are all used to help the plaintiff arrive at a specific figure. To combine the type and category of damages, there are:

- compensatory physical damages
- compensatory mental damages
- compensatory emotional damages
- compensatory financial damages

Consequential Damages

Consequential damages are harms that are not a direct result of the injury but a *consequence* of the harm. For example, a patient who is wheelchair-bound following an act of negligence may need to have a wheelchair ramp built onto his or her home. The costs associated with building that wheelchair ramp would be a consequence of the injury received from the negligent act. Consequential damages, however, do not include every conceivable item or issue that could potentially be tied to the accident because the court is only willing to reach so far in awarding consequential damages.

Sidebar

Expenses that a person will incur in the future, as a result of the harm, can also be included in compensatory damages. While it may not seem that providing future payments is compensatory, the plaintiff is being compensated for the damages that they will continue to occur into the future.

To combine the type and category of damages, there are:

- consequential physical damages
- consequential mental damages
- consequential emotional damages
- consequential financial damages

While consequential physical damages, mental damages, and emotional damages can occur, they are very rare. The most common use of consequential damages relate to consequential financial damages.

The two damages that we have discussed so far, compensatory damages and consequential damages are damages that have been received by the plaintiff. The last type of damages, punitive damages, is not related to the plaintiff at all, but is directed at the the defendant.

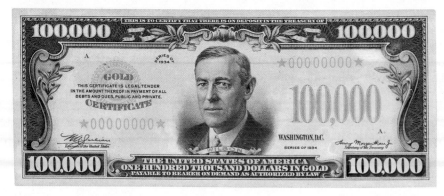

Tim Mainiero/Shutterstock

Punitive Damages

The name punitive is derived from the word *punish*, which is exactly what this category of damages is designed to do. Punitive damages are awarded to:

- punish the tortfeasor for their wrongful acts,
- send a message to others to let them know that if they act similarly, they can face the same or potentially more serious punishment, and

Understanding Your State

Some states place restrictions on the amount of punitive damages that are allowed in civil court cases. In addition, other limitations or caps have been placed on other categories of damages as well by different states. To understand what your state requires, check out the interactive map on the companion website.

Sidebar

One of the reasons you hear about multimillion-dollar jury awards on the news, is because—surprise—it's news! If it happened every day, in every court case, it would not be newsworthy. This should help alleviate the fears you might have regarding lawsuits, because multimillion-dollar jury awards do not occur in every case.

- provide the person wronged an amount of money that more than makes up for the injuries that were sustained, because the harm that was caused was so intolerable that the person should not have suffered in the first place.

Because punitive damages do not address *how* a plaintiff was harmed, they are not categorized as punitive physical damages, punitive mental damages, punitive emotional damages, or punitive financial damages because the focus of punitive damages is on the defendant, not on the plaintiff.

If you have ever heard about a multimillion-dollar jury verdict on the news, that amount is typically because punitive damages have been awarded. The other categories of damages, compensatory and consequential, rarely amount to the millions of dollars.

Court Case

Moskovitz v. Mt. Sinai Medical Center

69 Ohio St.3d 638, 635 N.E.2d 331 (1994)
Supreme Court of the State of Ohio

FACTS: Mrs. Moskovitz started seeing Dr. Figgie because of a mass on her ankle. As part of her diagnosis and treatment, Moskovitz was referred to numerous doctors and therapists. Throughout these consultations and treatments, several copies of Moskovitz's medical records were made. Moskovitz was eventually diagnosed with a rare metastatic cancer, and ultimately passed away. Prior to her death, Mrs. Moskovitz sued Dr. Figgie for negligence based on medical malpractice and failure to diagnose. Dr. Figgie claimed that Mrs. Moskovitz declined to have a biopsy done, a claim that was supported by copies of the patient's medical records that were provided by Dr. Figgie. However, prior to her death, Moskovitz disputed this claim stating that she never refused to have a biopsy performed.

During the discovery process, the Moskovitz's attorney sent subpoena ducus tecums to Dr. Figgie and the consultants and therapists that had provided treatment. Upon reviewing the records, the attorney noted that copies of Moskovitz's records provided by therapists did not match the records provided by Dr. Figgie. It was determined that, after making copies of the records for consultants and therapists, that Dr. Figgie had altered the original medical record, by inserting

a statement "As she does not want excisional Bx [biopsy] we will observe."

In the original trial, the jury found for Moskovitz, and awarded her compensatory and other damages. In addition, the jury added $3 million in punitive damages. Dr. Figgie appealed the assignment of punitive damages.

ISSUE: The issue that the court struggled with was "Were punitive damages, and the amount awarded, appropriate and proper on the facts of this case?"

RULE: "Actual malice, necessary for an award of punitive damages, is (1) that state of mind under which a person's conduct is characterized by hatred, ill will or a spirit of revenge, or (2) a conscious disregard for the rights and safety of other persons that has a great probability of causing substantial harm."

EMPHASIS: The court, in its written opinion stated, ". . . we reiterate that the purpose of punitive damages is to punish and deter." One of the issues that the court struggled to answer was how punitive damages are calculated. They stated; "Figgie's conduct of altering records should not go unpunished. We should warn others to refrain from similar conduct and an award of punitive damages will do just that." While the court readily admitted that there was no formulary to calculate how to arrive at a figure for punitive damages, they nonetheless reduced the punitive damages award to $1 million.

Sidebar
Many states have tried to cap the amount of punitive damages that a plaintiff is allowed to receive. The most common limitation is to punitive damages to three times the total of compensatory and consequential damages.

Mitigation

Before we leave the topic of damages, there is one more consideration that we need to discuss. Just because a person is injured by someone does not mean that he or she can sit back and rack up expenses. Instead, the law requires plaintiffs to affirmatively **mitigate** their damages.

> **mitigate:** to lessen, make less severe or less intense

The theory behind the mitigation requirement is that people should take what steps they can to minimize their suffering instead of allowing it to continue. For example, people who may have lost their jobs because of an injury cannot just sit back and collect what they would have earned for the rest of their lives. Instead, the court will require that they mitigate their damages by finding jobs that they can perform. A plaintiff who does not mitigate his or her damages may have compensatory or consequential damages decreased. This decrease is based on the amount a plaintiff could have mitigated his or her damages but failed to do so.

The words *negligence* and *malpractice* are often used interchangeably; sometimes correctly, sometimes not. Malpractice is negligence, but a special kind of negligence. Malpractice is used when referring to the negligence of a professional and how he or she has *practiced* that profession. Even though negligence and malpractice are the same thing, there are some differences in how each are analyzed. To fully understand malpractice, then, we first need to understand what negligence is.

> I have heard of negligence and malpractice. Is there a difference between the two?

Negligence

Now that we have reviewed some of the common torts, we can turn to the one tort that causes the most concern with healthcare professionals: the tort of **negligence.**

> **negligence:** when damages are caused by a breach of duty

Like the torts that we discussed previously, there are legal elements that need to be satisfied in order to determine whether negligence has occurred. The common law definition of negligence is:

damages that are caused by a breach of duty.

The legal elements required to satisfy a negligence claim are:

1. Duty
2. Breach
3. Damages
4. Causation

You may have noticed that the elements are not in the same order as the definition, like most of the other torts are. Because of how negligence is worded, the elements are not straightforward. Once we have reviewed the elements for negligence, the reason for this difference will become clearer.

Duty

Part of the reason the tort of negligence is one of the most commonly committed torts is because of the duty element. When addressing the element of duty, you are essentially asking: Does a person have a responsibility? If a person has a responsibility, then they have a duty. And while there are many different kinds of duty, such as ethical responsibilities or moral obligations, when analyzing negligence we are only concerned with whether a *legal* duty exists.

Suppose you are driving down the highway and see a car on the side of the road with a flat tire. Are you morally obligated to stop and offer assistance? Yes, but are you *legally* required to stop and offer assistance? No, you are not. The distinction is an important one to make. Even though there are all kinds of duties, responsibilities, and obligations, we cannot hold someone *legally* responsible unless there is a *legal* duty. When performing a legal analysis of negligence, we are not concerned with whether a duty exists, but only whether a *legal* duty exists.

Determining whether a legal duty exists is a legal question, requiring an interpretation of the law. Because the judicial branch is provided with the power to interpret the law, only the judiciary can answer questions of law. Regarding the car with the flat tire on the side of the road, if we allowed a jury to answer the question of duty, they might find someone responsible for not stopping and offering assistance. A person could then be found guilty, even though they had no legal duty to offer assistance.

While duty is a question of law, the remaining elements of negligence, breach, damages, and causation, are all questions of fact, which are left up to a jury to decide.

Breach

If a person has a legal responsibility (duty) and does not fulfill that obligation, they are in breach, commonly referred to as a *breach of duty*. To determine the element of breach, we ask: What did the person do, or not do, that they were suppose to? To make that determination you compare what the person was required to do with what actually occurred. If there is a difference, then the person is in breach.

Determining whether a person's actions were wrongful or not can sometimes be difficult. To help, the law uses the "reasonable person standard." The reasonable person standard asks

What would a reasonable and prudent person do in the same, or similar, situation?

If a person's actions are reasonable, then a person is not in breach. But if a person's actions are not reasonable, then they are in breach. The emphasis of the reasonable and prudent person is based on logical and intelligent actions, not on popular opinion.

Did you notice that the questions used to address breach and the reasonable person both use the word—*what*? Determining *if* a person has fulfilled an obligation is not the focus of breach, because *if* only requires a yes or no answer. Instead, when determining the element of breach, we have to isolate the specific action or inaction that the person has failed to perform.

There are three different ways a person can breach a duty: through malfeasance, misfeasance, and nonfeasance.

Malfeasance

Although the least common type of breach is through malfeasance, it provides us with a good foundation for us to discuss the other types of breach.

An example of malfeasance would be causing an accident when driving a vehicle without a license. Because the law requires a person to have a license when driving a motorized vehicle on the roads, operating a car without a license is unlawful. The focus of malfeasance is on the specific act performed—driving without a license—not on how the act is performed.

What would a reasonable and prudent person do in the same, or similar, situation?

teacept/Shutterstock

malfeasance: the performance of an unlawful act through wrongdoing or misconduct

Misfeasance

Misfeasance occurs when someone performs a lawful act, but the manner in which that act is performed is wrong.

The breach of duty by misfeasance is the most common type of breach. With misfeasance, the person is performing a legal act, but does so incorrectly. To continue our example, a licensed driver who causes an accident is breaching his or her duty of driving safely. The act itself—driving—is legal, but the person who caused the accident performed that action in a wrongful manner.

misfeasance: a lawful act, performed in a wrongful manner

Nonfeasance

A breach of duty usually occurs when a person performs an act. But, not acting—when you should—is known as nonfeasance.

An example of nonfeasance is a lifeguard who does not jump into a pool to save a drowning victim. Because the lifeguard has a legal responsibility to save a person's life, by not jumping in the pool to save the person, the lifeguard has breached his or her duty by nonfeasance.

nonfeasance: the failure to take action when action is required

Damages

The third element of negligence is damages. To determine whether this element has been satisfied or not, you simply ask: "What harms did the person suffer?" If you are able to list specific damages (harms, injuries) that a person suffered, then this element has been satisfied.

In determining the element of damages, we are only identifying *what* damages exist, not what the cause of those damages are. What caused the damages is the last element you identify in negligence; causation.

Causation

The last element of negligence to determine is causation (see Fig. 6-4). The causation element is asking: How were the damages caused? To understand how the causation element is analyzed, it may be helpful to go back to the definition of negligence: damages that are *caused by* a breach of duty. In order for the causation element to be satisfied, the damages must be caused by the breach of duty. To make this determination, we can use the definition of negligence as a formula, where we can plug in the specific information we obtained earlier.

Was the _____ *caused by* _____
         (Insert the specific   (Insert the specific
         type of damages)   action/inaction of breach?)

Previously, when we discussed the elements of damages and breach, we were asked to provide specific information and examples. It is this step in the negligence analysis where providing that specific information becomes relevant. In order to use the formula correctly, we have to plug in the specific information we obtained for damages and breach. To demonstrate, look at an example. Property owners have a responsibility (duty) to keep their sidewalk clear of obstacles, such as ice and snow. If they fail to shovel and de-ice their sidewalk, they have breached that duty. Suppose a person walking on the sidewalk slips on the ice and fractures his or her ankle. We can use that information to plug into our formula.

Was the <u>fractured ankle</u> *caused by the* <u>unshoveled, icy sidewalk</u>?

Yes! Since the fractured ankle was *caused* by the icy, unshoveled sidewalk, the causation element of negligence has been satisfied.

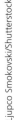

Now, suppose a person walking on the same sidewalk trips on his or her shoelaces and breaks an ankle. We can use that information to plug into our formula:

Was the <u>fractured ankle</u> caused by the <u>icy, unshoveled sidewalk?</u>

Because the fractured ankle was *not caused by* the icy, unshoveled sidewalk, the causation element has not been satisfied.

Of all of the elements in a negligence analysis, the element of causation can be the most difficult to prove. If a negligence lawsuit is unsuccessful, it is typically because the causation element has not been satisfied. Part of the difficulty in proving causation is that it typically involves complex issues where opinions about the causative factors of a person's damages are needed. To complicate matters, causation is a question of fact, answered by a jury. But most jurors do not typically have the knowledge and background needed to make the determination of causation on their own. To address the issue of causation, attorneys utilize expert witnesses.

Expert Witnesses

A witness called to the stand to testify can only testify to what he or she observed or did. Witnesses are not allowed to provide opinions about what they believe. The exception is a person who has been classified as an expert.

In order to be qualified as an expert witness, one has to meet certain legal requirements. While these qualifications vary from jurisdiction to jurisdiction, the most common are an advanced degree, several years of practice in that particular field, and some type of recognition by their peers (such as publishing professional articles, teaching in academia, or participating in research). A person who has been classified as an expert is allowed to testify about his or her opinions. The most common use of expert witnesses is to testify about the element of causation in negligence trials.

While the use of expert witnesses is commonplace to address the issue of causation, there is an exception where no expert witness is needed to testify about the element of causation.

> **Sidebar**
>
> Expert witnesses are unlike other witnesses at trial. They are testifying as witness to their area of expertise, not to the events that are the focus of the trial.

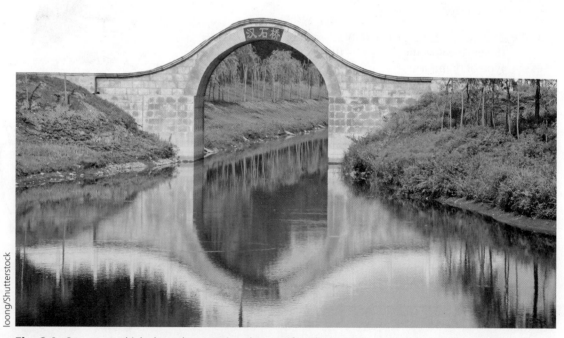

loong/Shutterstock

Fig. 6-4. One way to think about the causation element of negligence is to picture it as a bridge. The causation element brings together the elements of breach and damages.

res ipsa loquitur

All of the torts that we have discussed thus far, require that all of the elements of the tort be satisfied by evidence or testimony. But, there is one noted exception; when ***res ipsa loquitur*** exists.

The use of *res ipsa loquitur* removes the need to determine whether causation exists. To explain, suppose a patient comes into the hospital complaining of abdominal pain for the past few hours that is growing in intensity. On taking a medical history, the patient has been relatively healthy and has only had one surgical procedure in his life, when his appendix ruptured five years ago. An abdominal X-ray determines that the patient has a surgical sponge inside his abdominal cavity. There can be only one place and one situation to explain where the surgical sponge came from—the appendix surgery the patient had five years ago. Because of the existence of the surgical sponge, there is no need to determine whether the causation element exists, because the existence of the surgical sponge *speaks for itself*.

> ***res ipsa loquitur:*** "the thing itself speaks"; a legal theory whereby the mere occurrence of an event infers causation

Malpractice

As the name indicates, malpractice occurs when an error is caused by how a professional *practices*. Because of the additional education, training, and experience that professionals have, the standards that we use to determine a professional's negligence are different than that of negligence (see Table 6-3 for a detailed comparison). When a professional commits negligence, it is referred to as malpractice instead of negligence; which is often referred to as common negligence. The elements used to determine whether malpractice has been committed or not are the same as negligence.

1. Duty
2. Breach
3. Damages
4. Causation

Duty

In a malpractice case, the first element to be decided is whether a professional duty exists or not. Any time that a medical practitioner/patient relationship has been established, the healthcare provider has a legal duty to that patient. For example, any time you report to work, you have a legal duty to any patient that is present in your institution. Or, if you are working in a doctor's office, you have a legal duty to any patient that comes into the office to see the doctor.

Breach

Determining the breach of a person's duty in a malpractice case is the same as how breach is determined in a negligence case. You compare what responsibility a person has with what actually happened. Fortunately, making that determination is easier in malpractice than it is in a negligence case. To determine how a person has breached his or her duty, we only need to look at the professional Standards of Care.

Standards of Care

All healthcare professions have a Standard of Care that are written by their professional organization. To determine what responsibility (duty) a professional has, we can look at their Standards of Care published by the professional organizations.

Sidebar

When you call a medical office or hospital you will commonly get a recording: "If you have a medical emergency, please hang up and dial 9-1-1." Part of the reason for this message is because of the duty element of negligence. If the staff answers the phone and starts asking you medical questions, they are establishing a patient/healthcare provider relationship and could also be establishing the duty element of negligence.

Concept Connection

Malpractice and Standards of Care

The Standards of Care published by professional organizations are not only used to help define the profession, but also to indicate how a person must practice in his or her profession.

Concept Connection

Medical Records and Malpractice

The patient's medical records indicate what medical treatment has been provided and the patient's response to that treatment. In determining the element of breach, we look at the patient's medical records to determine what was actually done. This lends credence to the legal principle, "If it wasn't written down, it wasn't done," because the medical records will be the sole determinant of what care was provided.

Legal Alert! When a person steps outside of his or her scope of practice, which Standard of Care is utilized to determine breach? For example, if a nursing assistant prescribes medication, do we utilize a nursing assistant's standard of care or a doctor's standard of care? Because the law requires that we know what our scope of practice is, it holds us accountable to stay within that scope of practice. If we step outside of our scope of practice, we will be held accountable for the professional standards that we step into. Meaning, if a nursing assistant prescribes medication, the law will utilize the Standards of Care of a physician to determine what a person should do, not the Standards of Care of a nursing assistant.

Medical Records

When determining breach, we compare what a person is supposed to do and what actually happened. What a person is supposed to do is found in the Standards of Care. What actually happened is found in the patient's medical records. A patient's medical record is used to demonstrate what care has been provided to the patient and the response to that care. Therefore, the medical record will tell us what actually occurred. We can then compare the medical records to the Standards of Care to determine if there are any discrepancies. If there are, then a breach has occurred.

As with negligence, a person can be in breach in one of three different ways, either through malfeasance, misfeasance, or nonfeasance.

Malfeasance

The most common occurrence of malfeasance in a malpractice claim occurs when a healthcare professional steps outside of their scope of practice. For example, only doctors, physician assistants, and nurse practitioners can prescribe medications. A nursing assistant who prescribes medications is operating outside of his or her scope of practice, and thus committing malfeasance. The act is illegal because the law does not authorize nursing assistants to prescribe medications.

Misfeasance

The most common examples of misfeasance in a healthcare setting is failing to provide the correct type of care and/or performing technical skills adequately. With misfeasance the care provided is lawful, but the manner in which that care is provided is incorrect. An example of misfeasance would be performing surgery on the wrong body part. Performing surgery is legal, if the surgeon is licensed to do so, but operating on the wrong body part is misfeasance because it was done in a wrongful manner.

Nonfeasance

Nonfeasance occurs when a person does not act when the law requires them to. For example, when we administer medications, we need to monitor patients to make sure that they do not have an allergic reaction. If we fail to monitor patients after administering medication, we are committing nonfeasance, because our standards of care require us to monitor them. Other examples include not answering patient call lights or disregarding machine alarms.

Damages

Damages, under malpractice, are the same as the damages that occur with negligence. Remember, in determining the damages element of malpractice, we are only listing what damages the patient has. How or why those damages occurred is determined in the causation element of malpractice.

Causation

Just like negligence, malpractice requires that a person's damages be *caused by* a breach of professional duty. In malpractice, the same formulary is used as was used for negligence:

Was the _____ caused by _____?
          (Insert the specific   (Insert the the specific action/
          type of damages)   inaction of breach)

To demonstrate, we can look at an example. John has had insulin-dependent diabetes for several years. During one of his hospital stays, a nurse forgets to administer a dose of his morning insulin. During the afternoon, a check of John's blood sugar indicates a higher than normal level of the patient's blood sugar. The nurse administers a dose of insulin to correct the problem. A few months later at a follow-up visit with his doctor, it is discovered that John has diabetic retinopathy. Did the nurse who forgot to administer one dose of insulin *cause* the diabetic retinopathy?

To use our formulary:

Was the <u>diabetic retinopathy</u> *caused by* <u>the missing dose of insulin</u>?
    (Insert the specific   (Insert the specific action/
    type of damages)   in action of breach)

Diabetic retinopathy is the result of long-term exposure of the retina to high levels of sugar. Forgetting one dose of insulin is not the *cause of* diabetic retinopathy. Now look at a similar situation with a different result.

John has had insulin-dependent diabetes for several years. During one of his hospital stays, a nurse forgets to administer a dose of his morning insulin. During the afternoon John is found to be short of breath and has to be transferred to the intensive care unit (ICU). It is discovered that John developed ketoacidosis (a condition that occurs when the body cannot use glucose for energy because of the lack of insulin). Because of the severity of John's condition, he has to spend three days in ICU recuperating. Did the nurse who forgot to administer the dose of insulin *cause* John's damages?

Using our formulary:

Was the <u>ketoacidosis</u> caused by the <u>missing insulin dose</u>?
    (Insert the specific   (Insert the specific
    type of damages)   action/in action of
                    breach)

Yes! The ketoacidosis was *caused by* the missing insulin dose. Because the missing insulin dose *caused* the damages, the causation element of malpractice is satisfied.

After reading this section, you might be saying to yourself, how are you supposed to know whether a certain action has caused damages or not? The

Court Case

Schopp v. Our Lady of the Lake Hospital Inc.

739 So.2d 338 La.App 1 Cir 1999
Court of Appeals Louisiana, First Circuit

FACTS: In August 1993, Sophie Schopp fell in the bathroom of her home striking her head. She was not found until 5 hours later when her home health aide arrived in the morning. She was taken to the Emergency Room at Our Lady of the Lake Hospital and admitted for observation. During a radiology examination, an x-ray cartridge fell and hit Schopp on the head. There is conflicting testimony concerning how far the x-ray cartridge fell and what injuries Schopp received. A CT scan showed that Schopp had a large subdural hematoma (bleeding in the brain). Doctors performed a craniotomy to remove the blood and relieve the pressure in her head. While Schopp initially improved, her health deteriorated and she died 14 days later. Her family filed suit against the hospital and the x-ray technicians. The jury found for Schopp and her family.

While this emphasis of this appeal concentrated on procedural issue, one aspect relevant to our current discussion was the testimony of the different experts. The plaintiff's expert witness testified that the patient's death was caused by the x-ray cartridge falling on Schopp's head. The defense's expert witness testified that the patient's death was caused by the patient's fall at her home.

ISSUE: At issue in this case was whether one of the expert witnesses who testified was qualified to give a medical opinion.

RULE: The court stated that the jury believed the plaintiff's expert witness over the defendant's expert witness. Because the issue of causation is a question of fact, to be answered by a jury, the court deferred to the jury verdict and which expert witness they believed.

EMPHASIS: The importance of this case, for our present purposes, demonstrates how difficult the causation element can be in some cases and how expert witnesses are utilized. During medical malpractice cases, you will always have contradictory expert witness testimony, which ultimately boils down to which expert the jury finds more believable or more credible.

TABLE 6-3

Comparing Negligence and Malpractice

Elements	Negligence	Malpractice
Duty	Determined Only by a Judge	Determined Only by a Judge
Breach	Malfeasance Misfeasance Nonfeasance Reasonable Person Standard	Malfeasance Misfeasance Nonfeasance Standards of Care and Medical Records
Damages	Compensatory • Physical • Mental/Emotional • Financial Consequential • Physical • Mental/Emotional • Financial (most common) Punitive	Compensatory • Physical • Mental/Emotional • Financial Consequential • Physical • Mental/Emotional • Financial (most common) Punitive
Causation	Expert Witness *res ipsa loquitur*	Expert Witness *res ipsa loquitur*

mffoto/Shutterstock

answer will typically require a medical opinion, where, like negligence, an expert witness will be called to the stand to offer an expert opinion.

> **What happens if I get sued for malpractice? Is there anything that I can do?**

Just because a person has filed a lawsuit does not mean that the lawsuit will be successful. In order for a plaintiff to prevail in court, he or she must provide evidence and testimony proving all of the elements of the claim. A patient bringing a malpractice lawsuit is required to provide evidence that duty, breach, damages, and causation exists. A plaintiff who is unable to provide adequate testimony or evidence to prove all four of the elements, has not met his or her burden of proof, and will not be successful in a lawsuit.

The fear of lawsuits is a very valid concern to healthcare practitioners. If a lawsuit is filed against you, do not lose hope! The law allows a defendant an opportunity to address the evidence and testimony that is provided by the plaintiff, and to give their own testimony and evidence to the court. In addition, there are legal defenses that a defendant can use to help them in their case.

Legal Defenses

A person who has been sued has the right to present evidence and testimony that will refute a plaintiff's claim. There are three different ways that defendants can mount a defense against a lawsuit. They can:

- refute the allegations made in the lawsuit,
- try to diminish what they are responsible for, or
- escape responsibility completely.

Refuting the Allegations

The first and maybe most obvious way to defend against a civil lawsuit is by opposing the plaintiff's claims. Refuting the allegations would be similar to saying, "I did not do anything wrong!" Two defenses can be used to refute the plaintiff's allegations in a lawsuit, the denial defense or the assumption of the risk defense.

The Denial Defense

The use of the denial defense is similar to saying that you did nothing wrong. But instead of just denying the allegations outright, the denial defense will address a specific element of the law. For example, if health-care worker who is going to utilize the denial defense in a malpractice lawsuit will, in his or denial, want to address one of the four elements of negligence: duty, breach, damages, or causation (see Table 6-4).

Assumption of the Risk

As the name implies, the assumption of the risk defense is stating that the plaintiff *assumed the risks* involved. When we provide care to a patient, we are required to obtain their consent, whether it is a general consent for treatment or a specialized consent form. When obtaining a patient's consent, the law requires that we provide specific information regarding what risks are involved, for example, the possible complications a patient might have, what the outcome is anticipated to be, what alternatives are available, and what would happen if the treatment is not provided. This legal requirement is to ensure that patients are making an *informed* decision and providing *informed* consent. A patient who has provided informed consent has *assumed the risk* concerning those outcomes.

Emergency Defense

One of the most commonly known defenses is the emergency defense, which is also referred to as Good Samaritan laws.

The name Good Samaritan comes from the parable of a traveler who was attacked by bandits and left for dead on the side of the road. A stranger came along and not only dressed his wounds but provided him with food, clothing, and lodging. The parable is used to teach us that we should be encouraged to provide assistance to those in need. But despite our best efforts to try to help someone, we cannot always be assured of a positive outcome. For example, a man witnessed a car accident and noticed that the car had caught on fire. He raced over to the car and pulled the unconscious woman to safety before the car exploded. Unfortunately, even though he saved the woman's life, she ended up paralyzed because of a fractured spine. Does the injured woman have a right to sue her rescuer for her injuries?

When situations like this arose in the courts, the legislature stepped in and created Good Samaritan laws. The idea behind creating the emergency defense was to encourage people to provide assistance in an emergency. And, if they did, that they would not have to fear a lawsuit if something bad happened. But the emergency defense is not a blank slate either, and certain conditions apply.

Even though an emergency may exist, that does not mean that you can commit mistakes. Once you have taken it upon yourself to respond to an emergency, you are thereby creating a duty element, which you cannot breach. As a trained medical professional, you have advanced training and knowledge that an average citizen does not have. For example, an average citizen may not know to secure someone's neck before moving them out of a wrecked car. But, as a trained

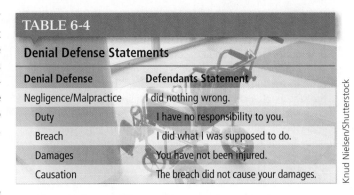

TABLE 6-4

Denial Defense Statements

Denial Defense	Defendants Statement
Negligence/Malpractice	I did nothing wrong.
Duty	I have no responsibility to you.
Breach	I did what I was supposed to do.
Damages	You have not been injured.
Causation	The breach did not cause your damages.

Knud Nielsen/Shutterstock

 Sidebar

Because the causation element of malpractice can be difficult to prove sometimes, a plaintiff's attorney will not usually file a negligence lawsuit until he or she has consulted with an expert witness about causation. If the expert hired does not believe that causation exists, there may be no reason to proceed with filing a lawsuit.

The Ethics of Law
Expert Witnesses

The law does not limit the number of expert witnesses an attorney can consult with. But should there be? What if an attorney consults with an expert witness and their opinion is contrary to what supports their case? For example, a plaintiff attorney consults with an expert witness who does not believe that the causation element has been satisfied. So, that person consults with another expert witness, and another expert, and another until they find one who will testify that the causation element has been satisfied. Is that fair?

• Should the law limit the number of expert witnesses that a person is authorized to consult with?

Legal Alert! The courts have specifically stated that patients cannot assume the risk of medical malpractice. Asking patients to consent to the possibility of malpractice removes the legal requirement of duty that we have to patients to provide the required care.

Concept Connection

Emergency Defense and Reasonable Person Standard

When a healthcare professional voluntarily offers medical assistance in an emergency, the courts will use a variation of the reasonable person standard to scrutinize their actions. The court will ask: What would a reasonable and prudent healthcare worker with the same training, education, and experience do in the same or similar emergency situation.

Beyond the Scope

There are questions, nuances, and requirements for using the diminishing responsibility defense, such as joint and several liability, that are beyond the scope of this text. For more information the reader is directed to outside resources.

medical professional, basic lifesaving techniques teach us that without securing the neck, a patient could become paralyzed. The law is not going to require that you carry around medical equipment, but it will hold you accountable to the training and experience that you have as a healthcare professional.

One common area of confusion regarding the emergency defense is when it applies. The emergency defense is not utilized simply because an emergency exists. Instead, it can only be utilized if there is no pre-existing duty to provide assistance. For example, a doctor who works in the emergency room or a paramedic working on an ambulance cannot utilize the emergency defense simply because they responded to *an* emergency. If we look back at the definition of the emergency defense, it provides a condition of "a person who *voluntarily* renders assistance." If a healthcare worker already has a pre-existing duty to provide emergency assistance, their actions are not voluntary, but legally required, so the emergency defense would not be available to them.

Diminishing Responsibility Defenses

There are defenses available that defendants can use to diminish their responsibility: the contributory negligence defense and the comparative negligence defense.

A defendant who uses either the contributory negligence defense or comparative negligence defense is making the assertion that the plaintiff, in some way, is partially responsible. And, because the patient is partially at fault, the defendant should not be held wholly accountable.

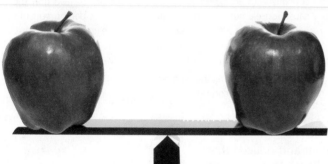

- When using the contributory negligence defense, the defendant is claiming that the plaintiff *contributed* to his or her damages.
- When using the comparative negligence defense, the defendant is claiming that both parties committed negligence, but by *comparison*, the plaintiff's negligence was worse than the defendant's negligence.

Escaping Liability

Due to technicalities in the law, there are times when lawsuits cannot be brought before the court—regardless of whether the plaintiff has a legitimate claim or not. While the courts may loathe the thought of a person escaping liability entirely, they will not hesitate to follow the law. There are two technical defenses: *res judicata* and the Statute of Limitations.

res judicata

The term *res judicata* literally means "a matter judge." Possibly the easiest way to describe and understand *res judicata* is to compare it to its criminal counterpart, double indemnity. A person who has been found not guilty of a crime cannot be retried for that same crime in a later trial. *Res judicata* is essentially the same thing, but utilized for civil litigation. Once an issue has been litigated in a civil court, that

Court Case

Clyde F. Deal v. L. John Kearney

851 P.2d 1353 (1993) Supreme Court of Alaska

FACTS: On September 16, 1984, John Kearney was involved in a life-threatening accident. He was taken Kodiak Island Hospital's emergency room. Because of his injuries, the ER doctor consulted with Dr. Clyde Deal, the surgeon on call for the hospital that day. Dr. Deal determined that Kearney would not survive the trip to Anchorage, Alaska, and took Kearney to the operating room, performing a ten-hour surgery. Following the surgery Dr. Deal gave written and verbal orders to the nursing staff. One of those orders was to arrange for a medivac flight transfer to an Anchorage hospital by 12:00 noon on September 17, 1984. But, for reasons undisclosed in the trial transcripts, Kearney was not medivaced until 5:00 pm on September 17, 1984. Upon his arrival at the hospital in Anchorage, Kearney was in critical condition. He underwent additional surgery, and eventually had his right leg amputated at the hip and his left leg amputated at the knee.

Kearney filed suit, alleging, among other things, that Dr. Deal was negligent in not arranging for the transfer. Or, if such an order was actually given, negligent in not following up to ensure that the transfer was complete. The delay in transfer, Kearney claimed, resulted in this loss of circulation in his legs,

and ultimately the amputations. In defending the lawsuit, Dr. Kearney claimed that he was immune from being sued under the Good Samaritan law.

ISSUE: Can Dr. Kearney use the Good Samaritan law as a defense in the lawsuit?

RULE: The court held that "… the immunity provided by the Good Samaritan statute is unavailable to physicians with a pre-existing duty to respond to emergency situations." The trial court, in denying Dr. Kearney's use of the Good Samaritan law, stated two reasons. First, Dr. Kearney was under a pre-existing duty to provide emergency care. As the on-call surgeon for the emergency room, he had a pre-existing duty to respond to a surgical emergency. Second, at issue in the negligence lawsuit was the appropriateness of follow-up care following surgery. The court concluded that when the surgery was completed, Dr. Kearney was no longer responding to an emergency, but was instead Kearney's treating physician.

EMPHASIS: This lawsuit demonstrates the use of the Good Samaritan law in the healthcare setting. It also demonstrates that the emergency defense (Good Samaritan law) cannot be used for healthcare professionals who have a pre-existing duty to respond to emergencies.

same issue cannot be relitigated in another civil lawsuit. Meaning, a defendant can be sued over and over again for the same mistake.

Statute of Limitations

The other technical defense is the Statute of Limitations. The Statute of Limitations sets a deadline for when a person can file a lawsuit. A person who waits too long to file a lawsuit, regardless of having a valid claim or not, will be unable to proceed to trial. But why would the courts put a limit on the time frame a person is allowed to file a lawsuit?

One reason for creating a Statute of Limitations is based on fairness to the parties involved in a lawsuit. A person should not have to worry about being sued long after an incident has occurred. Constantly worrying about being sued over something that you may have done 25 years ago is not the kind of swift justice that the law requires. While there are some crimes, such as murder, that do not have a Statute of Limitation applied to them, all civil infractions have a Statute of Limitations.

Another reason for creating a Statute of Limitations is based on the availability of evidence. Imagine that you are called to the witness stand, and asked what clothes you wore on your birthday 20 years ago? Or, what if you were asked to recall events that occurred on March 21st, 20 years ago? Would you be able to remember? Probably not.

Before we can use the Statute of Limitations as a defense, we have to determine what dates are used to measure the Statute of Limitations. There are two concepts associated with the Statute of Limitations that effect the start and stop dates of the Statute of Limitations; running and tolling.

Running On what date does the Statute of Limitations start? Most states have a Statute of Limitations of two years for negligence lawsuits. If an act of negligence occurred on March 21, 2011, a two-year Statute of Limitations would expire, or *run* out, on March 22, 2013. (The first day is not counted.)

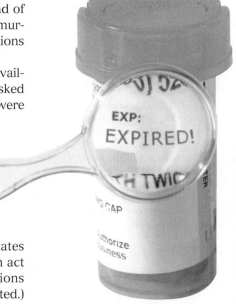

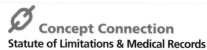

Concept Connection
Statute of Limitations and Civil Lawsuit
One of the steps in the path of a lawsuit includes the discovery of a wrong. If a person is not aware that a wrong has occurred, then there is no foundation for a civil lawsuit.

Concept Connection
Statute of Limitations & Medical Records
One of the guiding principles for determining how long we store and maintain medical records has to do with the age of majority and tolling under the Statute of Limitations.

Understanding Your State
All civil actions, including negligence and malpractice, have different Statute of Limitation periods and running and tolling requirements. To understand what your state requires, check out the interactive map on the companion website.

Any lawsuit filed after March 22, 2013 would be dismissed, because the Statute of Limitations has run. While the date an incident occurs starts the Statute of Limitations, there is one exception, and that is if the action goes undiscovered.

Suppose that a patient had surgery five years ago and the surgical team left a surgical sponge in the patient's abdominal cavity. Only if the patient develops problems will the patient know that a negligent act has occurred. If two years pass, and the patient does not find out about it, is he or she out of luck in regard to filing a lawsuit. No. The Statute of Limitations will not start until the patient discovers that the negligent act occurred. Upon the date of discovery of the wrong, the person has two years to file a lawsuit.

Tolling Most states set the age of majority at 18 years of age. That means that, under the law, a person cannot make legal decisions until they turn 18, which includes filing a lawsuit. But that does not mean that if a negligent act is committed on a child, they are out of luck. Tolling stops the Statute of Limitations clock, and tells us when it starts back up again.

If a negligent act is committed against someone under the age of majority, the Statute of Limitations starts on the day that the negligent act occurred (or was first discovered). But then, because of tolling, it automatically stops. The Statute of Limitations does not start again until the person reaches the

Court Case

Williams v. Kilgore

618 So.2d 51 (1992) Supreme Court of Mississippi

FACTS: On March 31, 1964, Gracie Williams underwent a bone marrow biopsy. During the procedure, the biopsy needle broke leaving a two-centimeter long section of the needle lodged next to her left iliac bone. Because Mrs. Williams was going to have surgery to remove a melanoma in her groin the next day, the doctor's decided that they would remove the needle fragment then. The operative report for the melanoma removal indicated that the needle fragment had also been removed. Following the surgery, when Mrs. Williams asked the doctor about the needle fragment, she was assured that the needle had in fact been removed. However, the needle was not removed and remained in Mrs. Williams hip.

In September 1985, Mrs. Williams was admitted to the hospital for back pain. An x-ray indicated the presence of the needle fragment in her hip. Upon discovering that the needle fragment remained in her hip, Mrs. Williams filed a lawsuit against the hospital and doctors, claiming negligence. The defendants requested that the case be dismissed because that Statute of Limitations had expired.

ISSUE Because the negligent act occurred in 1964, has the Statute of Limitations expired, barring Mrs. Williams lawsuit?

RULE "Applying our liberal analysis of the discovery rule . . . , we find that Mrs. Williams' claim is not barred by the statute of limitations." Because the needle fragment was not discovered until 1985, it is that date that is used to start the Statute of Limitations, not the date the incident occurred.

EMPHASIS Because Mrs. Williams was not aware that a negligent act had occurred until 1985, the date the negligent act is discovered is used to start the Statute of Limitations.

age of majority. Using the two-year Statute of Limitations for negligence and an 18 year-old age of majority as an example; if tolling occurs, the Statute of Limitations for negligence would expire on the person's twentieth birthday.

Burden of Proof

The burden of proof informs us who has the legal burden (requirement) of proving what they are claiming. For example, when a person files a lawsuit, he or she is complaining of having been harmed in some way. By filing the lawsuit, the person has the legal burden of proving his or her claim. This is accomplished by providing the necessary evidence and testimony to support that claim. While the burden of proof usually belongs to the plaintiff, that is not always the case. Sometimes, the defendant will have the burden of proof.

There are some who mistakenly refer to burdens of proof as switching or flipping between the plaintiff and the defendant. The burden of proof should not be thought of as belonging to a particular party in the lawsuit (plaintiff or defendant). Instead, the burden of proof belongs to the person who is making a claim. Our present discussion on defenses is a good example. If a defense is raised in a lawsuit, the person bringing that claim has the burden of proving of that claim. For example, if the Statute of Limitations is raised in a lawsuit, who has the burden of proving that the legal requirements exist? The person who is making the claim that the Statute of Limitations applies. By applying the burden of proof to the *person* who complains, not the party of a lawsuit, you will always be able to identify who has the legal burden of proving their complaint.

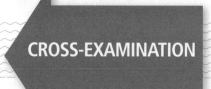

Make FALSE statements TRUE.

Rewrite the false statements below by replacing the bolded, italicized, and underlined word(s) to make it a true statement.

1. To classify torts by action, you have to understand the difference between ***negligence and malpractice***.

   _____

2. The law defines personal property, such as computers, furniture, and clothing as ***property***.

   _____

3. Strict liability torts are an example of ***professional*** liability.

   _____

4. In a negligence analysis, the reasonable person standard is used to address the element of ***causation***.

   _____

5. The doctrine ***respondeat superior*** is sometimes used to determine the causation element of negligence.

   _____

Circle Exercise

Circle the correct word from the choices given.

1. The use of restraints in healthcare can result in the commission of (**assault, battery, false imprisonment**).

2. Pain and suffering is classified as (**physical, mental/emotional, financial**) damages.

3. The category of damages that are not classified as physical, mental/emotional, or financial are (**compensatory, consequential, punitive**) damages.

4. Under the tort of negligence, the legal element of (**duty, breach, causation**) is only determined by a judge.

5. The feasances of negligence, malfeasance, misfeasance, and nonfeasance, address the element of (**duty, breach, causation**).

Matching

Match the numbered term to its lettered definition.

1. _____ chattel

2. _____ damages

3. _____ malfeasance

4. _____ misfeasance

5. _____ mitigate

6. _____ negligence

7. _____ nonfeasance

8. _____ *res ipsa loquitur*

9. _____ torts

A. a lawful act, performed in a wrongful manner

B. a person's belongings, other than land

C. a quantified amount of money used to demonstrate a loss or injury to a person or property

D. the area of civil law that addresses the harms a person receives, except for harms arising out of contract

E. the failure to take action when action is required

F. the performance of an unlawful act through wrongdoing or misconduct

G. "the thing itself speaks"; a legal theory whereby the mere occurrence of an event infers causation

H. to lessen, make less severe or less intense

I. when damages are caused by a breach of duty

Deliberations: Critical Thinking Questions

Question 1: One of the ways that torts are categorized is by a person's actions—whether the actions are intentional or unintentional. Which category do you think should lead to more severe legal punishment—those torts categorized under intentional actions or unintentional actions? Explain your answer.

Question 2: The element of duty, and whether it exists or not, is only determined by a judge. But even though a person may not have a legal duty, he or she might have an ethical or moral duty. Do you think that a person with a moral or ethical duty should still be held accountable under the law? Explain your answer.

Question 3: Expert witnesses are used to address the element of causation. Can an expert witness testify for the plaintiff in one case and the defendant in another? Do you foresee any problems with an expert witness who only testifies for plaintiffs or only testifies for defendants?

Question 4: There are three different ways that a professional can breach their duty of care, through malfeasance, misfeasance, or nonfeasance. Which of the three do you think is the most common type of breach in medical malpractice cases? Explain your answer.

Question 5: Why do you think that there is a different classification of negligence for professionals—that of malpractice? Should the analysis used to determine professional negligence (malpractice) be any different? Explain your answer.

Closing Arguments: Case Analysis

Patty is a patient care technician working in a busy physician's office. Mr. Smith has an appointment to get his blood pressure checked. The doctor recommends that Mr. Smith start on a new and different type of blood pressure medication than what he was taking before. The doctor, who left his prescription pad on his desk, goes to his office to retrieve it. While in his office, the doctor gets a call from the hospital next door, stating that his wife has been in a horrible car accident. The doctor rushes out the door and heads for the hospital.

Mr. Smith has been waiting for over an hour and is anxious to get home. Even though Patty has paged the doctor several times, he has not yet responded. Patty goes to the doctor's desk and notices Mr. Smith's chart. The chart is open with a prescription for Lisinopril on top of it. In the medical chart, the doctor's note indicates the he wanted to start Mr. Smith on Lisonopril, and lists the exact same dosage and frequency as what is on the prescription. While the prescription and doctor's note are exactly the same, the only thing lacking on the prescription is Mr. Smith's name.

Patty takes the prescription, writes Mr. Smith's name on the prescription and hands the prescription to Mr. Smith, telling him to call the office if he has any problems and to schedule a follow-up appointment. Mr. Smith stops by the pharmacy on his way home and

has the prescription filled. The next morning at breakfast, Mr. Smith takes the Lisinopril for the first time. About 10 minutes after taking the medication, Mr. Smith starts to feel funny and collapses. Mrs. Smith calls an ambulance, who rushes Mr. Smith to the hospital. In the emergency room, it is discovered that Mr. Smith had an allergic reaction to the Lisinopril. Because of the severity of the allergic reaction, Mr. Smith had to stay in the hospital for several days.

Question 1: Is Patty likely to be found guilty of malpractice? Perform a malpractice analysis, detailing each of the steps and how you arrived at your conclusions. (Note: We are only performing a malpractice analysis on Patty at this time and not on the doctor.)

Question 2: What about the doctor? Is he likely to be found guilty of malpractice? Perform a malpractice analysis, detailing each of the steps and how you arrived at your conclusions.

Question 3: If this case were to go to trial, are there any defenses that the doctor could use? What about Patty—are there any defenses that she can use? List each person, and what defenses they can use, separately.

The Briefcase

This section repeats the objectives from the beginning of the chapter and provides a summary of the most important concepts for each objective. Use this section as a quick review and to check your understanding of the chapter key points.

Objective 1: Identify the two different classifications of torts.
- Harms
  - Harm to the body (physical and mental)
  - Harm to personality (emotional)
  - Harm to property (financial)
  - Strict Harm
- Actions
  - Intentional torts
  - Unintentional torts

Objective 2: List the four different categories of harm.
- Harm to the body
- Harm to personality
- Harm to property
- Strict harm

Objective 3: Categorize the different torts according to their harm category.
- Refer to Table 6-2 on pg. 94.

Objective 4: Given the common law definition of a tort, list a tort's elements.
- Refer to Table 6-1 on page 92.

Objective 5: Describe the different types and categories of damages allowed by the courts.
- Types of Damages
  - physical damages
  - mental/emotional damages
  - financial damages
- Damage Categories
  - Compensatory Damages
  - Consequential Damages
  - Punitive Damages

Objective 6: Explain the concept of mitigation and damages
- To lessen the amount of damages.
- Only applies to compensatory and consequential damages.

Objective 7: Compare and contrast negligence and malpractice.
- See Table 6-3 on pg. 104.

Objective 8: Differentiate between misfeasance, malfeasance, and nonfeasance.
- malfeasance is an illegal act.
- misfeasance is a legal act performed the wrong way.
- nonfeasance is not acting when the law requires you to act.

Objective 9: List the defenses that are available to a defendant
- Refuting Allegations
  - Denial Defense
  - Assumption of the Risk
  - Emergency Defense/Good Samaritan laws
- Diminish Responsibility
  - Contributory Negligence
  - Comparative Negligence
- Escaping Responsibility
  - res judicata
  - Statute of Limitations

Maximize Your Success with the Companion Website

The Companion Website to this textbook contains materials that can help you better understand the concepts presented in this chapter. Go to www.myhealthprofessionskit.com to access:

- Sample Quizzes
- Web Links
- Games
- and more . . .

7

Professional Responsibilities

One of the overriding principles in healthcare is the right of the patient. Patients have a right to determine their own course of treatment, the right to deny treatment, and the right to privacy to name a few. While normally the patient's individual rights are paramount, there are times when the public's rights outweigh the rights of an individual. In this chapter, we will discuss the responsibilities that you have to the public, and when some of the exceptions to individual rights occur.

Jura publica anteferenda { privatis } Public rights are to be preferred over private ones.

MEASURE YOUR PROGRESS: LEARNING OBJECTIVES

After studying this chapter, you will be able to:

- Define what protected relationships are and explain why they exist.

- Explain why there is an exception to privacy rules and privileged communication.

- Categorize all public laws into one of three categories.

- Give an example of what vital statistics are and how they are used by public health officials.

- Compare and contrast endemic, epidemic, and pandemic.

- List what diseases and injuries a healthcare professional may be required to report.

- Provide examples of why the Medical Waste Tracking Act was enacted and what it accomplishes.

- Determine the difference between the different schedules of drugs classified by the FDA.

- Explain what responsibilities you have as a member of a healthcare profession to others in your profession.

KEY TERMS

endemic

epidemic

epidemiology

isolation

medical examiner

pandemic

privileged communication

quarantine

vital statistics

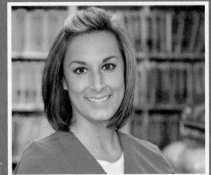
Judy Kennamer/Shutterstock

PROFESSIONAL HIGHLIGHT

Kim works as the office manager at a doctor's office. Prior to being promoted to office manager, she was a medical assistant in the same office. This gives her key insight into how the office runs. Kim gathers data and writes reports for the physicians in the office. She has to have an understanding of what reports are required and what information she must provide to various governmental agencies to ensure that the practice complies with the law. Without a thorough understanding of the professional responsibilities for all of the different professions in the doctor's office, Kim would not be able to maintain some of the professional responsibilities of the office staff.

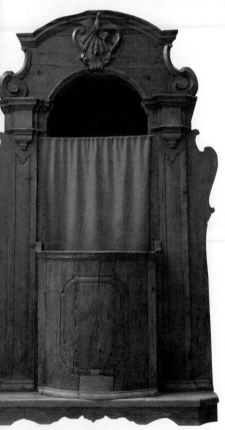

Mi.Ti./Shutterstock

T he short answer is yes. As a healthcare professional, you have a responsibility to many different people other than the patients you are providing care too. For example, while you have a responsibility to keep patient
information private, there are times when you will be required to disclose
patient information to select individuals or agencies. As we have seen,
the law is not always concrete, as there are a variety of exceptions to
the general rule; and sometimes exceptions to the exceptions. To help
you understand these exceptions, and the professional obligations
that you have as a healthcare professional, we can examine three
different categories:

- responsibilities to patient,
- responsibility to the profession, and
- personal responsibility.

Responsibility to Patients

When you provide patient care, your first and primary obligation is to the patient.
But, when providing care to one patient, does his or her medical condition or
the treatment that you provide affect other people? If it does, you may have a
responsibility to those people, even though they are not your patient.

Protected Relationships

Normally, the law requires the full disclosure of information in judicial proceedings. This requirement ensures that the parties involved in a lawsuit have
the pertinent and truthful information that is relevant to their case. In order to
obtain information attorneys use a variety of different tools, known as discovery. But there are times when a person cannot answer questions, not because
they do not know the answer, but because they are required by law not to
disclose information.

There are certain relationships that the law recognizes as *so important,* that
they are provided with special legal protection. Those relationships include
doctor/patient, priest/penitent, attorney/client, and husband/wife relationships. Because the nature of these relationships depends on open communication, any private conversation that occurs between these individuals is
considered **privileged communication**.

The reason that the court provides these specific relationships with special
protection is based on why the relationship exists. If confidential and private
information is an essential component to the existence of a relationship, without protecting that communication the reason for the relationship would be
destroyed. For example, the priest/penitent relationship exists, in part, so that
a priest can provide spiritual counseling and guidance to his parishioners. (The
privilege is not exclusive to priests; the privilege includes any religious leader,
such as ministers, reverends, and rabbis.) If parishioners feared
that what they said to a priest would be disclosed, it could destroy one of the underlying reason for the relationship, the providing of spiritual guidance.

The doctor/patient relationship is another example. Patients
need to feel comfortable telling doctors truthful and pertinent
information so that they can be treated appropriately. Failing to
disclose truthful and pertinent information could be detrimental to the patient's health.

Note that part of the definition of privileged communica-
tion says "cannot be used *as evidence* in civil and criminal trials." While the
limitations stems from laws related to the use of evidence at trial, it has been
extended to other areas as well. A doctor who is asked about a protected conversation he or she has had with a patient can politely refuse to answer, unless
ordered by a court of law to do so.

Concept Connection
Protected Relationships & Discovery
Two of the most common tools used during the discovery process are interrogatories and depositions. But
perhaps the most commonly used discovery tool in
medical cases is a *subpoena duces tecum.*

privileged communication: statements
made in private, during the existence of
certain relationships, that cannot be used
as evidence in civil or criminal trials

The law of privileged communications and special relationships present two unique problems we need to consider. First, the privilege is provided to doctors, not necessarily all healthcare providers. Whether additional healthcare professionals are provided with protecting privileged communication depends on the jurisdiction; as each have different requirements. In addition, the privilege may apply through extension to other healthcare providers even though not codified (written) in law. For example, if a doctor has a privileged communication with a patient, and then informs a medical assistant of that information in order for that person to provide care, that information, by extension, may apply to the medical assistant as well.

Second, there exists an exception to the rule of privileged communication. If information is obtained during a privileged communication that can cause harm to another person, we may be required by law to disclose that information to a third party. Consider the following court case.

Public Health

Typically, healthcare workers will take care of a select few patients in any given day. But healthcare professionals who work in public health have only one patient to take care of—the general public. By looking at the entire population as one individual patient, public health workers can concentrate on the healthcare needs of their patients. In addition, by thinking of the public as an individual patient, some of the exceptions that occur—when public rights override individual rights—might make more sense.

The main goal of public health is to take care of the health needs of the public, and in that way the public health worker is just like any other healthcare professional. When patients become sick or injured, they sometimes seek medical care. To determine what might be wrong with a patient, health

Court Case

Tarasoff v. Regents of the University of California

17 Cal. 3d 425, 551 P.2d 334, 131 Cal. Rptr. 14 Supreme Court of California (1976)

FACTS: Prosenjit Poddar, while attending the University of California at Berkeley as a graduate student, met Tatiana Tarasoff. Because of a kiss that occurred on New Year's Eve between Poddar and Tarasoff, Poddar thought Tarasoff wanted to enter into a romantic relationship with him. This feeling was not shared by Tarasoff, which she disclosed to Poddar. Feeling rejected, Poddar became severely depressed and started stalking Tarasoff. A friend of Poddor suggested that he seek psychological counseling, which he did at UC Berkeley's Cowell Hospital with Dr. Moore.

During a counseling session between Poddar and Dr. Moore, Poddar confided his intention to kill Tarasoff. Dr. Moore took the threat seriously, and alerted security, recommending that he be civilly committed as a dangerous person. But, when Poddar was detained by campus police, he appeared calm and rational, so Dr. Moore's supervisor ordered Poddar released and asked campus police not to subjected him to any further detention.

Two months later, on October 27, 1969 Poddar carried out his threat, stabbing and killing Tatiana Tarasoff. Tatiana's parents filed a civil lawsuit against the University of California (under *respondeat superior*) and campus employees including Dr. Moore, his supervisor, and campus police. The plaintiff's claim was that Dr. Moore had a duty to warn Tatiana about the danger imposed to her because of the threat made by Poddar.

ISSUE: The issue before the court was whether a therapist had a duty to warn Tarasoff of the danger even though she was not his patient; and would doing so be a breach of confidentiality and doctor/patient privilege?

RULE: The court ruled: "When a therapist determines, or pursuant to the standards of his profession should determine, that his patient presents a serious danger of violence to another, he incurs an obligation to use reasonable care to protect the intended victim against such danger."

EMPHASIS: While the Tarasoff case involved a therapist, after the ruling other healthcare professionals were concerned about how it might affect their profession. There are many important emphases and results of this case. The first emphasis this case demonstrates is how a judge determines the legal element of duty. The second emphasis demonstrates the concept of *respondeat superior*. The third emphasis is how the court used the Standards of Care specifically mentioning them in the court's ruling. And fourth, one of the main results of this case, was the creation of what is known as a Tarasoff Warning.

If a healthcare professional determines that "a patient presents a serious danger of violence to another" they can send an anonymous warning to that person to ensure that they are in compliance with the Tarasoff ruling. And, by issuing the Tarasoff Warning anonymously, they are protecting the confidentiality of the patient and maintaining the doctor/patient relationship.

professionals will gather information and look at the patient's signs and symptoms. Public health officials do the same thing. They gather information and look at the signs and symptoms of their patient in order to determine what might be wrong. But how they gather that information and obtain their patient's signs and symptoms is different. Public health officials obtain the signs and symptoms of their patient through information provided to them by healthcare providers. There are certain situations, medical conditions, or information that you might obtain from the patients that you provide care to that you will be required to provide to governmental agencies, such as public health officials. Public health laws will provide the details to help you identify when those situations occur, identify what those medical conditions are, and what information you need to report. Public health laws fall into one of three categories:

- Law of Populations
- Disease and Injury Prevention
- Police Powers

Law of Populations

In order to get a better idea of who their patient is, public health officials need to gather information regarding their patient. To provide a baseline for them to work with, they obtain information in the form of **vital statistics**.

While vital statistics provide much more than medical information, the basic vital statistic information utilized by public health officials relate to the occurrence of births and deaths.

Births

Every time a child is born, a Certificate of Birth form is completed and filed with the appropriate state agency; typically, the Secretary of State's office. Certificate of Birth forms (see Fig. 7-1) contain a variety of information, such as the name of the child, the names of the child's parents, and the date, time, and location of where and when the birth occurred. There is a difference between the Certificate of Birth forms that are filed with the state, and Birth Certificates that are given to the parents of newborns.

All states in the United States require that a Certificate of Birth be issued for any live birth, whether that birth occurs in a hospital or at home. Some states do not require Certificates of Birth for children that are stillborn or miscarried, but others do. In addition, some states require both a Certificate of Birth and a Certificate of Death for children who are stillborn or miscarried.

Public health officials will use the information contained on Certificates of Birth for a variety of different reasons. For example, if public health

vital statistics: the information gathered by governmental agencies related to births, marriages, divorces, and death that occur in a population

Meder Lorant/Shutterstock

Concept Connection
Vital Statistics and Certification
One of the reasons for certification that we mentioned was to verify the presence of predetermined requirements. When a healthcare institution issues a birth certificate, it is verifying that a child has been born.

Understanding Your State
The law of privileged communication differs from jurisdiction to jurisdiction. To determine whom the law applies to in your state, check out the map of the United States on the companion website.

Beyond the Scope
Sending out a Tarasoff letter is not something that should be taken lightly. Because the requirements for sending Tarasoff letters are complex, a person contemplating a Tarasoff letter should consult with legal experts before doing so.

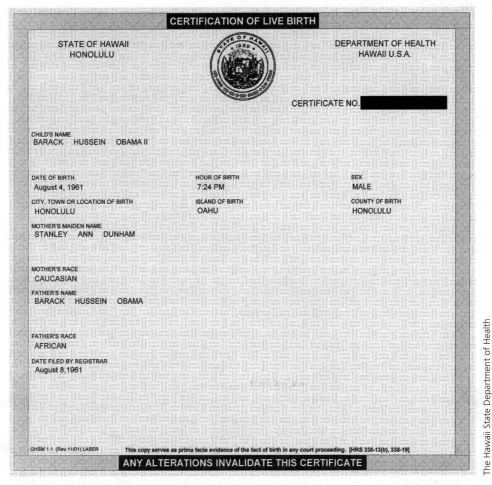

CERTIFICATION OF LIVE BIRTH

STATE OF HAWAII
HONOLULU

DEPARTMENT OF HEALTH
HAWAII U.S.A.

CERTIFICATE NO.

CHILD'S NAME
BARACK   HUSSEIN   OBAMA II

DATE OF BIRTH	HOUR OF BIRTH	SEX
August 4, 1961	7:24 PM	MALE
CITY, TOWN OR LOCATION OF BIRTH	ISLAND OF BIRTH	COUNTY OF BIRTH
HONOLULU	OAHU	HONOLULU

MOTHER'S MAIDEN NAME
STANLEY   ANN   DUNHAM

MOTHER'S RACE
CAUCASIAN

FATHER'S NAME
BARACK   HUSSEIN   OBAMA

FATHER'S RACE
AFRICAN

DATE FILED BY REGISTRAR
August 8, 1961

OHSM 1.1 (Rev.11/01) LASER   This copy serves as prima facie evidence of the fact of birth in any court proceeding. [HRS 338-13(b), 338-19]

ANY ALTERATIONS INVALIDATE THIS CERTIFICATE

The Hawaii State Department of Health

Fig. 7-1. After a highly publicized debate over whether President Barack Obama was a naturally born citizen of the United States, he released his Certificate of Birth to the general public.

officials notice an increase number of babies born to teenage mothers, they might utilize that information to increase teen pregnancy awareness programs or allocate additional funding to pediatric clinics that provide healthcare to young mothers.

Deaths

In addition to information about births, public health officials gather information about deaths as well. When a person passes away, a Certificate of Death is completed and sent to the appropriate state agency; again, typically the Secretary of State's office. If the death occurs in a hospital, the attending physician completes the Certificate of Death. Some of the information that the attending physician will be asked to fill out on the Certificate of Death are what the cause of death was and if there were any contributing factors. For deaths that occur in a hospital, this information may be easy to determine. For example following a heart attack or heart surgery, the cause of death might be cardiac arrest. But sometimes the cause of death is not readily identifiable or known. When the doctor is unsure why a death occurred, he or she may ask that an autopsy be performed. Autopsies are performed by a licensed

Understanding Your State

Each state has different requirements for Certification of Birth. To find out what your state requires, check out the companion website for links to your state.

The Ethics of Law

Birth Certificate Information

When a child is put up for adoption, some states allow the birth mother to keep her identity confidential. As part of the adoption process, judges will seal the Certificate of Birth and issue a duplicate, in which the birthparents' names are not contained on the Certificate of Birth. An adoptive child who wants to obtain information about his or her birth parents will be unable to do so because the record has been sealed.

- Can you think of any medical reasons it might be important to know who an adoptive child's biological mother or father is?
- Should a birth mother be given the right to keep that information private over the rights of the child?

medical examiner: a medical professional whose responsibility is to determine the cause of death and gather forensic evidence

physician known as a **medical examiner** to determine what the cause of death was and if there were any factors contributing to the death.

When a medical examiner performs an autopsy, they are gathering information concerning both the cause of death and the manner of death. The information obtained is included on the Certificate of Death, a copy of which is provided to public health officials.

The manner of a person's death, determined by the medical examiner relates to why the person died, whether from natural causes or from the commission of a crime. If the death has been caused by the commission of a crime, the medical examiner will notify appropriate law enforcement agencies.

Any death that occurs outside of a hospital is automatically referred to the medical examiner's office. After the referral, the medical examiner will determine whether an autopsy needs to be performed or not.

The information that is contained on the Certificate of Death can provide vital information to public health officials. For example, if public health officials see a rise in diabetic related deaths, they might ask doctors to perform diabetic screenings on all of the patients that come into the office, regardless of whether they have been diagnosed with diabetes or not.

Sidebar

A common area of confusion is the difference between a medical examiner and a coroner. Coroners are elected officials, and even though a medical license is not always required to hold the position, most do. The coroner system was developed in medieval England and brought to America during the early colonial period. Of the 13 states that still have coroners today, they exist mostly in rural counties and communities and typically serve as a liaison with other medical examiners within the state.

Disease and Injury Prevention

One of the main areas that public health officials concentrate on is the prevention of disease and injuries. There are certain diseases that always exist within populations or geographical locations. Examples include influenza, the common cold, or chicken pox. Diseases that are always present, in some degree, within a population are known as **endemic** diseases.

endemic: a disease that is always present, to some degree, in a population or location

The key part of the definition of endemic disease is that it is always present within a population. If you have ever heard some say "it's been going around" when referring to a disease, that disease is probably an endemic disease. Endemic diseases exists because of the way they are passed from one person to another, and are never completely eradicated. This route of infection is part of what makes an endemic disease always present within a population. The number or frequency of infections from endemic diseases is predictable as well. While the number of people infected will fluctuate, public health officials still monitor endemic diseases. If they see a drastic increase in the number of people infected by an endemic disease, public health officials will investigate to identify any likely cause to determine if any corrective action needs to be taken.

Sidebar

The literal meaning of the word *endemic* is "within the population." The prefix *en-* means "within," and the combining form *dem/o-* means "people" or "population. With the suffix *–ic*, meaning "pertaining to," the word *endemic* means "pertaining to within a population."

Within public health organizations, there are specialists that work to identify, track, and prevent disease. This specialized field of disease study is known as **epidemiology**. Most of the diseases that epidemiologists study and monitor are communicable and contagious diseases that have a significant impact on health. When looking at communicable and contagious diseases, epidemiologists attempt to determine:

epidemiology: the study of the characteristics, determination, frequency, and distribution of a disease

- what the pathogen is,
- where the pathogen comes from, and
- how a person becomes infected.

Part of the reason that epidemiologists monitor diseases is to identify potential outbreaks and to prevent the emergence of an **epidemic**.

epidemic: the occurrence of disease in greater numbers than expected, or the development of disease in a shorter than normal time frame

If an endemic disease occurs in greater frequency than expected, it can cause an epidemic. In order for an outbreak to be classified as an epidemic:

- the disease has to occur in greater numbers than what are normally seen,
- there is an emergence of a non-endemic disease,
- a disease's rate of infection or susceptibility has changed, or
- any disease that has lethal or devastating consequences has been discovered.

Identifying an epidemic will help public health officials to determine the cause, and to take appropriate measures. Sometimes, those measures might include a boil water order or ordering a quarantine of a person or location.

While monitoring epidemics, one of the concerns that public health officials have is whether an epidemic can become **pandemic**.

Pandemic diseases occur in more than one population, and typically result from an infection being transmitted from one population to another. The majority of diseases that are at risk for developing pandemic consequences are those diseases that are highly contagious and/or deadly. In order to combat the existence of epidemics and pandemics, public health officials require healthcare providers to report suspected infectious diseases.

Reportable Diseases

There are certain diseases that pose the greatest risk for causing epidemics and pandemics. The World Health Organization (WHO), a part of the United Nations, is a global public health agency. Among other things, WHO monitors disease outbreaks and tracks the occurrence of epidemics and pandemics around the world. WHO requires the reporting of patients that have been diagnosed, or are showing symptoms of:

Anthrax	Plague
Avian influenza	Polio
Cholera	Relapsing fever
Crimean-Congo Hemorrhagic fever	Rift Valley fever
Dengue hemorrhagic fever	SARS
	Severe Acute Respiratory Syndrome
Ebola virus	Smallpox
Hepatitis	Tularaemia
Influenza	Typhus
Lassa fever	Yellow fever
Marburg Hemorrhagic fever	

In the United States, the national public health organization is the Centers for Disease Control and Prevention (CDC). The CDC works in conjunction with

 Concept Application

Epidemics

In 1993, public health officials saw an alarming increase in the number of *Escherichia coli* infections in the western Pacific states. During their investigation, they determined that most individuals who had been infected had eaten at a Jack-in-the-Box fast food restaurant. Epidemiologist determined that the hamburger being served by Jack-in-the-Box had been infected with *E. coli* during the slaughtering process. In all, four children died and hundreds of people became sick from eating the contaminated and undercooked meat. At that time, it was the largest and deadliest epidemic of *E. coli* in American history.

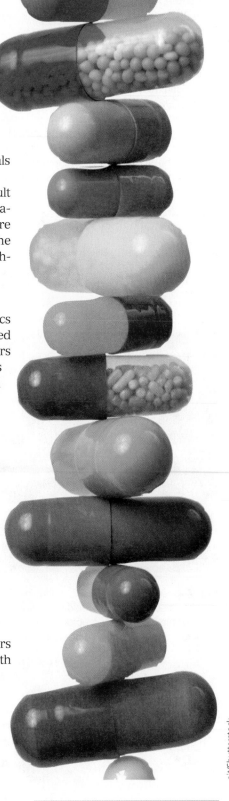

ajt/Shutterstock

pandemic: the occurrence of disease in many different populations or geographical locations

✔ Concept Application

Concert Attendees and Hepatitis

In 2003, the MMWR reported a drastic increase in the number of Hepatitis A cases in young adults in several southern states. Upon investigating this increase, public health officials determined that many of those who were infected with Hepatitis A had camped at a summer concert and used outdoor bathroom facilities (Porta-Johns). The CDC and local health departments worked with concert promoters and waste disposal companies to improve sanitation at these events. In addition, concertgoers who had attended these events in the past were notified about their risk of exposure to Hepatitis A through public service announcements, news organizations, and healthcare providers.

WHO to gather information related to reportable diseases. Because of the occurrence of past epidemics, or the potential for epidemics, in the United States, the CDC has added to WHO's list of reportable diseases to include:

Botulism

Hantavirus

HIV

Rabies

Tuberculosis

Every week, the CDC publishes information regarding these and other diseases in the MMWR (Morbidity and Mortality Weekly Report). The information published by the CDC in the MMWR is used by local public health officials and healthcare providers to serve as a tool to help them investigate, track, and prevent epidemics and pandemics.

Medical Waste

In the 1980s and 1990s healthcare institutions saw a dramatic increase in the amount of medical waste they were producing. In part, this increase was due to the occurrence of epidemics, such as tuberculosis and HIV. In order to destroy the pathogens that exist in medical waste, so as not to infect others, that waste

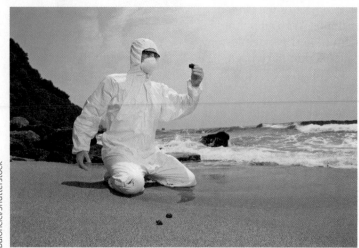

must be incinerated at high temperatures. The cost associated with not only incineration, but packaging and transporting of medical waste created huge financial burdens to healthcare organizations already feeling the pinch of financial constraints.

During this same time period, there were a number of incidences where medical waste was washing up on U.S. beaches, causing great public health concerns (see Fig. 7-2). Because the source of the medical waste could not be identified, nor what infectious agents might be contained in the waste, public health officials closed several beaches and issued boil water orders in many counties.

The outrage over the illegal dumping of medical waste prompted Congress to write the Medical Waste Tracking Act. The Medical Waste Tracking Act:

- provides definitions for what medical waste is,
- determines how waste should be managed, transported, and disposed of, and
- provides enforcement provisions.

Fig. 7-2. On August 13, 1987, a garbage slick, 30 miles wide, containing both medical and household waste was discovered off the East Coast. Some of the waste washed up on the shores prompting many beaches in New York and New Jersey to be closed to the public.

Reportable Injuries

In addition to diseases, there are certain types of injuries that healthcare providers must report to governmental agencies. But unlike diseases, the required reporting of injuries is not made to public health officials, but to law enforcement agencies instead.

Abuse Abuse, both physical and psychological, is an unfortunate but all too common occurrence in society today. While anyone can be the subject of abuse, the main three groups that suffer from abuse in our society are children, spouses, and the elderly. As healthcare providers, we will often be the first to encounter and/or identify abuse.

Many victims of abuse are very reluctant to inform health-care providers about the abuse. A common story told by abuse victims is that they tripped and fell down the stairs or walked into a door. But if the mechanism of injury does not match the story the patient gives us, we have to be concerned about whether abuse has occurred or not. For example, a Colles' fracture is a specific type of fracture to the distal radius (forearm bone), most commonly received when the hands are put out in front of a person to break their fall. If a patient informs you that they fell, but have a different type of fracture, other than a Colles' fracture, you might want to think about the possibility of abuse.

When we take care of patients, if injuries or illnesses are suspicious, we are required by law to report the *suspicion* of abuse to governmental agencies. The word *suspicion* is emphasized here, because that is exactly the requirement we as healthcare providers have and the extent to which we are obligated to act—reporting the suspicion. As healthcare providers, we are not members of law enforcement or crime investigators. Therefore, we do not take an active role in determining whether actual abuse has occurred or not. Our responsibility is only to report the *suspicion* of abuse to the appropriate law enforcement or governmental agencies.

While the list of professionals required by law to report suspected abuse varies from state to state, all states have identified healthcare workers as one of the professions required to report suspected abuse. In all states in the United States, the failure of healthcare workers to report suspected abuse can result in the healthcare professional being charged with a misdemeanor.

Legal Alert! Any time that you talk to abuse victims, you have to especially careful. One of the dangers that we have to think about is whether our interactions might cause more harm, further abuse, or the abuse to escalate. To allow an abuse victim to return home with spousal abuse pamphlets or printed woman's shelter information might actually be placing the patient in harm's way.

Court Case

People v. Davis

126 Cal.App.4th 1416, 25 Cal.Rptr.3d 92 (2005)
Court of Appeal of the State of California Fourth Appellate District Division Two

FACTS: In April 2000, an argument over a chair occurred between two patients at Vista Pacific Center, a long-term care facility that offers psychiatric services. After the patients were separated, Certified Nursing Assistant Gregory McMillan, approached the patients. Even though McMillan was told that everything was all right, McMillan ordered one of the patients, to his room; walking behind him and continually shouting "Go to your room!" At one point, McMillan hit the patient on the shoulder, spun him around, grabbed him around his neck and forced him to the floor. A nurse testified that McMillan's "manner was very threatening and aggressive. He was rigid, staring at the victim, pointing at him, and talking in a loud tone of voice." After the incident the patient was examined by a doctor and psychiatrist, both of whom determined that there were no injuries (either physical or mental) as a result of the incident.

An incident report was completed and ultimately forwarded to Deborah Davis, a licensed administrator for Vista Pacific Center. Although McMillan was fired, Davis decided not to report the incident as abuse to appropriate officials. She stated that she decided not to report the incident as abuse because the patient did not have any injuries. Part of her rationale was that a prior incident, described in professional publications, had been determined by the Department of Health not to constitute abuse. Davis was charged, and convicted, for failing to report abuse under the state's mandatory reporting law. Davis appealed her conviction. She stated that because "she determined that the allegation of abuse was unfounded, based on her experience and training, she did not entertain a reasonable suspicion and therefore had no duty to report the incident as suspected abuse."

ISSUE: Can a person use their training and experience to determine whether abuse has occurred to identify when reporting is required?

RULE: "[T]he Act does not permit a mandated reporter to investigate and determine that no abuse occurred, as defendant contends. On the contrary, the existence of such circumstances triggers the mandatory duty to report the circumstances to a designated outside agency."

EMPHASIS: This case demonstrates what the responsibility of mandatory reporter is, to report the suspicion of abuse; nothing more. The court, in its written opinion clarified that "[t]he duty to investigate and the authority to determine whether abuse actually did occur are vested in outside agencies."

Crimes and Other Activity As with abuse, healthcare providers are sometimes the first people to know about criminal activity as well. If a patient has been the victim of a crime or involved in a crime, you may be required to notify appropriate law enforcement agencies. Some common examples include gunshot wounds, stabbings, rape, car accidents, and animal bites. Because the reporting requirements vary from state to state and even from location to location, you should check your institution's policies and procedures and state laws to determine if you are required to report and what those reporting requirements are.

Police Powers

The last classification of public health laws have to do with the police powers provided to public health officials. While rarely used, they allow law enforcement and public health officials to take extraordinary measures to prevent disease and injuries. For example, if a train carrying hazardous materials derails in your community, a mandatory evacuation order may be issued by public health officials and law enforcement. If such an order has been declared, law enforcement can enter people's property and homes and, if necessary, forcibly remove them. Alternatively, if a person is suspected of having a highly contagious disease, the law allows that person to be **quarantined** and/or public health officials to take appropriate measures to ensure that the public's health is not endangered (see Fig. 7-3).

While the use of quarantine is rare, it is something that public health officials have utilized in the recent past. Since 9/11, Anthrax scares have surfaced around the United States. People who are exposed to suspected anthrax are typically placed in quarantine. However, instead of spending days in quarantine, they typically only spend minutes or hours in quarantine until decontamination procedures have been completed. The use of quarantine should not be confused with the use of **isolation**.

One way to remember the difference between isolation and quarantine is to focus on the reason for the procedure. The focus of isolation procedures is on the healthcare worker so that they do not transfer disease from one patient to another or transfer disease to themselves. Quarantines, on the other hand, are used to contain a disease so that it is not released to the general public.

quarantine: imposed isolation, most often used to contain individuals with highly contagious and/or deadly diseases

isolation: the measures taken to prevent the spread of disease, either from patient to patient or from patient to healthcare worker

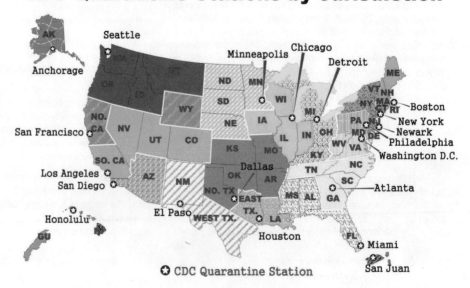

CDC Quarantine Stations by Jurisdiction

✪ CDC Quarantine Station

Fig. 7-3. The CDC maintains quarantine centers around the nation.

Court Case

In Re Eric Halko on Habeas Corpus

246 Cal. App.2d 553, 54 Cal. Rptr. 661 (1966)
District Court of Appeal of California, Second Appellate District, Division Four

FACTS: After Eric Halko was diagnosed with pulmonary tuberculosis, he received a six-month quarantine order from the Department of Public Health confining him to Mira Loma Hospital. One month later, he deserted the hospital in violation of the quarantine order. He was subsequently arrested, tried, and convicted of violating the Health and Safety Code of California and sentenced to jail. Prior to serving his jail sentence, however, he was served by the Department of Public Health with another six-month quarantine order, to be served in the security ward of Mira Loma Hospital. He subsequently received three additional quarantine orders, each one for six-months; totaling 24 months in all. Claiming that he was being unlawfully detained, Halko filed a habeas Corpus petition asking the court to order

his release. Halko's claim was that he was being deprived of his liberty without due process of law.

ISSUE: Is subjecting a person to consecutive quarantine orders, without a judicial questioning or determination, a deprivation of a person's liberty?

RULE: "The preservation of the public health is universally conceded to be one of the duties devolving upon the state as a sovereignty, and whatever reasonably tends to preserve the public health is a subject upon which the legislature, within its police power, may take action."

EMPHASIS: One of the questions raised in this case was the legislature's authority to write quarantine laws. The court in reviewing the quarantine law determined that it had a reasonable and rational basis to write and pass such laws. But, it also stated "On the other hand, a person quarantined without reasonable grounds is entitled to relief by habeas corpus." While rarely used, public health officials do have the right to institute quarantine measures.

Responsibility to the Profession

In addition to the responsibilities that you have to your patients and the public, you will also have certain responsibilities to your profession as well. Part of these professional responsibilities are outlined in your profession's Standards of Care and Code of Ethics. No matter which healthcare profession you enter, part of your professional responsibilities will be to maintain the integrity of the profession. This requirement not only applies to you and how you conduct yourself, but to other members of the healthcare profession as well. While there are many aspects to this professional integrity requirement, the most serious are the illegal and/or unethical behavior of other healthcare professionals.

Impaired Professionals

One of the challenges that we face working in the healthcare environment is how we personally deal with the tragic issues that we face on an almost daily basis. The pain and suffering of patients, exposure to death and dying, and some of the horrors that our patients go through can take their toll on a healthcare provider. Unfortunately, there are times when some healthcare workers resort to taking drugs or consuming alcohol in order to deal with those challenges. While we have little control over what healthcare workers do in their off-duty hours, if the effects of using drugs and alcohol affect a person's ability to perform their job, we have a professional and legal responsibility, to our patients and our profession, to report those individuals. We cannot allow impaired healthcare workers to jeopardize the care that is provided to patients or risk the safety of the workplace.

Controlled Substances

The abuse of drugs is not limited to those considered illegal, such as cocaine and heroin. Prescription drugs can also be abused, even though they may have been prescribed by a healthcare provider. Because some medications have the potential for chemical dependency, the federal government through the Food and Drug Administration (FDA) and the Drug Enforcement Agency (DEA) controls their use. The Controlled Substance Act regulates the manufacturing, importing, possession, use, and distribution of substances that are classified into one of five categories, known as schedules.

Court Case

Crabtree v. Dodd

No. 01A01-9807-CH-00370 (Tenn.App. 08/17/1999)
Tennessee Court of Appeals

FACTS: The Tennessee Medical Association has an Impaired Physician Program overseen by the Impaired Physicians Peer Review Committee. Dr. John Crabtree was a general surgeon licensed in the state of Tennessee. In addition to his surgical duties, Dr. Crabtree was also an original shareholder in State Volunteer Mutual Insurance Company that offered malpractice insurance for healthcare providers.

Within a six-month period, Dr. Crabtree was arrested twice; once for public drunkenness and another for driving under the influence. Cookeville General Hospital, where Dr. Crabtree had staff privileges, sent a request to the Impaired Physicians Program asking them to evaluate Dr. Crabtree for alcohol impairment. Because he believed that he was already receiving appropriate and adequate treatment, Dr. Crabtree refused to participate in the program.

The medical director for the Impaired Physicians Program, Dr. Dodd, was so angry with Dr. Crabtree's refusal to participate in the impairment program, "Dr. Dodd threatened Dr. Crabtree with the loss of his malpractice insurance and his medical license if he refused to participate."

A few months later, Dr. Crabtree was arrested again for driving under the influence. Cookeville General Hospital notified Dr. Crabtree that they were taking formal action against him. In addition, State Volunteer Mutual Insurance Company informed Dr. Crabtree that they were reviewing his insurability for malpractice insurance.

After Dr. Crabtree completed a rehabilitation program, an extensive after-care contract was developed that outlined the requirements and contingencies to which Dr. Crabtree had to adhere. This after-care contract was part of the Impaired Physician Program and required by Cookeville General Hospital as a condition for re-applying for staff privileges. After conferring with his attorney, Dr. Crabtree decided not to sign the after-care contract. A few months later, State Volunteer Mutual Insurance Company sent a letter to Dr. Crabtree notifying him that his malpractice insurance had been terminated. Dr. Crabtree filed suit against Dr. Dodd, medical director of the Impaired Physician Program. "Dr. Crabtree contended that he and Dr. Dodd had a physician-patient relationship and that Dr. Dodd's divulgence of confidential matters known as a result of this relationship was unlawful, intentional, and malicious. Dr. Crabtree asserted that as a result of Dr. Dodd's malfeasance, State Volunteer terminated and refused to renew Dr. Crabtree's medical insurance." Dr. Dodd successfully petitioned the court to have the case dismissed. Dr. Crabtree filed an appeal.

ISSUE: Was the trial court correct in dismissing Dr. Crabtree's complaint? And, did Dr. Dodd breach the patient/doctor relationship through malice or bad faith?

RULE: "As incentive for the medical profession to undertake professional review, . . . peer review committees must be protected from liability for their good-faith efforts. To this end, peer review committees should be granted certain immunities relating to their actions undertaken as part of their responsibility to review, discipline, and educate the profession." The appellate court affirmed the trial court's decision.

EMPHASIS: This case demonstrates how important the issue of impaired professionals is. In addition, it demonstrates the responsibilities that we have as members of the profession to maintain the integrity of the profession by reporting impaired professionals.

- Schedule I controlled substances have a high potential for abuse and no medically approved use by the FDA. Examples include GHB (gamma-Hydroxybutyric acid), known as the date-rape drug; MDMA (3, 4-methylenedioxynmethgamphetamine), or Ecstasy; and marijuana. No prescriptions for Schedule I drugs may be written by any healthcare provider.

- Schedule II controlled substances have a high potential for abuse and a medically accepted use that has been approved by the FDA. Examples include Ritalin, Methadone, and morphine. Prescriptions for Schedule II drugs may only be written by healthcare providers who have obtained a DEA number.

- Schedule III controlled substances have a potential for abuse, but not as high as Schedule I and II drugs. They also have a medically accepted use approved by the FDA. Examples include anabolic steroids, ketamine, and hydrocodone. Prescriptions for Schedule III drugs may only be written by healthcare providers who have obtained a DEA number.

- Schedule IV Controlled Substances have a low potential for abuse and an accepted medical use. Examples include Valium, Phenobarbital, and Lomotil. Prescriptions for Schedule IV drugs may be written by any licensed healthcare provider authorized to write prescription by their state. (Prescribing Schedule IV drugs does not require a DEA number.)

- Schedule V Controlled Substances have a medically approved use, but have a low potential for abuse and limited physical and psychological dependence. Examples include codeine, Lyrica, and Pyrovalerone. Prescriptions for Schedule V drugs may be written by any licensed healthcare provider authorized to write prescriptions by their state.

Personal Responsibility

In addition to the professional responsibilities that you have to the entire profession, you also have a professional responsibility to yourself. While you may be hoping that you will be done with all of the studying, training, and education when you graduate from your program, that is not the case. In fact, when you graduate, your education and training has only just begun. When you start working, you will be constantly learning new things. New medical procedures will be developed, new technology invented, surgical and medical procedures may change, and yes, even the law may be amended or changed. Because of all of the changes that occur within society, medicine, science, and the law, you have a responsibility to keep current on the latest information that relates to your profession and how you practice medicine.

Even though staying current is a professional responsibility, and something that you should do on your own, most states have a continuing education requirement for credentialed healthcare professionals. In order to renew your license or certification, you may be required to complete Continuing Education Units (CEU) when you apply for renewal. To find out what your requirements are, check with your state's medical board.

> **Concept Connection**
> **Scheduled Drugs and Medical Marijuana**
> According to federal law, no healthcare provider can write prescriptions for Schedule I drugs, as they have no FDA *approved* medical use. However, many states have passed medical marijuana laws, despite the fact that the federal government classifies marijuana as a Schedule I drug. What the future holds for medical marijuana laws is unclear, as certain legal and ethical issues have yet to be resolved.

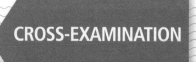

Make FALSE statements TRUE.

Rewrite the false statements below by replacing the bolded, italicized, and underlined word(s) to make it a true statement.

1. Privileged communication stems from the existence of ***professional responsibilities***.

   _____

2. A ***coroner*** performs autopsies to determine the manner and cause of death.

   _____

3. An endemic disease that increases in frequency is known as a ***pandemic***.

   _____

4. The ***Centers for Disease Control and Prevention***, a part of the United Nations, is the global public health agency.

   _____

5. With a special DEA number, prescriptions can be written for ***Schedule I*** drugs.

   _____

Circle Exercise

Circle the correct word from the choices given.

1. Vital statistic laws are an example of (**law of populations, disease and injury prevention, police power**) public health laws.

2. Diseases that exist in small amounts of a population are called (**endemic, epidemic, pandemic**) diseases.

3. Under the (**law of populations, disease and injury prevention, police power**) public health laws have the right to quarantine individuals.

4. Reportable injuries are made to (**public health officials, law enforcement agencies, professional organizations**).

5. The failure to report the suspicion of abuse can result in a healthcare worker being charged with (**felony, misdemeanor, civil penalties**).

Matching

Match the numbered term to its lettered definition.

1. _____ endemic

2. _____ epidemic

3. _____ epidemiology

4. _____ isolation

5. _____ medical examiner

6. _____ pandemic

7. _____ privileged communication

8. _____ quarantine

9. _____ vital statistics

A. a disease that is always present, to some degree, in a population or location.

B. a medical professional whose responsibility is to determine the cause of death and gather forensic evidence.

C. imposed isolation, most often used to contain individuals with highly contagious and/or deadly diseases.

D. statements made in private, during the existence of certain relationships, that cannot be used as evidence in civil or criminal trials.

E. the information gathered by governmental agencies related to births, marriages, divorces, and death that occur in a population.

F. the measures taken to prevent the spread of disease, either from patient to patient or from patient to healthcare worker.

G. the occurrence of disease in greater numbers than expected, or the development of disease in a shorter than normal time-frame.

H. the occurrence of disease in many different populations or geographical locations.

I. the study of the characteristics, determination, frequency, and distribution of a disease.

Deliberations: Critical Thinking Questions

Question 1: The main vital statistics that public health officials use are information related to births and deaths. In addition, public health officials gather information on the number of divorces. Why would this information be beneficial to public health officials? Can you think of any other vital statistic information that might be relevant to public health? Explain why.

Question 2: Some states only provide protection to doctor and patient communication. Do you think that this protection should include any healthcare profession? Explain your answer.

Question 3: A woman who is six months pregnant comes into the emergency room following a fall down the steps at her home. During the initial examination, a strong odor of alcohol is detected and a lab test verifies that she is legally intoxicated. Because the patient is pregnant and intoxicated, is that a form of child abuse? Should you report this as child abuse, as part of the mandatory reporting requirements?

Question 4: Most people are aware that healthcare professionals face mandatory reporting requirements. While the purpose for mandatory reporting is to identify and stop abuse and to provide assistance, can these type of laws also be a hindrance? For example, if a parent physically abuses a child, and knows if they take the child to the ER that they are going to be reported, what are the chances that the parent will seek medical help for their child? What suggestions do you have to help combat this problem?

Question 5: At a party, you notice that a nurse you work with is on the back porch smoking marijuana. Even though she is not impaired when she shows up to work the next day, do you have a responsibility to report her even though it occurred off duty?

Closing Arguments: Case Analysis

You just started working in Dr. Jones's office as a medical assistant. One of the patients today is a Registered Nurse who works in the Pediatric Unit of the local hospital. After the doctor's examination, he writes an order for some lab work. Because he wants to receive the results before he sends the patient home, he asks you to walk the sample over to the laboratory. You pick up the blood and urine samples and double-check the order to make sure that they match. As you are looking at the laboratory order, you notice that it is a request for a benzoylecgonine level, used to detect the presence of cocaine metabolites.

Question 1: You are concerned that the patient, a Registered Nurse, is taking cocaine. Do you have the right to question the doctor about the patient taking cocaine? Can the doctor tell you? Can you look in the patient's medical records to find out?

Question 2: Even if the Registered Nurse admitted to the doctor that she utilized cocaine, that discussion occurred during a privileged communication. But does that stop the doctor from reporting the nurse for taking an illegal substance? Regardless of your answer, even if the doctor cannot report, are you allowed to notify the hospital that the nurse is taking illegal substances?

Question 3: What if the doctor brings you a package of white powder, which he says is cocaine that a patient gave him, and asks you to dispose of it? How would you do so? Is this something that you should call the police about?

The Briefcase

This section repeats the objectives from the beginning of the chapter and provides a summary of the most important concepts for each objective. Use this section as a quick review and to check your understanding of the chapter key points.

Objective 1: Define what protected relationships are and explain why they exist.
- Special relationships that the law recognizes.
- Confidential and private communications is an important component to the relationship.

Objective 2: Explain why there is an exception to privacy rules and privileged communication.
- The public health
- Harm or danger to others.

Objective 3: Categorize all public laws into one of three categories.
- Law of Populations
- Disease and Injury Prevention
- Police Powers

Objective 4: Give an example of what vital statistics are and how they are used by public health officials.
- Certificate of Births: Track the number of live births, miscarriages, and stillborn deliveries.
- Certificate of Death: Track the number, cause, and manner of death.

Objective 5: Compare and contrast endemic, epidemic, and pandemic.
- endemic: diseases that always exist in small numbers.
- epidemic: diseases that occur in greater numbers than expected.
- pandemic: diseases that affect multiple populations.

Objective 6: List what diseases and injuries a healthcare professional may be required to report.

- Diseases: See pgs. 119–120.
- Injuries: Abuse, Crime

Objective 7: Provide examples of why the Medical Waste Tracking Act was enacted and what it accomplished.

- Illegal dumpling of medical waste represented a health risk to the public.
- Provides definitions for what medical waste is.
- Determines how waste should be managed, transported, and disposed of.
- Provides enforcement provisions.

Objective 8: Determine the differences between the different schedules of drugs classified by the FDA.

- Schedule I: cannot be prescribed.
- Schedule II: high potential for abuse, has a medically accepted use approved by the FDA. Requires a DEA number to prescribe.

- Schedule III: high potential for abuse, but not as high as Schedule II. Also has a medically accepted use approved by the FDA. Requires a DEA number to prescribe.
- Schedule IV: low potential for abuse and an accepted medical use. Anyone authorized to write prescriptions can prescribe.
- Schedule V: medically approved use, low potential for abuse, limited physical and psychological dependence. Anyone authorized to write prescriptions can prescribe.

Objective 9: Explain what responsibilities you have as a member of a healthcare profession to others in the profession.

- Reporting illegal and unethical behavior.
- Substance Abuse
- Impaired Professionals

Maximize Your Success with the Companion Website

The Companion Website to this textbook contains materials that can help you better understand the concepts presented in this chapter. Go to www.myhealthprofessionskit.com to access:

- Learning Tools, Games, and more
- Sample Quizzes
- Related Links
- Understanding Your State

PEARSON
myhealthprofessionskit™

PART 2 MEDICAL ETHICS

Why is the study of ethics included with the study of law? Aren't they two separate things?

The second half of this text discusses ethics and how ethics relates to healthcare and medicine.

Yes, the law and ethics are two separate topics. But the study of law includes ethics and the study of ethics includes the law. Both the study of law and ethics is an important part of your career. And while ethics can be more fun to study than the law, there is an important reason the law is discussed first. Part of making an ethical decision includes taking into consideration all of the alternatives. For example, is your ethical decision legal; or what are the legal consequences of your ethical decision? Without a full understanding of what the law is and how it is used, you cannot make sound ethical decisions.

But now that we have discussed the law, we can use what we have learned to understand if the ethical decisions we make are legal. One of the features of this half of the text is called the "Law of Ethics," which identifies the legal answers to some of the ethical dilemmas we will discuss. The law is concerned with "doing what is right," while ethics is concerned with "doing the right thing." As we will see throughout this part of the text, not all legal decisions are ethical, and not all ethical decisions are legal.

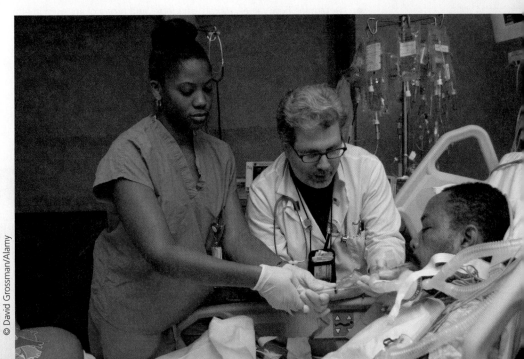

© David Grossman/Alamy

8

Introduction to Ethics

As a healthcare professional, you will be faced with making some difficult ethical decisions. Unlike the law, where others will make the decisions for you (lawyers, judges, jury, etc.); with ethics you will be asked to be the decision maker. One of the reasons ethical decisions are difficult to make is because you will struggle with determining, to whom is it good? Is it for the benefit of yourself, your patient, the greatest number of people, or something else entirely? In this chapter, we will discuss what ethics are and the principles involved with ethics.

MEASURE YOUR PROGRESS: LEARNING OBJECTIVES

After studying this chapter, you will be able to:

- Define what ethics is.

- Compare and contrast values and morals.

- List the four approaches that are used to ascertain morals.

- Differentiate the concepts of etiquette and protocol.

- List the three different types of etiquette and protocol.

- Describe what makes beliefs different from other concepts.

- Define the difference between dilemmas and conflicts.

- Identify a conflict or dilemma, if provided with a scenario.

- Determine how values, morals, etiquette, and protocol are used in ethics.

KEY TERMS

beliefs

conflict

dilemma

ethics

etiquette

morals

protocol

values

virtue

cui bono { To whom is it good?

PROFESSIONAL HIGHLIGHT

Seiko is a manager at the local hospital, and serves as the president of the hospital's ethics committee. The ethics committee meets regularly to discuss ethical situations that have arisen, and to decide a course of action. Without a thorough understanding of what ethics is, Seiko would be unable to advise fellow employees about how to resolve ethical dilemmas.

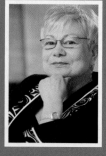

StockLite/Shutterstock

Ethics is sometimes defined simply as moral philosophy. But that simple definition does not help much when trying to understand what **ethics** is.

The formal definition does not necessarily help us either, without a full understanding of the concepts included in the definition. Because the definition of the word *ethics* includes the concepts of values, morals, conducts, and beliefs, we need to explain each one of those to understand how they help to determine the definition of ethics.

> **What is ethics exactly, and where did it come from?**

Values

What a person **values** can be hard to identify because it is different for everyone.

The concept of value addresses the question "*Does it matter; and if so how much?*" If it is something that matters to you, then it is of value to you. If is something that is important to you, then it is something that you value. But that only addresses one part of the question—*does it matter?* To determine the other part of the questions, *and if so how much?*, try to think of value as money.

On a shopping trip to the electronic store, you discover that two items are on sale for the same price: 1) a DVD featuring the director's cut of the latest award-winning foreign language film; and 2) a CD collection of the top 100 Hip Hop songs of the past decade. Which item you choose to purchase, if any, indicates how much that item is worth to you. Not everyone will value the same thing or place the same amount of value on the same things.

ethics: values that are used to determine moral conduct or beliefs

values: the measurement of worth or importance

Morals

The concept of values is not the only concept that people can disagree on. In addition to values, some may have differing thoughts about what is right and wrong. The concept of **morals** addresses the question "*What is right and what is wrong?*"

We obtain our morals from the same environmental factors that contribute to the development of our values (see Fig. 8-1). Culture, ethnicity, class structure, and social standing all play a role in how our values and morals are shaped. There are four different principles of morals: moral absolutism, moral universalism, moral nihilism, and moral relativism.

morals: the determination of right and wrong

Fig. 8-1. Many of the stories told in Aesop's Fables contained moral lessons that children could learn from.

Moral Absolutism

With moral absolutism, things are viewed in absolutes. Something that is wrong is always wrong, and something that is right is always right. If something was wrong only some of the time, moral absolutists would argue, demonstrates the flaw that it was wrong to begin with (see Fig. 8-2). For example, moral absolutists might believe that *all* killing is wrong—regardless of the circumstances: killing during war is wrong, the use of the death penalty is wrong, and euthanasia is wrong.

Moral Universalism

Moral universalism takes a universal approach to right and wrong. Rights and wrongs apply equally to

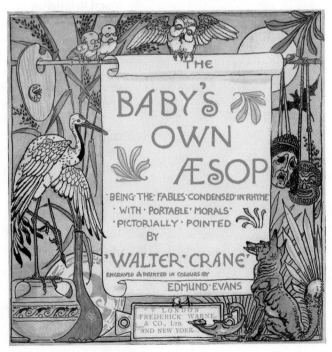

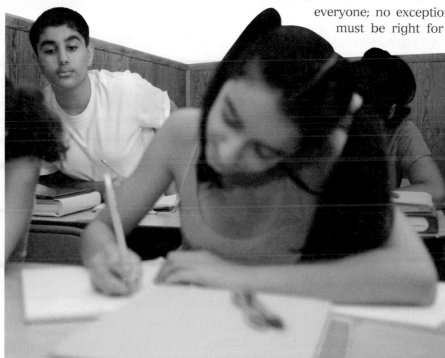

GG Pro Photo / Shutterstock

Fig. 8-2. Cheating is usually considered wrong under any circumstances. Can you think of a time when cheating is OK?

everyone; no exceptions are made. What is right for one must be right for everyone, and in contrast what is wrong for one person has to be wrong for everyone.

Moral universalism is different from moral absolutism in that the focus is on the person, not the situation. To compare, let us look at the debate concerning medical marijuana. A moral universalism argument would be: if marijuana is legal for some, then it has to be legal for everyone. Absolutism would argue that marijuana is an illegal drug and is wrong for everyone.

Moral Nihilism

The word *nihilism* comes from the *Latin* word *nihil* which means "nothing." But do not get confused by thinking that nihilists believe that nothing is right or wrong. Instead, nihilists believe that we as human beings are unable to make a determination of what is right and wrong. In order to make an accurate determination of what is right and wrong, a person needs to completely remove all emotion and beliefs from his or her thought processes. And, because of our human nature, we are unable to completely remove emotion and beliefs, leading nihilists to believe that we are unable to make a determination of what is right and wrong. A common statement made by someone who adheres to moral nihilism is *"You do not have the right to make that decision."*

Moral Relativism

Moral relativism is based on the idea that someone else cannot determine what is right and wrong for another individual. Only individuals can decide what is right and wrong for themselves. Determining what is right and wrong, moral relativists believe, is based on the unique experiences a person has had and the situations that they have faced. Only people who have had the same experiences or faced the same situations can determine whether something is right or wrong. When you take into consideration such things as age, gender, class, culture, ethnicity, and religion, every individual is unique and therefore no one else will ever have the same experiences as another person. Moral relativists believe that those experiences and viewpoints are *relative* to that person only, and therefore others are unable to pass judgment on what is right or wrong for another person. Moral relativism is sometimes used when discussing the issue of abortion.

Virtue

The four moral principles that we discussed are not static; meaning that a person will not subscribe to only one principal for all moral arguments. For instance, a person may subscribe to moral universalism for one moral issue and use moral relativism for another moral issue. Which moral principle a person chooses is a demonstration of their **virtue**.

virtue: the pursuit of moral excellence

For the most part, we all try to do the right thing. And while people may disagree about what is right and wrong, the decision-making process for either side is the same, striving for virtue. We all, for the most part, want to make the right decision. And just as morals play a role in how our virtue is developed, so too do culture, ethnicity, class structure, and social standing.

Two additional contributing factors in developing our morals, values, and virtue are the concepts of etiquette and protocol.

Sidebar

Ever wondered which fork to use? Initially, the number of utensils at a place setting demonstrated to a guest the number of courses that were going to be served. (Three forks and three spoons meant six courses; the knife was not counted.) Starting on the outside working in, courses are served in a particular order, so that a person would always know which utensil to use.

Etiquette

The use of **etiquette** was initially designed as set of rules that people could follow if they found themselves in unfamiliar surroundings.

etiquette: the manner of behavior, determined by custom, that is used in social, official, or professional interactions

While the precise origins of etiquette are unknown, some of the early forms of etiquette were developed by Louis XIV (king of France from 1643 to 1715). Louis XIV provided codes for the people he trusted, such as a gesture or specific words. A person performing the right movement, such as a curtsey, or who knew the password to gain entrance to the royal premises, was not considered to be a threat to the king. Etiquette has since evolved and today is more commonly referred to as manners, such as saying please and thank you, utilizing proper table manners, or excusing yourself after you burp. There are three different settings that will determine the type of behavior you are expected to have: social etiquette, official etiquette, and professional etiquette.

Social Etiquette

Social etiquette determines the behavior that is utilized when we interact with society. For example, if we are walking down the street, we do not push other people out of our way. Instead, we either walk around them or say excuse me, allowing them to step to the side. The purpose of social etiquette is to allow members of society to interact with each comfortably, and with certain boundaries. By conforming to social etiquette, everyone will know how to act toward others, and how we can expect others to act toward us.

Official Etiquette

Official etiquette determines the behavior that we are expected to utilize when we interact with officials, such as law enforcement, politicians, and dignitaries. For example, when a judge enters a courtroom, you will hear the court office call out *"All Rise!,"* in response to which everyone in the courtroom is expected to stand up. Standing when the judge enters the room is done to demonstrate the respect that you are giving to the judge and the judicial proceedings.

Professional Etiquette

Professional etiquette dictates the behavior that is used when we interact with people in a professional setting. For example, as healthcare practitioners, when you walk into a patient's room, which do you think would be more acceptable:, *"Hi, Sweety. I'm your therapist today"* or *"Hello, Mrs. Smith. I am the therapist that was assigned to take care of you today"*?

Professional etiquette determines how we are expected to act in a professional capacity. This allows people who interact with us in a professional capacity to know what to expect as well.

Protocol

While etiquette is determined by custom, **protocol**, is determined by an authority figure.

protocol: the manner of behavior, determined by authority, that is used in social, official, or professional interactions

Note: the only difference between the definition for etiquette and that for protocol is the replacement of the word *custom* for *authority*. Under protocol, an authority figure has determined the conduct that is required in order to achieve a certain result. To explain, we can look at the three different types of protocol: social protocol, official protocol, and professional protocol.

Social Protocols

Social protocols are the rules that have been written by an authority figure that we are expected to follow when in social situations. The best example of a social protocol is the law. Laws are written by an authority figure—the legislature—that we are required to follow when we interact with other members of society. If we do not follow these social protocols, we face the consequences. Those consequences can include being removed from society (for violating criminal laws) or being reprimanded by the courts (in the form of adjudication of a civil lawsuit).

Official Protocols

Official protocols are also rules written by an authority figure. They differ from laws because they do not address interaction with and between society's members. Instead, official protocols are the instructions that we need to follow in order to obtain a specified result. For example, if a person wants to obtain public assistance, there is a process that he or she must follow. That process may include filling out an application and demonstrating financial need. Official protocols are written, so that everyone knows what steps they are required to follow so that they can achieve that specific goal.

Professional Protocols

Professional protocols are the rules that you are required to follow when operating in a professional capacity. The rules or protocols you are required to follow are outlined in your profession's Code of Ethics. Each profession

---

Court Case

Edmund G. Brown Jr., Governor of California, et al., Appellants v. Marciano Plata et al.

Supreme Court of the United States No. 09-1233 (October Term, 2010) Argued November 30, 2010. Decision May 23, 2011

FACTS: In this case, the Supreme Court was asked to address "serious constitutional violations in California's prison system" that had remained uncorrected by the state of California. This case is the combination of two separate class actions in Federal District Courts. (Coleman v. Brown, addressing prisoners with serious mental disorders; and Plata v. Brown, addressing prisoners who have serious medical conditions.) This appeal asks the Supreme Court to remedy two ongoing violations of the Cruel and Unusual Punishments Clause of the Constitution, by the state of California, Edmund Brown governor.

The prisons in California are over-crowded, housing almost double the number of occupants the prisons were designed to hold. Due in part to over-crowding and staffing shortages, prisoners with serious medical conditions were not receiving adequate medical care. "[I]t is an uncontested fact that, on average, an inmate in one of California's prisons needlessly dies every six to seven days due to constitutional deficiencies in the [California prisons'] medical delivery system."

Pursuant to the Prison Litigation Reform Act of 1995 (PLRA); the plaintiffs Coleman and Plata asked the court to order the state of California to rectify the issue of inadequate medical care and over-crowding. The trial court agreed with the plaintiff's arguments, and ordered that the state of California either release an estimated 37,000–46,000 prisoners or build additional facilities. (But because of financial difficulties encountered by the state of California, it was unlikely that they would be able to build additional facilities.) The state of California, expressing concerns about public safety, appealed the decision.

ISSUE: Is prison over-crowding contributing to inadequate healthcare, a violation of a prisoner's constitutional rights?

RULE: "The court below did not err in concluding that over-crowding in California prisons was the 'primary' cause of the continuing violations of prisoners' constitutional rights to adequate health care."

EMPHASIS: While the actual issue in this case was the authority of a three-judge panel to order that California reduce the number of prisoners in correctional facilities, it is the implications of the decision that are more on point with our current discussion. The court was faced with outcomes, neither of which are desirable; 1) ordering the release of prisoners, or 2) allowing prisoners to suffer, and even die, as a result of inadequate medical care.

has at least one professional organization that will publish a Code of Ethics. These codes will inform you of the required protocols that need to be followed when operating in a professional capacity. The same professional organization that publishes the Code of Ethics is likely to be the same organization that will publish your profession's Standard of Care.

Beliefs

Even though we are provided with guidelines for how to conduct ourselves, there are times when we cannot readily explain why we value something over another, or why we believe something to be right or wrong. For some of those times, we rely on our **beliefs**.

In science, we utilize facts to determine what we know to be true. Under the law, we use facts, evidence, and testimony to determine what is true in a court of law. But with beliefs, we base truth on emotion or feelings instead of tangible proof. Beliefs are most commonly associated with religion, where we accept things as being true, even though we may not have tangible evidence to support it.

beliefs: what a person holds to be true, or rules that are followed that are not based on tangible proof

Revisiting Ethics

Now that we have thoroughly described the concepts used to define ethics, take another look at the definition of ethics.

ethics: values that are used to determine moral conduct or beliefs.

Ethics is how we determine what is important to us (values), and how we use what is important to us (values) to determine what is right and wrong (morals). Part of how we determine what is right and wrong (morals), is influenced by how we interact with others (conduct—etiquette and protocol), which may not necessarily be based on tangible proof (beliefs).

During your healthcare career, you will be faced with numerous dilemmas (see Fig. 8-3). As part of your professional duties, you may be asked to resolve those dilemmas or to avoid conflicts if they arise. Now that we have a more precise understanding of what ethics is, we can look at the different situations that occur regarding ethics; conflicts and dilemmas.

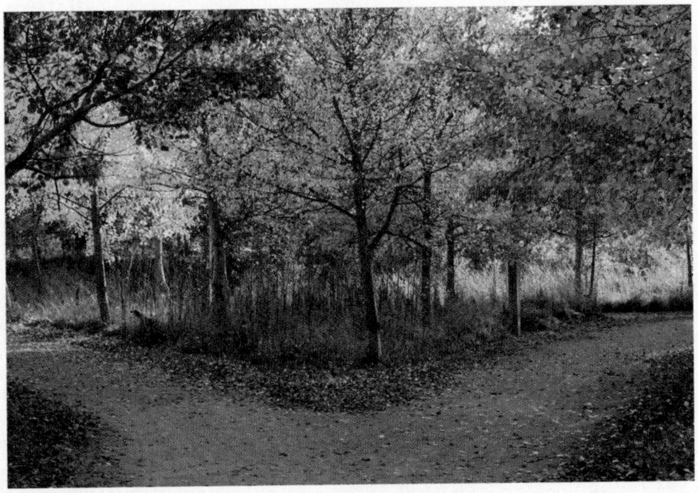

Fig. 8-3. Ethical decisions are hard to make because there is often more than one right answer or neither answer is desirable. The difficulty lies in making a decision.

costall/Shutterstock

Conflicts

Many times, the words **conflict** and dilemmas are used interchangeably, when they are really different things.

We can tell the difference between conflicts and dilemmas by looking at the problem itself. If the reason we are having a problem is because of how the problem was *created*, that problem is a conflict. Conflicts occur when there are competing interests, which create incompatibility between two different things. For example, a doctor being asked to treat his or her own family has a conflict. The conflict occurs between caring for a loved one and how that may interfere with the doctor's medical judgment. Conflicts create the problem; dilemmas, on the other hand, occur after the problem has been created.

conflict: when opposing forces of incompatibility exist at the same time or place

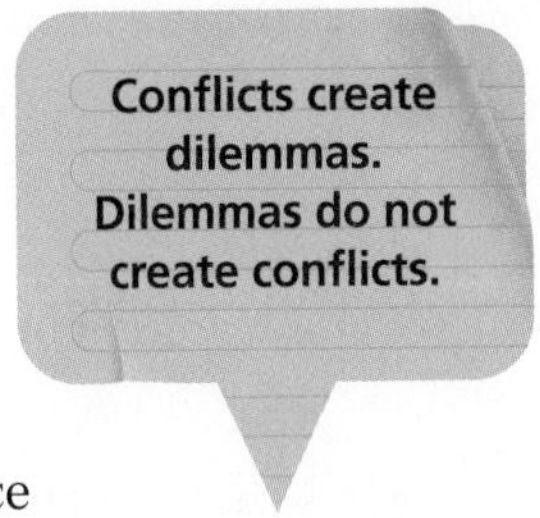

> **Conflicts create dilemmas. Dilemmas do not create conflicts.**

teacept/Shutterstock

Dilemmas

When taking exams, most students prefer multiple choice questions over fill-in-the-blank questions. Part of the reason is that with multiple choice

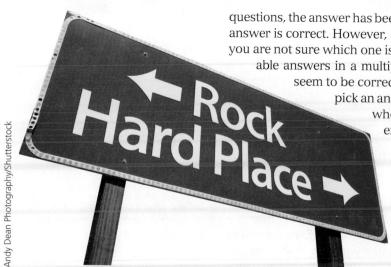

Andy Dean Photography/Shutterstock

questions, the answer has been provided for you; you just have to choose which answer is correct. However, sometimes after looking at the available answers, you are not sure which one is correct. Or, sometimes after reviewing the available answers in a multiple choice question, none of the answer choices seem to be correct. But, in order to do well on the test, you have to pick an answer. Being faced with choosing a correct answer, when you are unsure which one is correct, is a perfect example of a **dilemma**.

To face a dilemma is commonly referred to as being stuck between a rock and a hard place. No matter which way you turn, you are going to face difficulty. But despite this difficulty, you still have to make a decision. When dilemmas exist, part of the reason the decisions are difficult is because of competing concepts. Your concept of what is right and wrong might be conflicting with what you are supposed to do.

dilemma: a problem for which all outcomes are either equal or all outcomes are undesirable

Emotions

Emotions play a large role in ethics, and how we approach and decide conflicts and dilemmas. Understanding what the different emotions are, may help us understand not only why we make the decisions that we do, but why other people might make decisions that they do, especially if they are opposite of ours.

Psychologist Robert Plutchik believes that there are eight basic emotions: anger, anticipation, disgust, fear, joy, sadness, surprise, and trust (see Fig. 8-4).

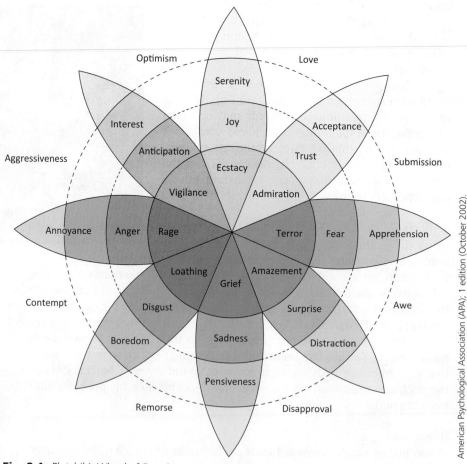

Fig. 8-4. Plutchik's Wheel of Emotion.

American Psychological Association (APA); 1 edition (October 2002).

And, with each of the basic emotions, a polar opposite emotion: anger/fear, disgust/trust, surprise/anticipation, and joy/sadness. Any of these basic emotions can be expressed in different ranges of intensity. For example, fear can be expressed simply as apprehension; or on the other extreme, as sheer terror. In addition to the eight basic emotions, there are eight additional emotions that exist when basic emotions are combined. For example, the emotion of love results from combining the basic emotions of joy and trust.

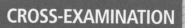
Make FALSE statements TRUE.

Rewrite the false statements below by replacing the bolded, italicized, and underlined word(s) to make it a true statement.

1. There are two principles underlying the understanding of **_etiquette_**, values and morals.

   _____

2. There are four different approaches to **_values_**: absolutism, nihilism, relativism, and universalism.

   _____

3. Both etiquette and **_ethics_** are used in the different situations we encounter in life: social, official, and professional.

   _____

4. If a problem exists because of how it was created, that problem is a **_dilemma_**.

   _____

5. Something that is not based on tangible evidence is known as **_morals_**.

   _____

Circle Exercise

Circle the correct word from the choices given.

1. In some dictionaries and text ethics is defined simply as (**consequential**, **moral**, **reasoning**) philosophy.

2. Protocol is a manner of behavior determined by (**authority**, **custom**, **law**).

3. The measurement of worth or importance is known as (**morals**, **protocol**, **values**) ethics.

4. The purpose of (**official etiquette**, **professional etiquette**, **social etiquette**) is to allow members of society to interact with each comfortably, and with certain boundaries.

5. The word virtue is closely associated with the concept of (**etiquette**, **morals**, **values**).

Matching

Match the numbered term to its lettered definition.

1. _____ beliefs
2. _____ conflict
3. _____ dilemma
4. _____ ethics
5. _____ etiquette
6. _____ morals
7. _____ protocol
8. _____ values
9. _____ virtue

A. a problem for which all outcomes are either equal or all outcomes are undesirable.

B. the determination of right and wrong.

C. the manner of behavior, determined by authority, that is used in social, official, or professional interactions.

D. the manner of behavior, determined by custom, that is used in social, official, or professional interactions.

E. the measurement of worth or importance.

F. the pursuit of moral excellence.

G. values that are used to determine moral conduct or beliefs.

H. what a person holds to be true, or rules that are followed that are not based on tangible proof.

I. when opposing forces of incompatibility exist at the same time or place.

Deliberations: Critical Thinking Questions

Question 1: The principle of moral nihilism is that humans cannot remove their basic emotions to make a determination of right and wrong. Do agree or disagree with this, explain why? If we adhere to premise of nihilism, how is right and wrong determined?

Question 2: Every business, including healthcare, has a list of policies and procedures that must be followed. Are policies and procedures an example of social protocols or professional protocols? Explain your answer.

Question 3: Think of the last time you were involved in a situation that you thought was unfair. Try to explain what the other person's viewpoints were, and why they might have that viewpoint.

Question 4: Initially the rules of etiquette were developed to make someone comfortable in uncomfortable surroundings. Unfortunately, however, some of the rules of etiquette are misused today—not to make a person feel comfortable in unfamiliar surroundings, but to look down on people who do not know the rules. Why do you think that is?

Question 5: There is an unwritten rule in healthcare, that healthcare providers should not provide medical care to family members. Why do you think that rule exists? What about close friends? Should the same rule and reasoning apply?

Closing Arguments: Case Analysis

A large part of a cardiologist's practice involves inserting pacemakers. Dr. Jones is a cardiologist who only uses pacemakers manufactured by the Acme Company. None of the other cardiologist who work at the hospital utilize Acme's pacemaker. All of the other physicians decide which pacemaker to use depending on the patient's medical condition, and which equipment will best serve their needs.

Dr. Jones is not only a cardiologist, but is a major stockholder in the Acme Company, serving on the board of trustees. In addition, he consistently lectures around the country for the company about the benefits of Acme's products, receiving a large stipend every year.

Question 1: Does Dr. Jones have conflict or a dilemma? Explain your answer.

Question 2: As the president of the medical board, you have been asked to address the issue regarding Dr. Jones' use of Acme pacemakers. Describe what ethical principles might be involved (values, morals, etiquette, and protocol) and how those principles might influence what you decide to do.

Question 3: Does Dr. Jones have the right to decide which pacemaker should be used on a patient, or is that something that should be dictated by the patient's individual needs? Explain your answer.

The Briefcase

This section repeats the objectives from the beginning of the chapter and provides a summary of the most important concepts for each objective. Use this section as a quick review and to check your understanding of the chapter key points.

Objective 1: Define what ethics is.
- System of principles and conduct
- Addresses values
  - individual
  - group
  - society
- Addresses morals
  - individual
  - group
  - society

- Etiquette— behavior by custom
- Protocol— behavior by authority
- Beliefs

Objective 2: Compare and contrast values and morals
- Values
  - worth
  - importance
- Morals
  - right
  - wrong
- Similarities
  - concepts used to that define what choices we make
  - used to understand how ethical decisions are reached

Objective 3: List the four approaches that are used to ascertain morals.

- Moral absolutism
- Moral nihilism
- Moral relativism
- Moral universalism

Objective 4: Differentiate the concepts of etiquette and protocol.

- Similarities
  - both are manners of behavior
- Differences
  - etiquette is based on custom
  - protocol is based on authority

Objective 5: List the three different types of etiquette and protocol.

- Both are used in different aspects that we face in life:
  - social etiquette and social protocol
  - official etiquette and official protocol
  - professional etiquette and professional protocol

Objective 6: Describe what makes beliefs different from other concepts.

- Beliefs are accepted as truth
- Beliefs are not based on tangible evidence

Objective 7: Define the difference between dilemmas and conflicts.

- Conflicts occur because of creation of the problem.
- Dilemmas occur when resolution to a problem is required.

Objective 8: Identify a conflict or dilemma, if provided with a scenario.

Objective 9: Determine how values, morals, etiquette, and protocol are used in ethics.

- The words values, morals, etiquette, and protocol are included in the definition of ethics.
- The concepts of values, morals, etiquette, and protocol define what ethics is.

Maximize Your Success with the Companion Website

The Companion Website to this textbook contains materials that can help you better understand the concepts presented in this chapter. Go to www.myhealthprofessionskit.com to access:

- Sample Quizzes
- Web Links
- Games
- and more…

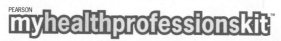

9

Ethical Decision-Making

Throughout your professional career, you will be faced with making choices every day. Sometimes, the choices that you make will be dictated by the patient's medical condition. But other times, which course of action you need to take will not be as clear cut. With ethics, there are typically two or more correct answers, making the decision-making process a little more difficult. In this chapter, we will discuss ethical decision-making, which asks you to consider whether it is correct or not.

MEASURE YOUR PROGRESS:

After studying this chapter, you will be able to:

- Explain the difference between the three different branches of ethics.

- List the nine different ethical principles used in ethical decision-making.

- Identify which ethical concepts: values, morals, conduct, or beliefs, are used for each of the nine ethical principles.

- Discuss the reasons the Potter Box is used to in ethical decision-making

- List the four steps that are used in the Potter Box.

- Describe the problems that each step of the Potter Box addresses.

- Given a scenario, work through the steps of the Potter Box to help you reach a decision.

- Explain why the Potter Box step Loyalties may affect ethical decision-making.

- Summarize why using the Potter Box will not give you an actual answer.

KEY TERMS

altruism

applied ethics

beneficence

consequentialism

deontology

egoism

meta-ethics

normative ethics

utilitarianism

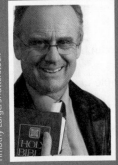

Timothy Large/Shutterstock

PROFESSIONAL HIGHLIGHT

Keith is the hospital chaplain for a large healthcare institution. He not only counsels patients and families during times of crisis, but also is available to hospital employees. As a chaplain, Keith is often consulted to provide insight and opinions about some of the complex ethical issues that arise in the healthcare environment. Keith calls on a combination of his skills, training, and expertise to assist in analyzing and deciding ethical issues. Without a thorough understanding of how ethical decisions are made, Keith would not be able to provide the insight he, and those in his position, are often asked for.

How you approach and decide an ethical issue is up to you. Unfortunately, there is no predetermined analysis that is going to get you to the right answer; because in ethics there are no correct answers. The decisions that you make, at the time you make it, with the information you have will be the correct decision. But that does not necessarily mean that it is the correct answer for everyone involved.

When you are faced with an ethical dilemma, you can only use the tools, resources, and knowledge that you have at the time the dilemma presents itself. But even though there are no predetermined answers for ethical dilemmas, there are some steps you can take to make sure that you are considering everything and weighing all of the available options.

But before we get to the actual ethical decision-making process, it is important to understand some of the ethical principles and theories that are used in the process.

Ethical Principles and Theories

Ethical principles are used every day, by every person, to make a variety of different decisions. Sometimes, we make ethical decisions automatically, without having to stop and think about them. Other situations cause us to pause, to consider the ramifications of our actions, or to decide which course of action to take. For example, if you are driving a car and come to a stop sign, you automatically stop your vehicle. While you have a choice *not to* stop, your concepts of right and wrong—and possibly the fear of getting a ticket or causing an accident—cause you to stop. But what if you come to a traffic light, and when the light turns green and the person in front of you does not move. Do you beep your horn to get their attention, do you lay on your horn and yell at them to move, or do you wait patiently for them to notice?

To better understand the different theories and principles that are used in ethics, we can start by examining the three branches of ethics: meta-ethics, normative ethics, and applied ethics.

meta-ethics: a subcategory of ethics that defines what ethics is and the contributing factors that define ethical principles

Meta-ethics

The process involved in trying to determine what ethics is, a branch of philosophy known as **meta-ethics**.

Meta-ethics is concerned with the foundations of defining *what* ethics is. Meta-ethics asks questions like: *What is good, what is bad, what is right, and what is wrong?* The answers that we strive for with meta-ethics attempt to determine the human nature of morals and values.

Normative Ethics

Normative ethics is concerned with understanding *how* a person makes a decision. There are nine different ethical theories that a person might use to determine *how* an ethical decision is made: altruism, beneficence, consequentialism, deontology, egoism, justice, least harm, respect for autonomy, and utilitarianism. At the end of a short discussion of these theories, Table 9-1 presents a comparison of the key elements.

TRINACRIA PHOTO/Shutterstock

normative ethics: a subcategory of ethics that defines how ethical decisions are made and the factors that contribute to ethical decision-making

altruism: concern for the welfare of others; an obligation to benefit others

Altruism

The word **altruism** is derived from the French word *altruisme* (*autrui*) meaning "other people."

The concept of altruism comes from the belief that other people are more important than the individual. To demonstrate that importance, a person must make a personal sacrifice that benefits others. Helping others, without personal sacrifice, altruists believe, does not demonstrate the importance of others over yourself. While there are different levels of personal sacrifice, an example of altruism is donating a kidney to a stranger.

Ethical concepts and altruism:

- Values: Values are the main ethical concept utilized in altruism. Altruistic viewpoints give value to others, rather than themselves. What is important to an altruistic person is other people's needs.
- Morals: Morals play a role in altruistic thought, that by helping others, they are doing what is right. Not helping others, by personal sacrifice, would be wrong because you are placing your needs above those of others.
- Conduct: The ethical principle of conduct is not addressed in altruism. While there are social etiquette or professional protocols that describe helping others, they do not do so by mandating personal sacrifice. (See *beneficence*.)
- Beliefs: The ethical concept of beliefs may be a factor in altruistic thinking. A person may believe that they have to sacrifice of themselves in order to truly give of others.

Beneficence

Like altruism, **beneficence** involves helping others, but in beneficence there is no individual sacrifice.

beneficence: an action that is used to help other people

The focus of beneficence is to recognize that others in society are in need of help and/or may not be as well off as you are. Beneficence demonstrates awareness of the inequality provided by social structures. An example of beneficence is the humanitarian organization Doctors Without Borders that provides medical care in underdeveloped countries. (A person who volunteers his or time and services to Doctors Without Borders—because of the personal sacrifice—is exhibiting altruism. The existence and function of the organization—providing medical care to the less fortunate—is an example of beneficence.)

Ethical concepts and beneficence:

- Values: Values are a part of beneficence because those that subscribe to beneficence think that it is important to help other people.
- Morals: Morals is the core ethical concept associated with beneficence. Helping other people, under beneficence, is the right thing to do. Not helping others would be wrong.
- Conduct: Conduct is a part of beneficence as it is customary (a type of protocol) to help others in need.
- Beliefs: The ethical principles of belief are not addressed in beneficence.

Consequentialism

With **consequentialism** a person considers the consequences before making a decision.

consequentialism: a decision-making process that uses the outcome to determine whether something is right or wrong

Consequentialism asks *"What is the end result?"* and uses that result to determine whether the action is warranted. If the end result is good, then the action to achieve that result must also be good. If the end result is bad, then the action to achieve that result must also be bad. For example, a consequentialist might argue that feeding a hungry child is a good result, even if it means stealing food from others. Consequentialism does not look at the act of stealing as right or wrong, but the result—the feeding of a hungry child—as the right thing to do.

Ethical concepts and consequentialism:

- Values: Because the focus of consequentialism is on the result, value is not attributed to consequentialism.
- Morals: Morals is the only ethical concept associated with consequentialism. The only way to determine what is right and wrong is by looking at the consequences.

- Conduct: There are no ethical principles of conduct associated with consequentialism.
- Beliefs: Beliefs are not a part of consequentialism.

Consequentialism reverses the normal process involved in applying ethical concepts. Arguments could certainly be made to support a consequentialism decision, but the use of those principles comes after the fact, not before. With consequentialism, ethical concepts are not used to reach a decision but used after a decision has been reached.

Deontology

deontology: the use of duty and rules to determine an outcome

The word **deontology** is derived from the word duty.

It is duty, or responsibility, that guides the determination for making decisions under deontology. Unlike consequentialism, deontology is concerned with the action and not the result. Performing your duty is always right and not performing your duty is always wrong, regardless of what the outcome might be. The rationalization is that through the creation of duty, good and bad have already been considered. If something were bad, then a duty would not exist. Military rules are an example of deontology thinking.

Ethical concepts and deontology:

- Values: Values are utilized as a rationalization because it is important to perform your duty and fulfill your responsibilities.
- Morals: Under deontology, what is right and wrong has already been determined, so morals are not factored into deontological thinking.
- Conduct: The ethical principle of conduct is the key concept utilized in deontological thinking. By following duty, deontology thinkers are applying the rules that society and authority figures have determined are important, whatever form that may be.
- Beliefs: Beliefs do not play a role in deontological thinking, because we are not asking people to accept something without tangible proof.

Egoism

egoism: the use of individual self-interest

While altruism and beneficence focus on others, the exact opposite is the ethical principle of **egoism**, which concentrates on the benefit of the person instead of others.

Instead of taking others into consideration others, with egoism the only thing that is considered is oneself. Only my best interest is important or what benefits me is used to make decisions. There is no regard to how things will affect other people, because they are not a factor in the equation. An example of egoism is a person who talks during a movie.

Ethical concepts and egoism:

- Values: Values is the key ethical concept utilized with egoism, in that the only thing of value is what is important to that person.
- Morals: Egoism defines morals, in that what is best for a person is right and what does not benefit the person is wrong.
  - Conduct: The ethical concept of conduct does not factor into egotistical thinking. Rules are disregarded if they go against what is best for the egoist.
  - Beliefs: Beliefs may play a role in rationalizing egotistical thinking but do not factor in what decision is made.

Justice

The word *fair* is often substituted for the word *justice*, and helps a person to determine what is right and wrong.

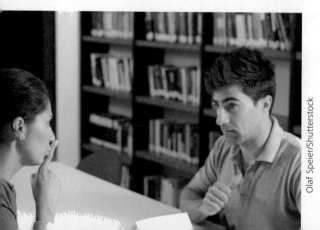

Olaf Speier/Shutterstock

Under justice, what is fair is right and what is not fair is wrong. For example, two students do not show up to class to take a final exam. One student simply overslept, while the other was in the hospital emergency room at the time of the exam. Would allowing both students an opportunity to take the exam be fair, or should only the sick student be allowed?

Ethical concepts and justice:

- Values: The ethical principle of values is a part of determining ethical justice. Ascertaining justice is worthwhile and should be strived for.
- Morals: Morals is the core ethical concept used to determine justice. We utilize justice as the measure of what is right and wrong.
- Conduct: The ethical concept of conduct is used as a guiding principle to determine justice. Following the rules will help determine what is fair or just.
- Beliefs: Because people rationalize tangible things to determine justice, the ethical concept of beliefs is not utilized to determine justice.

Ethics Alert! While the word *justice* is commonly used in the legal arena, legal justice and ethical justice are not the same thing. Legal justice is concerned with actions, and ethical justice is concerned with results. An example of legal justice is how the courts ensure that the law is applied to everyone the same way, such as ensuring a fair trial. Ethical justice would be used to argue that all murderers should receive the same sentence, because to render different sentences to murderers would be unfair (some receive life imprisonment, others the death penalty).

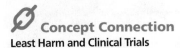

Concept Connection
Least Harm and Clinical Trials
The ethical concept of Least Harm is an essential component to the clinical trial process.

Least Harm

The least harm theory of ethical reasoning is best understood by the idea of the path of least resistance. If a solution provides no harm, then that is the right thing to do, and that particular course of action must be taken. If all of the available options cause some type of harm, the option that provides the least amount of harm is chosen. An example of the least harm principle is clinical trial procedure, where a manufacturer is trying to determine whether the side effects of a medication are worth the benefit of the medication.

Ethical concepts and least harm:

- Values: The ethical principle of values plays a part in the least harm principle, because it is an important not to inflict harm on others, or if harm is necessary, the least amount of harm possible.
- Morals: The ethical concept of morals is the core concept behind the least harm approach. As human beings we do not want to inflict harm, so the least amount of harm is the right thing to do.
- Conduct: The ethical principle of conduct plays a role in the least harm principles. Customary etiquette dictates that our actions should not harm others.
- Beliefs: Beliefs do not play a role in the least harm principle.

Respect for Autonomy

Autonomy is the concept of being able to make your own decisions and control your own destiny. Decisions should be made based on what allows people free reign over themselves and their bodies. The underlying principles that support this theory rationalize that only individuals know their own emotions, the life experiences they have encountered, and what is important to them. Any decision contrary to that would be discrediting their very existence. Respect for autonomy should not be confused with egoism. With egoism, it is the person's feelings, thoughts, and beliefs that drive the decision-making process. But with respect for autonomy, the focus is on a person's right to be included in decisions, and his or her decision is the option that is given the most weight. An example respect for autonomy is euthanasia and the right to die.

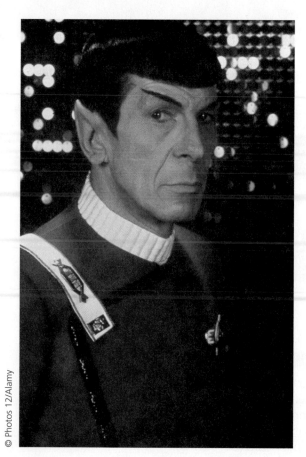

Fig. 9-1. In the *Star Trek* movie *The Wrath of Khan*, Spock states "logic clearly dictates that the needs of the many outweigh the needs of the few."

utilitarianism: providing the greatest good

applied ethics: a subcategory of ethics that uses ethical concepts and principles to reach an ethical decision

Ethical concepts and autonomy:

- Values: The concept of right and wrong play a role in respect for autonomy, because it is worthwhile or important to allow a person to control his or her own destiny.
- Morals: Morals is the core ethical concept associated with respect for autonomy. What allows a person to determine their own fate is right, and what does not is wrong.
- Conduct: There are no conduct ethical concepts associated with respect for autonomy.
- Beliefs: Beliefs play a vital role in respect for autonomy, as it addresses a person's soul.

Utilitarianism

Utilitarianism is based on providing the greatest benefit, whether that benefit is an amount or for the greatest number of people (see Fig. 9-1).

If provided with a list of options, whichever option benefits the most people is the one to choose. And by choosing that option, a right decision will always be made.

When we approach family members to consider organ donation, we utilize the concept of utilitarianism. By donating one person's organs, many lives can be saved.

Ethical concepts and utilitarianism:

- Values: The ethical principle of values is the core ethical concept utilized for utilitarianism. Helping the most people is important.
- Morals: Morals plays a role in utilitarian thinking, in that what benefits the most people is right and what does not is wrong.
- Conduct: Conduct does not play a role in utilitarianism.
- Beliefs: Beliefs do not play a role in utilitarianism.

Applied Ethics

So far we have discussed how ethics is defined and some of the principles that are used in the decision-making process. The next step is the application of those principles to real-life situations known as **applied ethics**.

TABLE 9-1

Ethical Concepts and Ethical Principles

	Values	Morals	Conduct	Beliefs
Altruism	Contribute	Core Concept		Contribute
Beneficence	Contribute	Core Concept	Contributes	
Consequentialism		Core Concept		
Deontology	Contribute		Core Concept	
Egoism	Core Concept	Contribute		
Justice	Contribute	Core Concept	Contributes	
Least Harm	Contribute	Core Concept	Contributes	
Respect for Autonomy	Contribute	Core Concept		Contribute
Utilitarianism	Core Concept	Contribute		

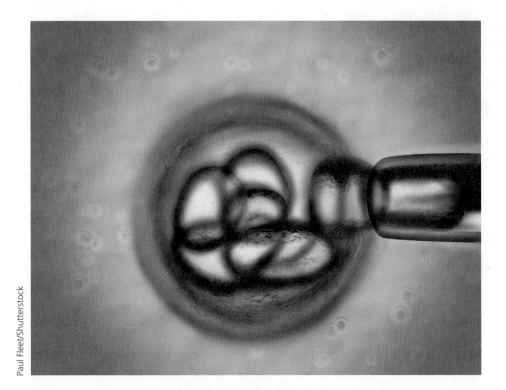

Paul Fleet/Shutterstock

Now that we have reviewed all of the tools that we need to actually make an ethical decision, the next thing we need to do is go through the process for decision-making. With the law, there is a specific format that must be followed. The law provides elements, which after they have been analyzed, will give us a specific answer to the legal question.

By performing a legal analysis, we can come up with a clear and precise answer to whether a person has broken a law or not. But with ethics, there is no format that is going to give you an exact answer. Ethical decisions differ from the law because of the:

- person making the decision,
- information available at the time the decisions is made,
- factors that are involved that created the dilemma or conflict, and
- current social, political, and cultural influence of the present day.

With the law, one person makes a decision—either the judge or the jury. But with ethics, there is no specific individual who will make ethical decisions. Instead, ethical decisions are made by anyone who faces a dilemma or conflict. In addition, the information that is available to make a decision differs between the law and ethics. With the law, rules of evidence dictate what information can and cannot be used to make a legal decision. But with ethics, there are no rules to determine what information can and cannot be used to assist in deciding ethical dilemmas.

While there is no specific process you can perform that will give you an exact answer to ethical dilemmas, there are some guidelines that you can follow to walk you through the decision-making process, an example of which is the Potter Box.

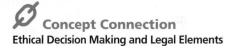

Concept Connection
Ethical Decision Making and Legal Elements
The use of the legal elements of law to perform a legal analysis is similar to utilizing ethical information to perform an ethical analysis.

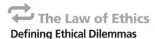

Sidebar
There are several different ethical decision-making models. While each has its own unique approach, steps, or requirements, most are variations of, or similar to, the model seen in the Potter Box.

The Law of Ethics
Defining Ethical Dilemmas
In order to define ethical situations, we sometimes have to talk to people other than the patient. Because of laws like HIPAA, discussing problems with people other than the patient has become problematic.

- Is there a way to resolve these issues?
- Can we talk to people about a patient's problem without the patient's authorization?
- What about people who are unconscious or in a coma; how do we determine whom we are authorized to talk to?

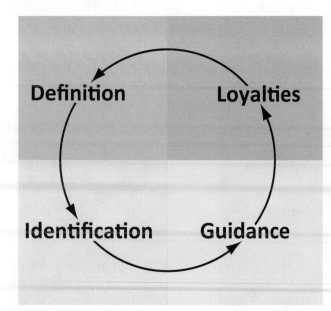

Fig. 9-2. The Potter Box diagram.

Ethical Decision Making: The Potter Box

The Potter Box was developed by Ralph B. Potter Jr., a professor of social ethics at Harvard Divinity School. The Potter Box was designed to address some of the most common problems people have when making ethical decisions. By using the Potter Box, you will not be wandering aimlessly through debates and discussions. Instead, following the process outlined in the Potter Box makes sure that you stay on track and address the issue (see Fig. 9-2). The Potter Box contains four steps:

1. Definition
2. Identification
3. Guidance
4. Loyalties

Step 1: Definition The first step in the ethical decision-making process is to define the dilemma. In this step you are identifying what the question is you are being asked to answer. By defining the question, we are also going to define the parameters that will guide our discussion. Without a clear understanding of what the question is, we may not address the issue or come up with a satisfactory answer. This is a common problem in ethical debates—because many ethical dilemmas are multi-faceted, and it is easy to get off topic. By defining the issue, you can make sure that you are addressing the problem and that the solution you come up with will solve the problem.

Step 2: Identification After you have defined the issue, the next step is to identify the ethical principles that are influencing the dilemma. By understanding what influences are contributing to the difficulty, you can better understand what the identifying issues are. You review the nine ethical principles and determine whether they are being used or not in order to identify the core issues involved. (When identifying whether an ethical principle is being used or not, there is no correct or incorrect answer. If you think an ethical principal is being used, then add it to your list for consideration.) In order to continue our discussion about how the Potter Box is used, we need an example scenario to determine which ethical principles apply. Consider the following:

Scenario

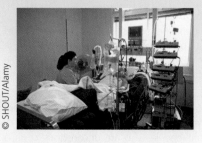

An 80-year-old widow suffers a stroke at home and is taken to the hospital. Because she had no advance directives, she was placed on a ventilator to support her breathing, and given medication for her blood pressure and heart function.

Our patient has two children, a daughter named April and a son named Zack. April has been living in the patient's home and caring for her for the past 10 years. April would like to continue life support to keep her alive as long as possible. Zack, is one year older than April but lives on the other side of the country. He talks with his mother once a month by phone, but has not actually visited her in over 5 years. Zack would like to remove life support to end his mother's pain and suffering so that she can die peacefully.

© SHOUT/Alamy

Now that we have a scenario to utilize, we list the nine ethical principles and make a determination as to whether they are being utilized in the dilemma.

- *Is someone using the ethical principle altruism?* Altruism may be a part of April's decision-making process, because she has given up part of her life by living with and caring for her mother.
- *Is someone using the ethical principle of beneficence?* Beneficence may be a part of Zach's thought process because he wants to help his mother's suffering by allowing her to die peacefully.
- *Is someone using the ethical principle of consequentialism?* While you may initially think that Zach is utilizing consequentialism, this ethical principle is not being used by Zach. Remember, with consequentialism the result (or consequences) is used to determine what actions are taken. Since the result, from Zach's position would be death, he would not be utilizing consequentialism. Instead, April may be using consequentialism because the end result—her mother's death—is what she is trying to avoid.
- *Is someone using the ethical principle of deontology?* Deontology may also be a factor here in two different respects. First, both April and Zach have a responsibility to their mother stemming from the parent/child relationship. But April has an added duty of that as a caregiver, having lived with her and cared for her for 10 years.
- *Is someone using the ethical principle of egoism?* Egoism could be contributing to some of the emotions involved in this scenario. Consider April's position; she may be scared about losing her mother, which may be contributing to her wanting to continue life support.
- *Is someone using the ethical principle of justice?* Justice is the concept of fairness. In this particular scenario it is hard to pinpoint a fairness principle that either April or Zach are using.
- *Is someone using the ethical principle of least harm?* Least harm is a driving force behind Zach's position, as he wants to stop his mother's suffering instead of prolonging it.
- *Is someone using the ethical principle of respect for autonomy?* If the mother had advances directives, indicating what her wishes were, respect of autonomy would be a consideration here. But because the mother does not have advance directives, and she is currently in a coma and unable to decide for herself, this ethical principle is not part of the equation.
- *Is someone using the ethical principle of utilitarianism?* Utilitarianism may be a factor in Zach's motives. Zach might be considering relief of both the suffering of his mother and the burden on his sister.

Listing each of the ethical principles and determining if they are being used provides a lot of insight into the dilemma. During the identification process, you may come up with some additional questions that you want to ask the parties that are involved; and that is OK. If you need to go back to the definition step to fine-tune the ethical question, you are able to do so. Once you have been able to identify the ethical principles that are being used in a dilemma, the next step is to prioritize them.

Step 3: Guidance The reason ethical dilemmas exist is because two or more ethical principles are competing with each other. If there were not at least two competing ethical principles, an ethical dilemma would not exist. In the guidance step, you ascertain which of the ethical principles you identified in Step 2 as the *guiding* principle. Regardless of the number of principles that are influencing a dilemma, by identifying the *guiding* principle, you can isolate the issues that are causing the dilemma.

In our scenario, Alice and Zach have different opinions regarding how to proceed with their mother's care. But of the principles that are being used, which ones do you think are the guiding principles underlying their thought process? To make that determination, review which principles they are using.

- Alice is possibly using the ethical principles of altruism, consequentialism, deontology, and egoism. Of the ethical principles being utilized by Alice, which do you think is the guiding principle supporting her position?
- Zach is possibly using the ethical principles of beneficence, deontology, least harm, and utilitarianism. Of the ethical principles being utilized by Zach, which do you think is the guiding principle supporting his position?

Note: Just because both Alice and Zach are using deontology does not mean that deontology is the *guiding* principle. In this step, we are not looking for similar principles but the main principle of each of the parties.

Even though there is no right answer, in order to continue our discussion on how the Potter Box works, we need to make some assumptions. Let us assume that Alice's guiding ethical principle is *consequentialism* and Zach's guiding ethical principle is that of *least harm*. In using consequentialism, Alice is concerned with the consequences of the decision, her mother's death. In using the least harm, Zach is concerned with the amount of suffering his mother is undergoing and wants to provide the option that gives the least amount of harm. Now that we have identified what the competing principles are, we can use those principles to help us define the ethical discussion and come up with a decision.

One of the problems with ethical decision-making is that during the process, it is easy to get off track, go on tangents, and discuss issues that are not going to resolve the dilemma. By identifying the guiding ethical principles, you are setting the parameters of the discussion that will lead you to a decision. But before we get to the actual discussion and decision of the dilemma, there is one last step in the Potter Box to complete.

Step 4: Loyalties The last step in the Potter Box is reviewing our loyalties. In this step, we are looking inward and not at the dilemma itself. By looking at our loyalties, we are identifying whether we have any biases, prejudices, or relationships that may hinder our decision-making ability. As a healthcare provider your loyalties are to your patients, and doing what is best for them. But as a mother or father, your loyalty is to your child or spouse. Can a mother who is also a physician provide objective ethical decisions for their own child? Do they have loyalties that may interfere with their ability to make a decision? If you identify loyalties that may interfere with the decision-making process, you have a responsibility to recuse yourself from the decision-making process.

Potter Box Summary:

1. Definition: What is the question?
2. Identification: What is impacting the problem?
3. Guidance: What is the driving ethical principle?
4. Loyalties: Is there anything that might interfere in the discussion or decision?

Reaching a Decision

Now that we have gone through the Potter Box, the next step is to reach a decision. If you are making this decision on your own, consider all of the information that you have gathered using the Potter Box. If you are making

Court Case

Italo Falcone v. Middlesex County Medical Society

162 A.2d 324, 62 N.J.Super. 184, 1960 NJ 40212
New Jersey Superior Court, Law Division

FACTS: In 1946, Italo Falcone received a Doctor of Osteopathy degree from the Philadelphia College of Osteopathy. At that time, the college was not an approved college by the American Medical Association (AMA). After graduating, he completed his one-year internship and three-year residency at Detroit Osteopathic Hospital, which also was not recognized by the AMA. Afterward, he submitted his application for licensure to the New Jersey State Board of Medical Examiners, and successfully passed the exam. He was granted a license to practice medicine and surgery by the state of New Jersey. After receiving his Doctor of Osteopathy license, Falcone attended the University of Milan, Italy; a school that was approved by the AMA. Because of his previous education, Falcone was given credit for the first three years of classes. He completed the fourth and final year at the University of Milan. Upon graduation, he was awarded a Doctorate of Medicine (M.D.) degree. Upon graduating with an M.D., Falcone completed an internship and residency in surgery.

In 1953, Falcone applied to the Middlesex County Medical Society as an associate member. His application only included information related to his Doctorate of Medicine degree, and did not mention his Doctorate of Osteopathy education. Falcone was granted with associate membership in the Middlesex County Medical Society. Falcone joined the medical staff at Middlesex General Hospital and St. Peter's Hospital; and was allowed to admit and treat patients. In order to be granted staff privileges, both institutions required membership in the Middlesex County Medical Society.

During his associate membership, members of the Middlesex County Medical Society learned that Falcone had only attended the University of Milan for one year, having been given credit for the first three years based on his osteopathic education. The medical ethics committee of the Middlesex County Medical Society reviewed Falcone's application, and decided not to renew his membership and removed his name from their membership roster. In part, the medical ethics committee's decision was based on a requirement that a person attend four years of medical school from an AMA approved institution. Because membership in the Middlesex County Medical Society was required to have staff privileges at Middlesex General Hospital and St. Peter's Hospital, both hospitals revoked Falcone's admitting privileges. Falcone filed suit asking that the courts to require the Medical Society to grant him membership.

ISSUE: At issue in this case was whether an organization had the authority to dictate and determine a right that was not granted to them. Essentially, was the Medical Society dictating, indirectly, the requirements for the practice of medicine in the state of New Jersey?

RULE: The court, in reviewing the case found "the defendant Middlesex County Medical Society, combined with the other component parts of the State Medical Society of New Jersey and the American Medical Association, has virtual monopolistic control of the practice of medicine." They ordered that the Medical Society grant membership to Falcone.

EMPHASIS: The court said only the state of New Jersey determines what the practice of medicine is, not the Medical Society. While this is an old case, it demonstrates some of the historical differences that occurred at one time in healthcare history, the difference between an M.D. and a D.O. The emphasis for our current discussion, however, is the decision-making process of the medical ethics committee. All members of the Middlesex County Medical Society's ethics committee were Medical Doctors (M.D.); none were Doctors of Osteopathy (D.O). Were there any loyalties that members of the ethics committee had that should have precluded them from making a decision?

this decision as part of a group, then discuss the issues between members of your group. (Note: if discussing the issue in a group, group members may not all have identified the same guiding principle, and that is OK. It is a good way to start the discussion, in an attempt to identify how everyone sees the issue.)

Making a decision may be the hardest part of ethics, because of the difficulties raised by the ethical dilemmas. If reaching a decision was easy, it would not be an ethical issue. But while the issues will not get any easier, the more you use the Potter Box, the process will.

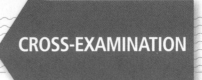

Make FALSE statements TRUE.

Rewrite the false statements below by replacing the bolded, italicized, and underlined word(s) to make it a true statement.

1. The process involved in trying to determine what ethics is a branch of ***law*** known as meta-ethics.

   _____

2. Like ***consequentialism***, beneficence involves helping others, but in beneficence there is no individual sacrifice.

   _____

3. The word deontology is derived from the word ***elderly***.

   _____

4. Ethical ***justice*** is the exact opposite of altruism and beneficence.

   _____

5. ***Least harm*** is the concept of being able to make your own decisions and control your own destiny.

   _____

Circle Exercise

Circle the correct word from the choices given.

1. (**Altruism, Beneficence, Utilitarianism**) is based on providing the greatest benefit, whether that benefit is an amount or for the greatest number of people.

2. The ethical principle of morals is the core concept used in (**consequentialism, egoism, utilitarianism**).

3. In the ethical principle of deontology (**values, morals, conduct**) does not play a role.

4. Of all of the concepts that contribute to the ethical principles, (**morals, conduct, beliefs**) is not one of the core concepts for any of the nine ethical principles.

5. The Potter Box is associated with (**meta-ethics, normative ethics, applied ethics**).

Matching

Match the numbered term to its lettered definition.

1. _____ altruism
2. _____ applied ethics
3. _____ beneficence
4. _____ consequentialism
5. _____ deontology
6. _____ egoism
7. _____ meta-ethics
8. _____ normative ethics
9. _____ utilitarianism

A. a decision-making process that uses the outcome to determine whether something is right or wrong.

B. a subcategory of ethics that defines how ethical decisions are made and the factors that contribute to ethical decision-making.

C. a subcategory of ethics that defines what ethics is and the contributing factors that define ethical principles.

D. a subcategory of ethics that uses ethical concepts and principles to reach an ethical decision.

E. an action that is used to help other people.

F. concern for the welfare of others; an obligation to benefit others.

G. providing the greatest good.

H. the use of duty and rules to determine an outcome.

I. the use of individual self-interest

Deliberations: Critical Thinking Questions

Question 1: Review the ethical principles listed in this chapter, and pick three. Write a few sentences describing a situation where you utilized the principles that you have chosen. Explain how those ethical principles were used.

Question 2: You have been asked to take part in an ethical discussion concerning whether a patient's life-support system should be removed. The children of the patient wish to be included in the discussion, or at least present when you discuss the issue with your peers. How would you respond to the children's request? Regardless of your decision, describe some of the problems that may arise from whatever decision you have chosen.

Question 3: The concept of moral nihilism is addressed when using the Potter Box. Which of the four steps in the Potter Box do you think is attempting to address the issue of moral nihilism? Explain your answer.

Question 4: Of the nine ethical principles, the concept of beliefs is the least frequently used concept to support the ethical principles. In addition, beliefs is not the guiding principle of any of the ethical principles. Why do you think that is? Explain your answer.

Question 5: With the law, rules of evidence dictate what information can and cannot be used to make a legal decision. But with ethics, there are no rules to determine what information can and cannot be used; but should there be? Would defining a list of rules to determine what information can and cannot be used to decide ethical issues help or hinder the process?

 ## Closing Arguments: Case Analysis

A 9-year-old girl named Ashley is severely physically and mentally disabled (functioning at the level of a three-month-old), and suffers from a variety of different medical conditions. Ashley requires around-the-clock care, which is provided mostly by her parents. Part of providing care for Ashley requires constant lifting, carrying, and moving her from the bed to a wheelchair and the bathroom. As Ashley matures, and her parents get older, providing physical care has become more and more difficult.

Ashley has been admitted to the hospital for elective surgery and medical treatments. The doctor has scheduled an elective hysterectomy (removal of the uterus), which will be followed by a treatment regime of large doses of estrogen. The goal of treatment is to stunt her growth and to prevent her from menstruating. By keeping Ashley small in stature, her parents will be able to continue lifting, carrying, moving, and providing her care. Members of the medical and surgical team have expressed concerns over the treatment and surgery and have brought the issue to the ethics committee for resolution. As a member of the ethics committee answer the following questions.

Question 1: Which of the ethical principles do you think the parents utilized when deciding whether to have the surgery or not? Explain your answer. (You can use one or more than one to explain your answer.)

Question 2: What about the doctor who is going to perform the surgery? Which ethical principles and theories do you think the doctor may have used in making the determination to perform the surgery and treatment? Explain your answer.

Question 3: Go through the steps involved in the Potter Box, come up with an answer to the question. Should the child be allowed to have the surgery, or should the surgery be cancelled?

 ## The Briefcase

This section repeats the objectives from the beginning of the chapter and provides a summary of the most important concepts for each objective. Use this section as a quick review and to check your understanding of the chapter key points.

Objective 1: Explain the difference between the three difference branches of ethics.
- Meta-ethics: what ethics is.
- Normative Ethics: how a person makes a decision.
- Applied Ethics: reaching an ethical decision.

Objective 2: List the nine different ethical principles used in ethical decision-making.
- altruism
- beneficence
- consequentialism
- deontology
- egoism
- justice
- least harm

- respect for autonomy
- utilitarianism

Objective 3: Identify which ethical concepts: values, morals, conduct, or beliefs, are used for each of the nine ethical principles.
- See Table 9-1 on page 146.

Objective 4: Discuss the reasons the Potter Box is used in ethical decision-making.
- To guide the discussion
- To provide a format to reach a decision
- To stay on topic

Objective 5: List the four steps used in the Potter Box.
- Define
- Identify
- Guidance
- Loyalties

Objective 6: Describe the problems that each step of the Potter Box addresses.
- Definition: ascertains what the question is. Allows you to isolate the question and stay on topic.
- Identification: determines which principles are being utilized. Allows you to stay on topic and not let corollary issues over-cloud the real dilemma.

Objective 6 (continued):
- Guidance: identifies the guiding principle. Helps you to isolate the issue each party has.
- Loyalties: considers bias and prejudice. Ensures that our individuality is not affecting the decision.

Objective 7: Given a scenario, work through the steps of the Potter Box to help you reach a decision.

Objective 8: Explain why the Potter Box step Loyalties may affect ethical decision-making.
- Removes bias and prejudice.
- Removes personal interest in the outcome from guiding the decision or influencing the outcome.

Objective 9: Summarize why using the Potter Box will not give you an actual answer.
- Ethical answers are not exact.
- Ethical answers differ from situation to situation and person to person.
- There are no right ethical answers.

Maximize Your Success with the Companion Website

The Companion Website to this textbook contains materials that can help you better understand the concepts presented in this chapter. Go to www.myhealthprofessionskit.com to access:

- Sample Quizzes
- Web Links
- Games
- and more…

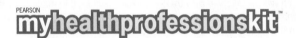

PEARSON
myhealthprofessionskit™

The Beginning of Life 10

The beginning of life can be a wonderful and exciting time. But despite this joyous occasion, many ethical issues arise at the beginning of life. One of the main controversies is determining when life begins. A scientific definition of life provides the requirements that science needs to determine when life begins, but that same definition may not suit the requirements for determining life for medical purposes. In addition, religious beliefs may conflict with either the scientific or medical definition of life which adds a different perspective to consider. In this chapter, we will discuss the ethical issue associated with the beginning of life.

MEASURE YOUR PROGRESS: LEARNING OBJECTIVES

After studying this chapter, you will be able to:

- List the ethical debates associated with fertilization.

- Describe the opponent's arguments to artificial insemination and in vitro fertilization.

- List the ethical debates associated with conception.

- Give an example of a legal problem associated with surrogacy.

- Describe the opponent's arguments to genetic screening.

- List the ethical debates associated with childbirth and childhood.

- Provide an example of how the Safe Haven law is used.

- Explain why the controversy over vaccines exists.

- Describe what The Best Interest of the Child is.

KEY TERMS

artificial insemination

electroejaculation

embryo

eugenics

fertilization

in vitro fertilization

neonate

surrogate

zygote

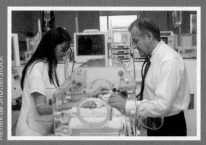

Reflekta/Shutterstock

PROFESSIONAL HIGHLIGHT

Anuja is a neonatal intensive care nurse who specializes in caring for premature babies. Anuja has been working in the neonatal ICU for several years and has encountered many different ethical dilemmas in her career. Anuja uses her knowledge of medicine and ethical principles to help her work through some of the complex ethical dilemmas that she faces.

Why does it seem like there are more and more debates concerning the beginning of life than in the past?

Many of the ethical debates that our nation is currently facing were never considered a few decades ago. This is due, in part, to advancements in the fields of science, technology, and medicine that have created never before conceived ethical issues. Part of the problem, which goes to the heart of some of these debates, is the approach that science takes: "What are we able to do?" This approach allows science to accomplish seemingly impossible tasks that were not possible before. However, providing answers to such questions has unintentionally caused ethical concerns because science sometimes does not stop to ask, "Even though we can, has anyone considered whether we should?"

Fertilization

Many couples desire to become pregnant and have children. Prior to advances in medicine, a woman's ability to become pregnant was left to chance. But as science evolved, techniques became available to assist in problems associated with **fertilization**.

fertilization: conception; the uniting of a female gamete (called an ovum) and a male gamete (called a spermatozoon)

The first step in fertilization is the release of a viable ovum from the ovary into the fallopian tube. In addition, a spermatozoon must travel through the reproductive system and survive long enough to reach the ovum in the fallopian tube. If any problem occurs with these processes, fertilization will not occur. If a couple is experiencing difficulties becoming pregnant, there are scientific procedures that can be utilized to assist in the process, depending on which part of the fertilization process a couple is having problems with.

Artificial Insemination

One of the most common difficulties associated with fertilization relates to the male gamete. If a spermatozoon lacks motility (the process of movement), it will not be able to make the necessary journey through the female reproductive system to join with the ovum in the fallopian tube.

If a couple is encountering difficulties becoming pregnant, one of the first techniques utilized is **artificial insemination**.

artificial insemination: the placement of sperm into the female reproductive system by means other than sexual intercourse

In artificial insemination, the male's sperm is collected and placed in a syringe-like apparatus (see Fig. 10-1). The procedure, however, has a time limitation (around 12 hours), as it must coincide with the female's ovulation cycle.

When artificial insemination was first used it had a few critics. Some felt that science was interfering with God's plan, and creating children when God had not intended them to be created. As the use of artificial insemination grew, so did the number of critics. When artificial insemination was first utilized, only a husband's sperm was used to fertilize his wife's eggs. But it was not very long before some people realized that being husband and wife was not a medical pre-requisite for using artificial insemination. Single women who desired to have a child but were not yet ready to get married, did not want to get married, or had not yet found a compatible spouse started utilizing donated sperm to have a child through artificial insemination.

Some religious organizations called up the state medical boards to establish guidelines for when artificial insemination could be performed by healthcare professionals. Specifically, they were requesting that medical professionals be authorized to perform artificial insemination only on married women using only their husband's sperm. The medical community argued that establishing such a policy would cause more harm than good—that people would resort to performing the procedure themselves, at home, using common household items. By doing so, they run the risk of contracting an infection or suffering from severe bleeding by perforating anatomical

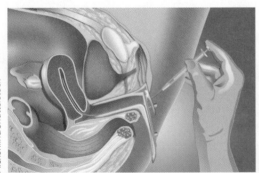

Alexonline/Shutterstock

Fig. 10-1. In artificial insemination a tube is inserted into the female anatomy and placed in the upper cervix, near the entrance to the fallopian tubes. The sperm is then inserted through the tube and deposited at the distal fallopian ostium (opening of the fallopian tube).

Sidebar

There are many old wives' tales associated with pregnancy. But where did the phrase "old wives' tales" come from? The phrase comes from the Old English word *wif* (which means "woman," not necessarily a married spouse); the plural form of *wif* is *wive*. An old *wif* would tell younger children fables to either encourage or discourage certain behavior. These stories were passed down from generation to generation and collectively became known as old wives' tales.

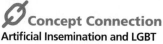

Concept Connection

Artificial Insemination and LGBT

Many gay and lesbian couples utilize artificial insemination to have children of their own. This is one of the unique ethical issues that the LGBT community faces.

structures from improper technique. Even though no state medical board adopted such a policy, artificial insemination critics still remain.

Sperm Collection

Part of the process involved in artificial insemination is the collection of male sperm. Typically, the donor provides a specimen on his own, just prior to the procedure. However, that is not the only way sperm can be collected.

Electroejaculation

Due to advances in medical procedures, sperm collection can occur through a process known as **electroejaculation**.

In an electroejaculation procedure, a probe is inserted into the anus, and placed near the prostate gland. A slight electric charge is applied to the probe, causing contraction of the prostate and pelvic muscles, resulting in ejaculation. The sperm sample is collected and can be used for artificial insemination. The procedure itself has been around for many years, and is common in the farming industry. But the practical use in humans did not come to light until recently.

electroejaculation: a medical procedure whereby an electrical charge is applied to male reproductive organs to obtain a sperm sample

Ethics Case

Nikolas Evans

Travis County Probate Court (April, 2009)

FACTS: On March 27, 2009, 21-year old Nikolas Evans was assaulted outside a bar in Austin Texas. After being taken to the hospital, and placed on life support, doctors determined that he was clinically brain dead. The medical team approached Nikolas' mother, Marissa Evans, about donating her son's organs. Marissa gave her consent for organ donation, but requested that prior to the organ procurement that her son's sperm be collected as well. Marissa stated that her son had always talked about having children of his own, and that with sperm collection a surrogate could be used to fulfill that wish and allow the legacy of Nickolas to live on through his child. The organ procurement team, however, did not have the equipment or procedures to honor such a request. The hospital, therefore, declined Marissa's request for sperm collection, but would proceed with the organ donation.

In order for the sperm to be collected and utilized, it must be obtained while the person is still alive, or within 24 hours after death. Because of the urgency and time limitation, Marissa contacted an attorney who filed court papers asking that Nikolas' body be preserved so that the electroejaculation procedure could take place while the sperm was still viable.

ISSUE: There are many ethical issues raised in this case. The first was whether a mother could consent to sperm donation. While

a parent has the legal right to donate his or her child's organs, does that consent include the donation of sperm? Second, can a mother authorize the fathering of a child posthumously, without the father's consent? And third, what effect will this have on the child, should one be conceived? The question that Marissa's attorneys argued was that the sperm must be obtained, so that these type of issue can be addressed. By not allowing for the sperm collection, irreparable harm would result because of the short time-frame for sperm collection to occur.

RULE: Part of the difficulty that the court struggled with was that there was no legal precedence for the posthumous collection of sperm. But, regardless, the probate court judge agreed with Marissa and granted her request. The judge ordered that Nikolas' body be preserved so that the electroejaculation procedure could be performed while the sperm was still viable. (Marissa located a urologist, who performed the procedure.)

EMPHASIS: Even though medical science evolves quickly, the law does not catch up as fast. While issues such as artificial insemination and abortion have been going on for years, there are always new and different ethical dilemmas that will arise as science advances.

(End note: Five people received Nikolas' organs. At the time of the publication of this text, a child has not yet been conceived utilizing Nikolas' sperm. Marissa is currently raising the funds she needs to pay for a surrogate.)

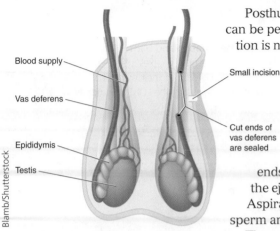

Blood supply

Vas deferens

Epididymis

Testis

Small incision

Cut ends of
vas deferens
are sealed

Blamb/Shutterstock

Fig. 10-2. A vasectomy involves the surgical removal of part of the vas deferens. Even after a vasectomy sperm production continues in the testicles. But it cannot be released because of the closed vas deferens.

in vitro **fertilization:** the fertilization of an ovum outside of the womb

Posthumous sperm collection is not the only time that electroejaculation can be performed; it can also be utilized in medical conditions where ejaculation is not medically possible, such as men who have a spinal cord injury.

Post-Vasectomy Sperm Collection

A vasectomy involves the surgical removal of a part of the vas deferens (see Fig. 10-2).

If a man has had a vasectomy and later decides that he wants to have children, there are two different medical procedures that can be performed. The first is a vasovasostomy, where the ends of the vas deferens are sutured back together again, allowing for the ejaculation of sperm. The second is Microsurgical Epididymal Sperm Aspiration (MESA), where a small incision is made in the epididymis and sperm and spermatic fluid aspirated and collected.

The main criticism of such techniques comes from within the medical community itself. Some doctors argue that only a vasovasostomy should be performed. Since MESA is a surgical procedure, if a pregnancy does not occur, the surgical procedure will need to be unnecessarily repeated. To minimize the number of surgical procedures, critics argue, a vasovasostomy should be performed because it only occurs once. Critics outside the medical community believe that once a vasectomy surgery has been performed, that men should not be allowed to change their mind later on in life.

In vitro Fertilization

In order for fertilization to occur, one factor that needs to be present is a viable ovum outside of the ovary. The most common problem that women face with fertilization is with ovulation, the release of an egg from the ovary. If ovulation does not occur, neither can fertilization. But medical science developed a process whereby eggs could be removed from the ovary and fertilized outside of the body through *in vitro* fertilization.

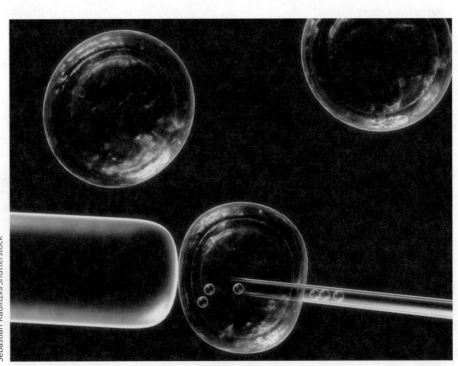

Sebastian Kaulitzki/Shutterstock

The process of *in vitro* fertilization involves collecting a woman's eggs from the ovary and removing them from the body. The eggs are placed in a special medium where the male gametes are added so that fertilization can take place. The combined medium is then returned to the woman's body so that the **zygote** can implant itself into the uterine wall.

In vitro fertilization is not a guarantee that pregnancy will occur, however. And, because of the way that *in vitro* fertilization works, there is no guarantee that only one zygote will be implanted. One of the most common problems associated with *in vitro* fertilization is multiple births.

zygote: a single cell that is produced by the union of an ovum and spermatozoon

Frozen Products of Conception

Ovum, sperm, and zygotes that are used for *in vitro* fertilization do not need to be implanted right away. If not utilized right away, they can be frozen and used for implantation at a later time. There are several reasons a person might have products of conception frozen. For example, a woman who has been diagnosed with cancer might want to have her eggs harvested before undergoing chemotherapy. After the treatment, if she is able to, she can become pregnant herself; or if she is unable to become pregnant, she can have the embryos implanted into a surrogate.

It is unknown how long products of conception can be frozen for and still be successfully utilized. One physician reported that sperm that had been frozen for 12 years had been successfully utilized in an *in vitro* fertilization pregnancy. As the length of time increases that products of conception remain viable, so do the legal complexities.

Sidebar

The term *in vitro* literally means in glass. When *in vitro* fertilization was first developed glass containers were utilized for fertilization. Although glass containers are not always used nowadays, the name stuck.

Sidebar

A growing number of female soldiers shipping out to Iraq or Afghanistan are having their ova frozen prior to leaving for overseas duty.

Ethics Case

Nadya Doud-Suleman

Bellflower California (January, 2009)

FACTS: On January 26, 2009, Nadya Denise Doud-Suleman gave birth to eight children by cesarean section. The octuplet birth was newsworthy, because it was only the second time in recorded history that eight children had been born from one pregnancy. The mother and children garnered national media attention, dubbing Ms. Doud-Suleman "Octomom." However, public attention quickly turned negative as more information regarding Ms. Doud-Suleman came to light. Shortly after the octuplet's birth it was discovered that not only did Ms. Doud-Suleman have six other children, all conceived through *in vitro* fertilization, but that she was a single mother living on welfare. Questions were raised about the mother's ability to care for all 14 of her children and the burden that she was placing on public assistance.

The physician who performed the *in vitro* procedure, Dr. Kamrava, became the focus of both social and medical scrutiny. In a statement, Dr. Kamrava's attorney stated "The question is—and society may not approve—but if it's satisfactory between patient and physician, that is something to be weighed very significantly."

ISSUE: Despite the public concerns, medical/ethical questions were raised as well. The California State Medical Board filed a formal complaint against Dr. Kamrava, alleging:

- gross negligence for the number of embryos implanted at one time,
- failing to refer Ms. Doud-Suleman for a mental health evaluation,

- failure to exercise "appropriate judgment,"
- failing to question Ms. Doud-Suleman's actions,
- repeated negligent acts by the excessive use of fertility drugs, and
- failure to keep adequate medical records.

The medical board is asking that Dr. Kamrava's license be revoked or suspended, and that he be required to pay for monitoring during his probationary period. In response to the allegations, Dr. Kamrava maintains that his actions were not negligent, because he was following his patient's wishes.

RULE: The state medical board revoked Dr. Kamrava's license to practice medicine. In announcing their decision, the medical board did not believe that probation provided the appropriate oversight needed to protect the public. Instead, that protection could only come from revoking Dr. Kamrava's license.

EMPHASIS: At the time Dr. Kamrava implanted the embryos into Ms. Doud-Suleman, there were no laws regulating the number of embryos that could be implanted. Instead, it was left up to the clinician to determine what was best for the patient. Despite the fact that no laws existed, there are still guidelines, based on sound medical practices, that dictate what a healthcare professional can and/or should do. This case is an example of how violation of a professional Code of Ethics can result in licensure suspension.

↻ The Law of Ethics
Childbirth After Divorce

When a couple undergoes a divorce, one of the issues that they may have to address is child custody. But what happens when there are frozen products of conception: either eggs, sperm, or zygotes? Because they are not yet children, no clear criterion has been determined as to how the courts should handle them. Typically, frozen products of conception are awarded to one party or the other. However, there are legal consequences involved in any decision that a court makes. For example, if after a divorce a woman is awarded custody of the zygote and undergoes artificial insemination or *in vitro* fertilization, is the ex-husband now fathering a child that he will be responsible for helping to raise and even possibly even having to pay child support for?

---

embryo: a fertilized ovum from 7 days after fertilization through 8 weeks gestation

---

surrogate: a woman who carries and gives birth to another person's child

---

⊘ Concept Connection
Surrogacy and Contract Law
One of the elements required to form a contract is the element of consideration. When surrogacy contracts are challenged in court, the most common contractual element at issue is the element of consideration.

Conception

Whether utilizing the natural method or assisted by science, conception occurs when the ovum and spermatozoon unite creating a zygote. If the zygote successfully attaches to the uterine wall, it will start to divide and grow and after seven days is referred to as an **embryo**.

While fertilization is one of the more common problems, carrying a child to term can be a medical problem for some women. They may have a medical condition that either causes spontaneous miscarriages, or being pregnant becomes detrimental, either to the health of the mother or the embryo.

Surrogacy

There are times when women are unable to carry a child of their own and may turn to a **surrogate** to carry and deliver that child for them.

The process for surrogacy is essentially the same as with *in vitro* fertilization. But once the eggs have been removed from the donor and fertilized, instead of being returned to the donor they are implanted into the uterus of another woman. The surrogate then carries the child to term and, upon delivery, the child is returned to the biological parents to raise.

When this concept was first conceptualized, the surrogate was typically a family member or close relative. However, nonrelatives were soon selected to act as a surrogate, which raised some important legal and ethical issues that society and the law needed to address.

If a nonrelative or stranger is a surrogate, the parties typically enter into a surrogacy contract. This usually involves a detailed description of what each party will be responsible for and how the process will work. For example, the contract will state that the surrogate must maintain a healthy environment during the pregnancy, and will attend any and all medical examinations requested by the OB/GYN doctor. The donor parents, in return, will pay for all medical expenses and upon delivery of the child pay a lump sum to the surrogate. But despite all good intentions, inherent problems arise. For example, what happens if the surrogate wants to keep the child as her own and refuses to give the child to the donor parents? In most instances, the courts will require the surrogate to hand over the child to the child's biological parents. In part, the court's decision is based on contract law, focusing on the element of consideration. Because the parties entered into a valid contract, the courts will enforce that contract.

Genetic Testing

Many surrogacy contracts include provisions requiring that the surrogate submit to genetic testing of the fetus. Genetic testing is typically performed after the sixteenth week of pregnancy. Through amniocentesis, the fetus's DNA is analyzed to determine not only the sex of the child, but whether the fetus has any genetic defects or carries risks for genetic defects diseases later on in life. There are literally hundreds of different genetic defects that can be ascertained through a genetic testing, such as Down Syndrome, sickle-cell anemia, Tay-Sachs, or Alzheimer's disease.

The controversy surrounding genetic testing is not with the procedure itself, but what is done with the information that is obtained from genetic screening. For example, Tay-Sachs is an autosomal recessive disorder that causes rapid deterioration of physical and mental capabilities through destruction of nerves. Symptoms usually start at 6 months of age and

The Law of Ethics
Ultrasound Boutiques

Another common test that is performed during pregnancy is an ultrasound. And while ultrasounds can provide valuable medical information, pictures of the developing baby can also be obtained. This is exactly what some have turned into a growing business. Over the past few years, ultrasound keepsake shops have opened up in shopping malls. Pregnant mothers can walk into a shop, have an ultrasound performed, and receive a picture or video of their child that they can share with loved ones. In addition, some shops offer T-shirts, coffee mugs, or key chains with the image imprinted on them. There is nothing stopping a woman from going into an ultrasound shop once a week to have an image taken.

The problem, however, is that these shops are not regulated by the medical boards, because the images are not being taken for medical purposes. But medical questions have arisen. What is currently unknown is what effects repeated ultrasounds might have on a developing fetus? In addition, what if there is something visible on an ultrasound that could constitute a medical problem, such as a fetal tumor? The technicians who perform these procedures are not authorized, and sometimes do not have the skill, to read and interpret images. But are mothers getting a false sense of security when they are not told of potential problems?

progress until brain death occurs (usually at four years of age). Because there is no cure for Tay-Sachs, nor is it treatable, the only available medical intervention is to alleviate pain and suffering. If it is discovered that a fetus has Tay-Sachs, a mother may decide to terminate the pregnancy instead of putting the child and the family through the pain and suffering associated with the disease.

What if it was discovered that the child had Down Syndrome, and the parents do not believe that they can adequately take care of a child with that condition? Or, to add more complexity to the situation, what if the child is being carried by a surrogate, and the biological parents discover that the fetus has Down Syndrome. They opt to terminate the pregnancy, but the surrogate does not want to and opts to keep the baby herself? There are no easy answers to some of these complex questions, as the law has not caught up with medical science yet. Critics of genetic testing, who commonly refer to it as genetic screening, argue that it is not right to have that information in the first place. These critics believe that the practice of genetic screening is a type of **eugenics**.

Eugenics is the process of utilizing science to selectively breed desirable traits, and also to deselect undesirable traits. Theoretically, it is believed that through the practice of eugenics and genetic testing virtually all genetic diseases could be eliminated. The practice of eugenics gained popular support in the early 1900s, but after it was associated with Nazi Germany, it quickly lost support within society and the scientific and medical communities.

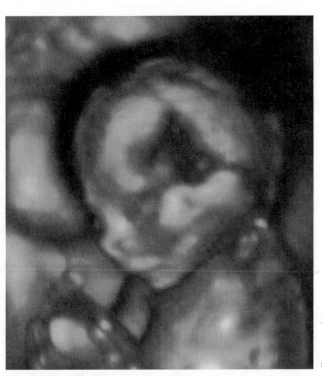

Shutterstock

eugenics: the process of applying selective breeding to humans

Childbirth & Childhood

Despite all of the problems that can occur with fertilization and pregnancy, children are conceived and born every day, most without fertility assistance. A newborn child, up to its first birthday, is referred to as a **neonate** (see Fig. 10-3).

Unfortunately, ethical dilemmas are not isolated to issues prior to birth, as there are several ethical issues raised during the first few years of a child's life.

neonate: a newborn from the time of birth until one year of age

⦿ Understanding Your State

Some states put limits on how old a child can be to meet the requirements of Safe Haven laws. In addition, different states dictate what locations will qualify as a Safe Haven site. To find out what your state's Safe Haven laws requires, check out the companion website.

⇄ The Law of Ethics
Safe Haven Age Limits

The initial purpose of Safe Haven laws was to protect newborns. But, because of word choices used in some state safe haven laws, the definition of the word *child* created problems. In Omaha, Nebraska, a woman surrendered her 17-year-old child to a safe haven site. Because of situations like this, most state legislatures are rewriting the Safe Haven laws to limit the age requirement allowed. But should they?

- Should Safe Haven laws be limited to only newborns?
- What about unwanted children that do not meet the definition of newborns? Is there a way to protect them as well?

Safe Haven Laws

Unfortunately not every child is a wanted child. Instead of going to a hospital to have the child, the child is born at home, in a hotel room, or in a back alley. After delivery, instead of taking the neonate to a hospital or placing it up for adoption, some people place the baby in a garbage dumpster or on the street, or worse yet kill and dispose of the baby. This phenomenon is most common with teenagers who have hidden their pregnancy.

To combat this growing problem, all states have passed laws allowing a mother to give up their children. Safe Haven laws allow any mother to bring a child to an emergency room, fire station, or police station, and surrender the baby. In addition, any parent who surrenders a child under the Safe Haven law is provided with immunity from prosecution (such as for child abuse, child neglect, or abandonment). Once a child has been received by a safe haven, the child is placed with child protective service, and then placed in a foster home and put up for adoption.

Safe Haven laws are not without complications, however. For example, what if after surrendering the child, the parent wishes to take the child back? Or, what if the father discovers that his child has been surrendered to a safe haven without his consent? Does the father have the right to get the child back?

Circumcision

Shortly after a male child has been born, the couple will be asked whether they want their child circumcised or not. Circumcision is a medical procedure whereby the foreskin is removed from around the head of the penis. While there are some rare medical conditions where circumcision is medically necessary, the procedure is usually performed for religious or cultural reasons (see Fig. 10-4).

There are those that disapprove of circumcision believe it is an unnecessary medical condition, and traumatizing to the child. In fact, some go as far as calling it genital mutilation. Opponents to circumcision state that it is a human rights violation and should only be performed when a person is old enough to make his own medical decisions.

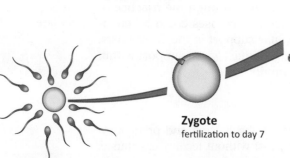

Neonate
birth to 1 year

Fetus
9 weeks to birth

Embryo
1 week to 8 weeks

Zygote
fertilization to day 7

Gametes
ova & spermatazoon

Fig. 10-3. The progression and nomenclature of pregnancy and childhood.

While the controversy surrounding circumcision continues, there are medically valid reasons for circumcision. Studies have been performed which indicate that males who have been circumcised have lower percentages of penile and prostate cancer. In addition, the study also showed that women married to circumcised men have lower rates of cervical cancer.

Vaccinations

The mere mention of vaccinations can conjure up some very strong emotions. There are those, some doctors included, who believe that vaccinations are not necessary and are even harmful to the body. Part of that belief comes from a 1998 study that was published in the British medical journal the *Lancet,* which mentioned a correlation between the MMR vaccine and autism. That study has since been retracted, sighting incorrect and contrary findings and flaws with the analysis. The CDC has released several reports stating that there is no casual link between vaccines and autism. However, despite all available studies, reports, and medical

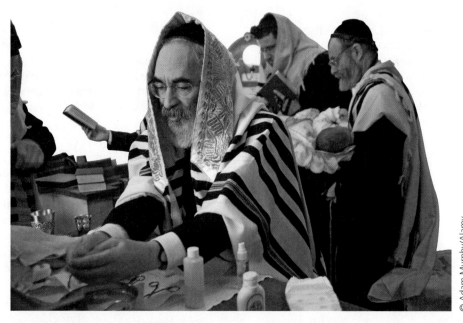

Fig. 10-4. A Mohel prepares for a Brit Milah (covenant of circumcision) on an eight-day-old Jewish boy.

© Adam Murphy/Alamy

Ethics Case

The Story of John/John

Winnipeg Mannitoba and Baltimore Maryland
April, 1966 to May 2004

FACTS: On August 22, 1965, healthy identical twin boys named Bruce and Brian were born to Mr. and Mrs. Reimer in Winnipeg, Mannitoba. At 6 months of age, the twins were diagnosed with phimosis, a condition whereby the foreskin cannot be fully retracted over the glans penis. Left untreated, it can result in repeated infections, penal scarring, and urinary problems. To correct the problem, doctors recommended that the boys undergo circumcision. Instead of performing a surgical excision, using a scalpel, the doctor opted to burn the foreskin off using a cauterization procedure. When the doctor performed the procedure on Bruce, the penis was mistakenly burned. The burn was so severe and extensive it was beyond surgical repair.

Concerned about his future happiness and sexual function, Bruce's parents took him to noted psychologist John Money at Johns Hopkins Medical Center, who specialized in gender identity. John Money believed that the best thing to do was for the child to undergo sexual reassignment surgery. The sex change operation was performed when the child was 22 months of age. The parents renamed Bruce, Brenda.

Money continued to treat and observe "Brenda" for several years, reporting updates in medical journals. (To preserve anonymity, Money referred to it as the John/John case.) Money believed that this was an ideal research study, because her twin brother could serve as a control group, and the monitoring of

Brenda could be utilized for research purposes to better understand the development of gender identity.

As Brenda reached adolescence, estrogen was provided to assist in the development of female breasts and other female attributes. Neither Money nor the parents told Brenda that he had been born a boy, about the circumcision, or the sexual reassignment surgery.

ISSUE: There are many ethical issues raised by this case. Was it appropriate for the parents to consent to sexual reassignment? Should the child have been told about the incident, and if so when? Was the research portion of Money's treatment and handling of the case appropriate?

RULE: Even though this case did not involved the courts, colleagues of Money were very critical of his handling of the case.

EMPHASIS: After many years of medical and psychological treatment, "Brenda" became depressed and refused to continue to see Money in Baltimore. After threatening suicide, and with the advice of an endocrinologist and psychiatrist, Brenda—at age 13—was finally told that he had been born a boy, about the circumcision, and that he had had sexual reassignment surgery. Afterwards, Brenda decided to call himself David and started living as a boy. He later underwent several surgeries, including a double mastectomy and two phalloplasty operations, and received testosterone injections. David lived as a male and got married and helped raise his step-children. On May 5, 2004, after separating from his wife, David committed suicide.

⇄ The Law of Ethics
Illegal Circumcision?

In May 2011, a group in San Francisco was successful in getting a measure put on the November 2011 California ballot. The measure, if passed by voters, would outlaw the performance of circumcision, punishable by a $1,000 fine or up to one year in jail. One of the main controversies of this proposal was that there were no religions exceptions written into the proposed law.

- Do you think that voters should have the right to vote on such a measure?
- Why do you think that this is such an important issue to some people?

◣ Sidebar

While circumcision is most commonly performed on boys, there is a type of circumcision that can be performed on girls. A clitorectomy is the surgical removal of the clitoris, and sometimes involves removal of, or partial suturing of, the external female genitalia. Although rarely performed, the most common and approved use is for cancer treatment.

Fig. 10-5. The CDC publishes a schedule of recommended vaccinations that children and adolescents should receive.

Dmitry Naumov/Shutterstock

findings, some people still hold to the belief that vaccines can cause autism.

The most recent vaccine debate has to do with the vaccine for the human papillomavirus (HPV), known to cause cervical cancer. The HPV virus is usually contracted through sexual intercourse. In order to combat the sexual transmission of HPV, the vaccine needs to be given before a person becomes sexually active. It is recommended that the vaccine be given to girls at the age of 9 to allow adequate time for antibodies to build up in the immune system. However, critics believe that vaccinating girls at such a young age is giving them license to engage in sexual intercourse (see Fig. 10-5).

Best Interest of the Child

Despite all of the difficulties that we face in deciding some of the ethical and legal issues related to the beginning of life, there are some legal guidelines utilized. All states in the United States have statutes collectively referred to as "The Best Interest of the Child" laws, to help decide some of the complex legal issues that relate to children. Initially, these laws were developed to help the courts determine placement and custody issues. However, their use has been expanded over the years to serve as a guide when deciding any legal issue that relates to children.

While there are variations between different states, some of the most common guidelines outlined in The Best Interest of the Child laws are:

- The importance of family integrity.
- The health, safety, and protection of the child.
- The importance of timely and permanent decisions.

Court Case

M.N. and V.N., Parents of B.N., An Infant v. Southern Baptist Hospital of Florida

648 So. 2d 769
Court of Appeal of Florida, First District (1994)

FACTS: The parents of an eight-year-old girl (who court records refer to as B.N.) brought their child to Southern Baptist Hospital of Florida. She was diagnosed with acute monocytic leukemia, severe anemia, and a low platelet count. Doctors recommended chemotherapy as the most appropriate treatment, which would also require blood transfusions. B.N.'s parents, Jehovah's Witnesses, refused to consent to the blood transfusions. The hospital filed an emergency petition with the court, asking them to grant the administration of chemotherapy and blood transfusions without the parents' consent. The parents argued that they did not want to consent to the treatment not only because of religious grounds, but because the treatment would cause undue suffering. The trial court ordered that the treatment could be started without the parents' consent. The parents appealed.

ISSUE: The issue before the court was under what circumstances could the court override a parent's wishes and what standard should be used to make that determination.

RULE: The court ruled that "the parents' wishes may be overcome when there is sufficient medical evidence to invoke the state's *parens patriae* authority, and to establish that the child's welfare will be best served by the disputed treatment." The court, in explaining its reasoning, stated, "the policy of advancing the best interests of the child is well rooted in this state and guides the courts in many diverse contexts."

EMPHASIS: While the best interest of the child standard is most commonly used in custody cases, it can be used in other issues related to a child's welfare. In this case, the appellate court ruled that the best interest of the child standard applies to deciding whether a parent's wishes for the refusal of medical treatment can be over-ridden.

Some common factors that are taken into consideration when making these decisions include:

- The emotional ties and relationships between the child and his or her parents, siblings, family, household members, or caregivers.
- The capacity of the parents to provide a safe home and adequate food, clothing, and medical care.
- The mental and physical health needs of the child.
- The mental and physical health needs of the parents.
- The presence of domestic violence in the home.

Sidebar

The FDA advisory panel recently recommended approval for the administration of the HPV vaccine for males. Providing the vaccine to males prevents the occurrence of genital warts but does not affect a man's ability to spread HPV to women or other men.

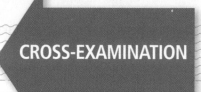
Make FALSE statements TRUE.

Rewrite the false statements below by replacing the bolded, italicized, and underlined word(s) to make it a true statement.

1. If a couple is encountering difficulties becoming pregnant, one of the first techniques utilized is ***electroejaculation***.

   _____

2. When ***surrogacy*** was first utilized, it had a few critics. Some felt that science was interfering with God's plan, and creating children when God had not intended them to be created.

   _____

3. In *in vitro* fertilization, the combined medium is then returned to the woman's body where the ***gamete*** will implant itself into the uterine wall.

   _____

4. If the zygote successfully attaches to the uterine wall, it will start to divide and grow and after four days is referred to as an ***neonate***.

   _____

5. ***Clitorectomy*** is a medical procedure where by the foreskin is removed from the head of the penis.

   _____

Circle Exercise

Circle the correct word from the choices given.

1. Artificial insemination attempts to correct problems associated with (**fertilization, conception, childbirth**).

2. Surrogacy attempts to correct problems associated with (**fertilization, conception, childbirth**).

3. A child referred to as a neonate involves a time-frame associated with (**fertilization, conception, childbirth**).

4. A study erroneously associated (**Down's syndrome, Autism, Tay-Sachs**) with vaccinations.

5. The importance of family integrity is stated as a reason for writing (**Safe Haven laws, Best Interest of the Child laws, surrogacy contracts**).

Matching

Match the numbered term to its lettered definition.

1. _____ artificial insemination

2. _____ electroejaculation

3. _____ embryo

4. _____ eugenics

5. _____ fertilization

6. _____ *in vitro* fertilization

7. _____ neonate

8. _____ surrogate

9. _____ zygote

A. a newborn from the time of birth until one year of age.

B. a fertilized ovum from 7 days after fertilization through 8 weeks gestation.

C. a medical procedure whereby an electrical charge is applied to male reproductive organs to obtain a sperm sample.

D. a single cell that is produced by the union of an ovum and spermatozoon.

E. a woman who carries and gives birth to another person's child.

F. conception; the uniting of a female gamete (called an ovum) and a male gamete (called a spermatozoon).

G. the fertilization of ovum outside of the womb.

H. the placement of sperm into the female reproductive system by means other than sexual intercourse.

I. the process of applying selective breeding to humans.

Deliberations: Critical Thinking Questions

Question 1: An insurance company has established a policy requiring pregnant females to undergo genetic testing prior to delivery. The rationale the insurance company gives is to financially prepare for any possible diseases the child might have. If a parent refuses to have the genetic test performed, the insurance company will deny payment regarding any disease the child may develop that could have been discovered by genetic testing. What are your thoughts? Is this something that the law should be allowed?

Question 2: A couple who had a child through a surrogate has not informed the child. There are no laws that require a parent to inform a child that they were born through surrogacy. What are your thoughts regarding a law requiring parents to inform their child if they were born through a surrogate, by artificial insemination, or in vitro fertilization? Explain your answer.

Question 3: You are the parent of a child who was born a hermaphrodite (a child that has the sexual organs of both a male and a female). The doctor mentions that surgery is possible to make the child anatomically male or female. Would you decide to have the surgery and assign the child as male or female, or decide keep the child a hermaphrodite? Explain your answer.

Question 4: Billionaire Bill, an 87-year-old, was admitted to the hospital following a stroke. He was pronounced dead, and you are prepping him for transfer to the funeral home. Bill's 25-year-old wife has come to the hospital asking doctors to perform an electroejaculation procedure. She hopes to collect sperm in order to become artificially inseminated and have Bill's baby. Bill's sons and daughters do not want another heir to his vast fortune have. They threaten to get a court order stopping you from performing the procedure, and rush to find a lawyer and a judge. However, even if they are successful, by the time a decision is reached, it will be too late, as the time to harvest the sperm will have expired. Bill's wife encourages you to have the procedure performed anyway, stating that if the court rules against her, the sperm can be destroyed. What should you do? Would you perform the procedure or not? Explain your answer.

Question 5: Mary has been pregnant three times, and has delivered three girls. For each child that she has had, within days of taking the child home, the father of the child has admonished both his wife and the child, because Mary cannot give him a boy. When Mary takes her child to the local hospital to drop her off under the Safe Haven law, the nurse on duty remembers her because she had previously dropped off her other two children under the Safe Haven law as well. What should the hospital do? Are there any actions that the hospital can take to prevent Mary from surrendering any future children?

Closing Arguments: Case Analysis

Peggy and Gary had been married for five years, and had been trying to have a child. They had undergone artificial insemination and in vitro fertilization, but each pregnancy had resulted in a miscarriage. Peggy and Gary decide that surrogacy was their best option and placed an advertisement in the local college newspaper.

Josephine, a 21-year-old college student, answered the advertisement. At the time, she was dating a man named Jerry who she loved very much and hoped to marry. But Jerry had recently broken up with Josephine. Hoping to trick Jerry into marrying her, Josephine agreed to be the surrogate for Peggy and Gary. Using Peggy and Gary's zygote, Josephine underwent in vitro fertilization and became pregnant.

During the pregnancy Josephine underwent routine medical examinations, as required by the surrogacy contract. During one of the examinations, a genetic screening test was performed and it was discovered that the child had Down Syndrome. Peggy and Gary did not desire to have a child with Down Syndrome and in accordance with the surrogacy contract paid Josephine to undergo an abortion. In addition, Josephine contacted Jerry, telling him that she was carrying his child. Not wanting to be a husband or father at a young age, Jerry paid Josephine for an abortion as well. He then transferred to another school in a different state.

As a college student who could use the cash, Josephine gladly took the money for the abortion. But because of religious reasons she did not have an abortion and carried the child to term. She never told Peggy, Gary, or Jerry that she delivered a child.

Unfortunately, being a single mother and college student was too much for Josephine. At three months, she took the child, whom she called Greg, to the local hospital and surrendered him under the state's Safe Haven law.

Question 1: Shortly after the child was surrendered, Jerry found out that Josephine had delivered a child, which he thought was his. Jerry's parents completed the paperwork necessary to adopt Greg, because they could not fathom the idea of someone else raising their grandchild. Should Jerry's parents be allowed to adopt Greg? Explain your answer.

Question 2: Shortly after the child's second birthday, Greg needed to have minor surgery to correct an intestinal problem. Part of the pre-surgery laboratory work involved determining the child's blood type. The blood typing indicated that it was biologically impossible for Jerry to have fathered Greg. Jerry and Jerry's parents are now suing Josephine. Should Josephine have to pay the amount of money it cost to raise and support Greg? Explain your answer.

Question 3: As part of her testimony in the lawsuit, Josephine discloses the truth about Greg and the surrogacy pregnancy. Although enraged, Jerry's parents felt it necessary to contact Peggy and Gary. When Peggy and Gary learn that their biological child had actually been born, they petitioned the court to have their child returned to them and to award them custody. How should the court decide? Should the child remain with Jerry's parents or be given to Peggy and Gary? Explain your answer.

The Briefcase

This section repeats the objectives from the beginning of the chapter and provides a summary of the most important concepts for each objective. Use this section as a quick review and to check your understanding of the chapter key points.

Objective 1: List the ethical debates associated with fertilization.
- Artificial insemination
- Electroejaculation
- *In vitro* fertilization
- Frozen products of conception

Objective 2: Describe the opponent's arguments to artificial insemination and *in vitro* fertilization.
- Playing God
- Creating children when God did not intend for children to be created

Objective 3: List the ethical debates associated with conception.
- Surrogacy
- Genetic screening
- Eugenics

Objective 4: Give an example of a legal problem associated with surrogacy.
- Contract law
- Returning child to biological parents
- Surrogacy visitation

Objective 5: Describe the opponent's arguments to genetic screening.
- Is it fair to have the information before hand?
- Increased use of abortion for undesirable traits

Objective 6: List the ethical debates associated with childbirth and childhood.
- Safe Haven laws
- Circumcision
- Vaccinations

Objective 7: Provide an example of how the Safe Haven Law is used.
- Children are surrendered to qualified facilities.
- Unwanted children can be surrendered without fear of prosecution.
- Prevents the abandonment or murder of children.

Objective 8: Explain why the controversy over vaccinations exists.
- Fear over autism
- Concern about injecting harmful substances into the body.

Objective 9: Describe what The Best Interest of the Child is.
- Law used to help define situations regarding children.
- Initially used for child custody and visitation rights.
- Utilized for a variety of different issues regarding children.

Maximize Your Success with the Companion Website

The Companion Website to this textbook contains materials that can help you better understand the concepts presented in this chapter. Go to www.myhealthprofessionskit.com to access:

- Sample Quizzes
- Web Links
- Games
- and more…

PEARSON
myhealthprofessionskit™

Death and Dying 11

Talking about the end of a person's life is never easy. And while there are things that we can do to prepare for the end, when the time comes we always wish we had more time, if only for a few minutes. Because of the unique nature of our work, as healthcare professionals, we deal with the possibility of patients dying almost every day. With death come unique issues and controversies that those working in the healthcare profession need to be aware of. In this chapter, we will talk about the ethical issues related to the end of life.

MEASURE YOUR PROGRESS: LEARNING OBJECTIVES

After studying this chapter, you will be able to:

- Describe the difference between clinical death and actual death.

- Explain how organ donation allocation works.

- List the order of people that the courts use under the law of intestacy.

- Give an example of what an advance directive is.

- Explain the difference between a healthcare proxy and a living will.

- Determine what type of care will be provided when a doctor writes a DNR order.

- Describe the type of care a patient who enters hospice will receive.

- Provide an example of the four different types of euthanasia.

- List the stages of grief as identified by Dr. Kübler-Ross.

KEY TERMS

advance directives

DNR

euthanasia

grief

healthcare proxy

hospice

intestacy

living will

palliative

in extremis { In extremity; at the end, often meaning near death.

PROFESSIONAL HIGHLIGHT

Jeff is a department manager for the cancer ward at a large healthcare institution. Because of the type of patients admitted to his unit, Jeff needs to be familiar with the issues related to death and dying. Using his knowledge of medicine and the issues related to death and dying, he can provide the medical care, counseling, and advice that his patients and their families need.

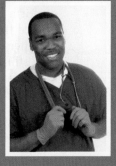

Karin Hildebrand Lau/Shutterstock

There are many different reasons end of life issues are brought to a court of law. When a judge is asked to intervene, the two most common issues have to do with whether life support should be removed and identifying which person is allowed to make the decision.

Part of the reason end of life issues make for difficult decisions has to do with the determination of when death occurs. Everyone can agree that when the body and body organs stop functioning, the person is no longer alive. The difficult issues arise around the matter known as clinical death.

> I've heard stories about court fights over removing a person from life support. Aren't there some guidelines that the hospitals and courts follow when issues like this come up?

Determination of Death

The Uniform Determination of Death Act (UDDA) was drafted by the National Conference of Commissioners on Uniform State Laws. The National Conference of Commissioners worked closely with the American Medical Association (AMA) and the American Bar Association (ABA) when drafting the UDDA.

It is important to note that the UDDA is not a federal law, passed by the U.S. Congress that applies to all states. Instead, the UDDA is a model that has been presented to each of the states that they can use in drafting their own, state legislation regarding the determination of death.

The UDDA model provides two different requirements for determining when death has occurred.

1. Irreversible cessation of circulatory and respiratory function, or
2. Irreversible cessation of all functions of the entire brain, including the brain stem.

Concept Connection
UDDA and State Autonomy
Each state in the United States has the authority to create laws that affect its own citizens, as long as there is no federal law that supersedes it. Since there is no federal law regarding the determination of death, each state is free to write its own laws.

Note the use of the word *or* at the end of the first condition. The inclusion of the conjunction indicates that only one set of criteria needs to exist, not both. In addition, note the use of the word *irreversible* in both of the conditions. When bodily organs cease to function, such as the heart, lungs, and brain, everyone can agree that death has occurred. The difficulty comes when bodily organs may still be functioning, but have been damaged to a point where they are beyond repair and cannot sustain life on their own. Medical science may be able to use machines or medicine to keep certain organs functioning, such as a respirator or pacemaker; but without their use those organs would not be able to function on their own. When irreversible conditions occur, it is commonly referred to as clinical death.

Doctors utilize different tests to determine when irreversible cessation occurs. For irreversible cessation of circulatory problems, the doctors will turn off the pacemaker and monitor the heart to see if it beats on its own. For irreversible cessation of respiratory problems, the doctors will turn off the respirator and see if the patient can initiate a breath on their own (referred to as the apnea test). To determine brain activity, doctors perform an electroencephalogram (EEG) to identify the electrical function of the brain. The outcome of these tests help doctors to determine whether a person has met the clinical definition of death, although they may still technically be alive. But it is this determination of clinical death that brings with it difficult issues, such as, when should life support be removed? Or, because some of the body is still functioning, is organ donation something that should be considered prior to removing the person from life support?

Organ Donation

Perhaps one of the most difficult situations a healthcare provider can face is informing family members that a loved one is clinically dead, and then asking about organ donation. If not done properly, it could appear that the healthcare provider is more interested in saving others than their loved one's life. Or, family members may feel that the medical team is giving up when they have not yet actually died. One approach is to demonstrate how their loved one can live through the life of others who will receive their organs. But that approach can itself be difficult. The difficulty associated with approaching family members has been made easier over the past few years with increased awareness and education about organ donation in the general public. However, approaching family members about organ donation should only be done by people who have been trained in discussing organ donation.

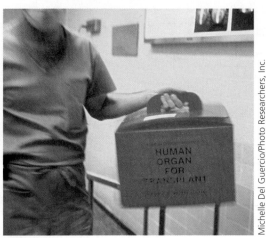

Despite the increased public awareness, the topic of organ donation has unique ethical problems. At one time, stories surfaced in the news about celebrities receiving organs over those who had been on the waiting list longer. To combat some of the growing ethical issues related to organ donation, Congress passed the National Organ Transplant Act (NOTA), in 1984. NOTA:

- established the United Network for Organ Sharing (UNOS),
- established the Organ Procurement and Transplant Network (OPTN),
- established a Task Force on Organ Transplantation, and
- banned the purchase or sale of human organs and tissues.

Organ Donation Waiting List

A patient in need of an organ is medically evaluated by his or her physician and a recommendation is made to the local transplant team. The transplant team, which in some hospitals is made up of the ethics committee, evaluates each patient. The team determines factors such as whether the person is a viable candidate for a transplant and how serious their medical condition is. If the patient is approved as an organ recipient candidate, his or her name and application are added to the organ donation waiting list maintained by UNOS (see Graph 11-1).

Organ Donation Allocation

Even though a patient is on the waiting list, there is no guarantee that he or she will receive an organ. If a potential donor has been identified, the patient's information is provided to UNOS. Using a computer program, UNOS provides a list of potential recipients to the hospital where the potential donor is located. Some of the contributing factors used to determine who potential recipients are include:

- donor and recipient blood type (including immune system identification)
- size of the organ being donated
- medical urgency of the recipient
- time spent awaiting a transplant
- distance between the donor and recipient

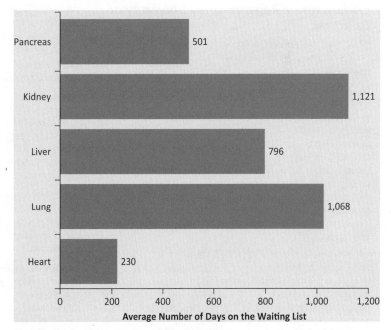

Graph 11-1. The average waiting period for organs in the United States. (Information tabulated from USON/OPTN published reports.)

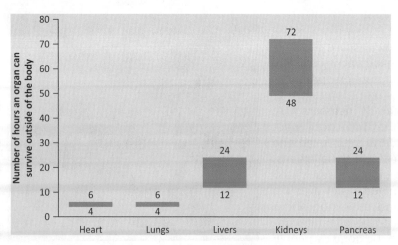

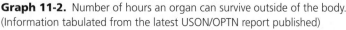

Graph 11-2. Number of hours an organ can survive outside of the body. (Information tabulated from the latest USON/OPTN report published)

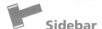
When patients who are on the waiting list are contacted and informed that a potential organ has been received, they typically only have a matter of minutes to report to the hospital (see Graph 11-2). Potential recipients are often required to carry beepers or cell phones with them 24 hours a day, 7 days a week, so that they can be notified when an organ becomes available.

A patient in need of an organ who is placed on the waiting list does not necessarily start at the bottom. Instead, there are criteria to prioritize where a patient is placed on the waiting list. For example, if two patients are waiting for a kidney transplant, and one patient only has a few days to live because dialysis is no longer working, that individual will be given priority over other patients on the waiting list.

Court Case

Elodie Irvine v. Regents of the University of California

57 Cal.Rptr.3d 500, 149 Cal.App.4th 994 (2007)
Court of Appeal State of California,
Fourth Appellate District Division Three

FACTS: Elodie Irvine was diagnosed with end-stage liver disease, a polycystic liver, and kidney disease. Doctors determined that because of the seriousness of her condition, she needed a liver and/or kidney transplant. In June 1998 the transplant team at the University of California at Irvine (UCI) Medical Center, evaluated her case and added her to the transplant. UCI notified the United Network for Organ Sharing (UNOS) requesting an organ and placing Elodie on the waiting list. After months turned into years, Elodie grew concerned. Doctors at UCI "continuously assured [her] that [she] was high on the priority list to receive a transplant due to [her] serious life-threatening medication condition."

After waiting for four years for a transplant, Elodie became discouraged and consulted with a doctor outside of UCI. Her new physician told her that waiting four years was unacceptable. He informed Elodie that the extended wait time was likely due to internal problems at UCI. In October 2002, Elodie transferred her transplant application to Cedar-Sinai Medical Center in Los Angeles. She received a liver and kidney two months later.

Elodie filed a lawsuit against UCI claiming medical negligence, negligent infliction of emotional distress, fraud, and conspiracy.

As part of the discovery phase of her lawsuit, UNOS responded to a letter from Elodie's attorney, indicating that UNOS had made offers to UCI of almost 40 different livers or kidneys. that potentially matched Elodie's criteria.

ISSUE: While this appellate case focused on procedural issues involved during the trial phase, the initial lawsuit was asking the court to determine whether UCI had "conspired to keep her low on the transplant list and granted priority to healthier patients to increase the percentages of successful transplantation and thereby attract more prestige, more patients, more profit and more research funding."

RULE: The appellate court remanded the case back to the trial court for a decision. However, after the appellate court's ruling the parties entered into a settlement agreement that include a non-disclosure clause. Therefore, the final outcome of this case is unknown.

EMPHASIS: While there are many issues and problems presented by this case, for our present discussion it demonstrates how the organ donation system works and how priority and the allocation of organs is suppose to be allocated. The more serious a person's medical condition, the higher on the donation list he or she is supposed to be.

Even if a patient has not made his or her wishes known regarding organ donation, the law will allow certain individuals to make that decision if the person is unable to. The Uniform Anatomical Gift Act (UAGA) provides, among other things, a list of people who can make decisions regarding whether a patient's organs will be donated. For example, a young adult may not have allocated their organs for donation, but following an accident, the youth's parents may be called on to donate their child's organs. Or, if the potential donor is married, the individual's spouse may be consulted about organ donation. Which persons are authorized to make such decisions is not arbitrary but based on preexisting law—the law of intestacy.

Intestacy

If a person dies without a will, how do the courts determine who inherits a person's estate, and if there is more than one person how the estate is divided? When a person dies without a will, the law utilizes the rules of **intestacy** to determine inheritance (see Fig. 11-1).

The law of intestacy compiles a list of people who will receive a person's estate. The list was created using two different factors:

1. Who would a person most likely designate as the recipient of their property if they had a will?

2. Which person would be the most deserving of a person's property?

Normally, when somebody writes a will, they leave the majority of their property to their current spouse. Those with children will typically leave a portion of their estate to their children as well. It is this logic that was used to develop the intestacy list. When using the law of intestacy, the first person a court looks to is the person's current spouse. If there is a spouse, then that spouse receives 100 percent of the person's estate. (The ex-spouses of those who are divorced or legally separated are not considered in the law of intestacy.) If there is no current spouse, the law will turn to any children a person may have. If there are three children, then the estate is divided into three equal shares. If there are no children, the law then turns to the person's parents, and so on, down the list of family members until a person is identified.

While the law of intestacy was developed for the courts to determine inheritance, it has been adopted for use in other situations as well. One of the most common uses of the list of intestacy is to determine who will make medical decisions if a person becomes incapacitated and does not have advance directives. For example, the courts will first turn to a person's spouse, or, if no spouse is present, to the person's children to make medical decisions. If no children are present (or they are not of the age to make a decision), then the courts will turn to the person's parents.

But even though the law of intestacy provides guidelines to courts and medical professionals, it is not without problems. Consider the Terri Schiavo ethics case.

When determining the distribution of assets for a person who dies without a will, the law of intestacy determines percentages. For example, if a widowed man dies without a will, and has four children, each child will receive 25 percent of his assets. But when the law of intestacy is used to make medical decisions, the answers are not as clear-cut. Returning to our example, if a widowed man is incapacitated and does not have advance directives, his children—all four children—are asked to make a decision. The law of intestacy does not give preferential treatment to one child over the other. Instead, it only designates which person(s) will make a decision. If more than one person

---

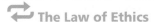

The Law of Ethics

Presumed Consent for Organ Donation

Most European countries have presumed consent laws regarding organ donation. Presumed Consent laws state that unless a person has specifically identified that their organs are *not* to be donated, any viable organ *will be* donated. While no state in the United States has adopted such a law, some state legislators are considering such a proposal to address the shortage of organs available in the United States.

- What do you think?
- Do you think that this is a law that should be considered in the United States?

---

intestacy: the division of property by descent and distribution, for individuals who die without a will

1. Spouse

2. Children

3. Grandchildren

4. Great Grandchildren

5. Great Great Grandchildren

6. Father/Mother

7. Brother/Sister

8. Nephew/Niece

9. Grandparents

10. Uncle/Aunt

11. Great Grandparents

12. Great Uncle/Great Aunts;
    First Cousin; Great Nephew/Niece

13. Great Great Grandparents

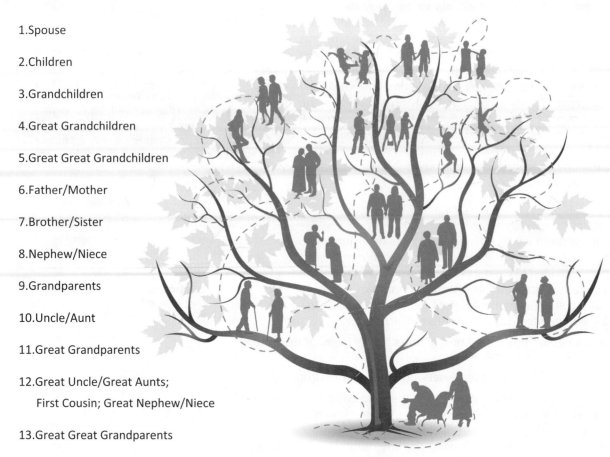

Fig. 11-1. The rules of intestacy are used by the court to determine the order of inheritance for a person who dies without a will, or whom the courts will look to when medical decisions need to be made and there are no advance directives.

Ethics Case

Terri Schiavo

St. Petersburg, Florida (1990–2005)

FACTS: On February 25, 1990, Terri Schiavo collapsed in her St. Petersburg, Florida, home. Although alive when paramedics arrived, she suffered extensive brain damage and was deemed to be in a persistent vegetative state. At the time that Terri collapsed, she did not have advance directives to indicate what her medical wishes were. In 1998, Terri's husband petitioned the court to have Terri's feeding tube removed, but was opposed by Terri's parents, Mr. and Mrs. Schindler. Terri's husband, Michael, testified that Terri would not want to be kept alive by artificial means. But Terri's parents disputed that claim by arguing that she was a devout Catholic and would not violate the church's position on suicide or euthanasia. A seven-year legal battle ensued, which included over 14 appeals. Even the governor of Florida, the United States Congress, President George W. Bush, and Pope John Paul II tried to intervene or weighed in with their opinions.

ISSUE: At issue in the case was the right of the spouse to make medical decisions over the rights of the parents. Because Terri had no advance directives, her wishes regarding medical treat-

ments and the sustaining of her life was unknown. Mr. and Mrs. Schindler tried to attack Michael Schiavo's rights as a spouse by raising unsubstantiated allegations of abuse, which they claim contributed to Terri's persistent vegetative state. In addition, by the year 2000 Michael was living with his girlfriend, whom he had fathered a child with. Terri's parents unsuccessfully argued that living with his girlfriend and fathering a child negated Michael's standing as Terri's spouse. But the courts determined that absent a divorce decree or legal separation, Michael was still considered Terri's spouse in the eyes of the law.

RULE: During the legal battle over Terri's life, her feeding tube was removed a total of three different times, but it was twice reinserted pursuant to court orders. The final removal of Terri's feeding tube came on March 18, 2005, and Terri expired on March 31, 2005—15 years after her initial collapse.

EMPHASIS: Although the law of intestacy was originally developed for use in determining how to distribute a person's assets, it is also utilized in other areas as well. While Terri's parents tried to intervene on her behalf, the courts deferred to the law of intestacy, giving Terri's husband the right to make the final decision.

exists in that category, then all members of that category are asked to make a decision. Returning to our example, all four children will be asked for a decision regarding end of life care. If all four children can agree on a decision, then that decision is carried out. But, if all four children cannot agree, then no decision is made, and the law of intestacy is no longer used. Instead, the children will have to fight each other in court, to determine which of the four should be appointed guardian.

Advance Directives

Like the name implies, **advance directives** provide *directions* to family and healthcare workers *in advance* of their death or incapacity.

By completing advance directives, a person details what their wishes are concerning life support, extraneous medical treatment, tube feedings, or length of time medical treatment should be continued. Advance directives can come in many different forms, but the most common is a living will.

advance directives: any document that provides instructions for patient care that is made by a patient before he or she becomes incapacitated

Living Will

If you become incapacitated and are unable to make medical decisions, you can still tell healthcare providers what your wishes are regarding the medical treatment and when treatments should be stopped. By creating a living will, you are indicating what you wishes are, while you are still alive and able to make decisions.

living will: a document detailing the situations and type of medical care a patient desires

There are very few requirements indicating what needs to be included in a living will. For the most part, living wills include:

- what medical treatments you want to receive
- the extent of medical treatments you want to receive (i.e., life support, feeding tubes)
- when you authorize removal of medical treatments
- who you designate to make decisions for you (if there are questions or situations not covered by your living will)—a healthcare proxy

Healthcare Proxy

As we saw with law writing, laws are not always interpreted by the judicial branch the way the legislature intended. The same holds true for any writing. For example, in writing your living will, you might mean one thing but people reading it might think of something entirely different. If you write a living will, and questions arise as to what you meant, or if situations arise that are not covered by your living will, who will interpret your meaning for you? A **healthcare proxy** is a person you designate to interpret your meaning and to make medical decisions for you, should you become incapacitated.

 Beyond the Scope

The rules used by the courts to determine who is appointed as guardian is completely different than the law of intestacy. Because guardian rules involve more complex issues, such as child custody, the complexities involved in guardianship are beyond the scope of this text. For more information regarding guardianship, the reader is directed to outside resources.

Understanding Your State

While all states recognize living wills, there are different requirements in each state that dictate what must be included in a living will. To see what your state requires, check out the map of the United States on the companion website.

healthcare proxy: a person designated to make medical decisions for someone who is incapacitated

The person you designate as your healthcare proxy should have a clear understanding of what your wishes are. If a healthcare proxy is designated, it negates the law of intestacy because the person whose care is in question has made his or her wishes known. (Remember, the law of intestacy is only used when a predetermination has not been made.) There are very few rules regarding who you can decide to be your healthcare proxy, as you can choose anyone you want. For example, even though you are married, you can designate your parents as your healthcare proxy. That would mean that your parents would make medical decisions despite what your spouse's wishes are. But even though there are few rules related to healthcare proxies, there are some noteworthy limitations. First, healthcare proxies are only allowed to make decisions regarding your medical care. They cannot make decisions regarding your finances, estate, or other matters. Second, the healthcare proxy is only utilized if you do not have advance directives or if situations arise that are not addressed by your advance directives. Meaning, if you have advance directives, those advance directives will be carried out. Third, there are no legal limitations on whom you can designate as a healthcare proxy except when healthcare workers are designated. Because of conflicts of interest, healthcare workers cannot be designated as healthcare proxies unless they are related by blood or marriage to the person making the designation. Meaning, you cannot serve as a healthcare proxy for your patients, but you can for your parents or spouse. Fourth, if the person whom you designate to be your healthcare proxy declines that responsibility, the law of intestacy replaces the healthcare proxy.

Do Not Resuscitate (DNR) Orders

The last advance directive, and probably the most commonly know type, is a DNR (Do Not Resuscitate) order.

DNR: an order written by the physician which indicates what medical treatments or procedures are not to be performed

If a patient is faced with impending death, he or she may request that the doctor sign a DNR order. A DNR order indicates what measures are to be withheld should a patient's condition warrant medical intervention and/or resuscitation. The most common type of procedures included in DNR orders are CPR, mechanical ventilation, and defibrillation.

One of the common misconceptions in the general public regarding DNR orders is that it means do not treat. Some people and patients are under the misconception that with a DNR order, healthcare providers will stop providing all medical treatment, including the administration of pain medication; which

Court Case

Lujan v. Life Care Centers of America

229 P.3d 970, 971-72 (2009) Colorado Court of Appeals, Division V

FACTS: In October 2006, Estella Lujan was admitted to a Life Care facility, Evergreen Nursing Home. Accompanying her was her son Alvin Lujan, who purported to act as Estella Lujan's legal representative, completing all of the admission paperwork. (Estella Lujan had been admitted to Evergreen a year earlier but discharged. During that earlier admission, because of her dementia, doctors determined that she was unable to make her own decisions. Doctors suggested that the family appoint a healthcare proxy, but the record does not indicate whether that was done on the previous admission.)

During her October 2006 admission, Estella Lujan died. Estella Lujan's daughter Kathryn Lujan, as representative of Estella Lujan estate, filed a lawsuit against Life Care Centers claiming, among other things, wrongful death due to a felonious killing. (The actual events surrounding Estella Lujan's death were not part of the trial transcripts.)

In response to the lawsuit, Evergreen moved to have the case dismissed because of a mandatory arbitration agreement that

had been signed by Alvin Lujan, as legal representative of Estella Lujan, as part of the admission paperwork in October 2006.

ISSUE: The issue that this court struggled with in this case was "whether Alvin Lujan, purportedly acting as a healthcare proxy, had the authority to enter into an arbitration agreement on behalf of Mrs. Lujan." They additionally had to decide "whether a decision to agree to arbitrate is a "medical treatment decision" that can be made by a healthcare proxy.

RULE: The court concluded that Alvin Lujan did not have the authority to enter into an agreement on behalf of Estella Lujan. In addition, they determined that a decision to arbitrate is not a "medical treatment decision" that can be decided by a healthcare proxy.

EMPHASIS: The importance of this case demonstrates what authority a healthcare proxy has and what type of decisions this individual can make. The court, in its written opinion stated: "The person selected to act as the patient's health care proxy should be the person who has a close relationship with the patient and who is most likely to be currently informed of the patient's wishes regarding medical treatment decisions." But that authority is limited to making medical decisions only.

is not the case. A DNR order only excludes the specific measures that are designated by the patient. While we will not perform CPR or defibrillate a patient, in accordance with a DNR order, we will continue to provide comfort measures and pain relief to those in need. As healthcare providers, we can do a lot to educate the public regarding DNR orders and to ensure people that we will continue to provide compassionate care to their loved ones.

Hospice

There may come a time when we have done all that we can for patients. Even though there may not be a cure for a patient's medical condition, there are still things that we can do to alleviate their pain and suffering by offering **hospice** services.

In hospitals, the care that we provide to patients is guided by their medical condition. But with hospice, the focus is no longer on their condition, but on patients and their families. The hospice philosophy approaches patient care by determining what we can do to alleviate the pain and suffering of the patient and of the patient's family in their loved one's final days. Instead of working toward a cure of the patient's disease using curative care, **palliative** care is provided instead.

The largest part of providing palliative care to hospice patients is with pain medication. The amount and quantity of pain medication that may be given to a hospice patient far exceeds what we would normally allow a patient to receive. The delicate balance that hospice workers have to maintain is between providing enough pain medication to relieve suffering without giving too much that it will hasten the patient's death.

Euthanasia

There are many medical conditions that cause patients to experience severe pain, both physically and psychologically. Sometimes, when the pain gets to be more than a patient can endure, the patient may seek out **euthanasia** as an alternative to end his or her suffering.

The problems associated with euthanasia are multifaceted. Are we allowing patients to commit suicide? Are we giving up on patients at a time when they need us the most? When should a person be able to decide that enough is enough? Should we only allow patients to die naturally, even though it means suffering in pain?

There are two different types of euthanasia; active euthanasia and passive euthanasia—each of which can be performed either voluntarily or involuntarily (see Graph 11-3).

Active and Passive Euthanasia

When most people think of euthanasia, they are thinking about active euthanasia. With active euthanasia, a person performs an action that causes or hastens a person's death. An example of active euthanasia is a person administering a lethal dose of medication. The key to active euthanasia is a person performing a particular action. And while active euthanasia may be what most people think about when they think of end of life assistance, there is another kind of euthanasia, called passive euthanasia. With passive euthanasia, a person does not perform particular actions, when such actions might be required, thus causing the death of another person. An example of passive euthanasia is not performing CPR when a person's heart stops. (Not performing CPR on a person with a valid DNR order is not passive euthanasia. Not performing CPR on a person who does not have a DNR order is passive euthanasia.)

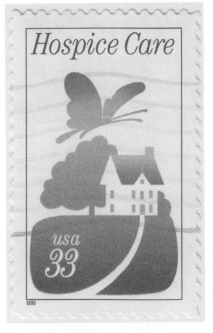

akva/Shutterstock

hospice: an ideology related to caring for patients and their families when facing the end of life

palliative: an approach to patient care where comfort measures and pain relief are provided instead of trying to cure a patient's disease or medical condition

euthanasia: the ending of a person's life either voluntarily or involuntary, either by taking measures to end that person's life or not performing measures that would save the person's life

The Law of Ethics

For-Profit Hospice

Initially, hospice facilities were run by volunteers and nonprofit agencies. But after Medicare and Medicaid provided reimbursement for the services provided by hospice facilities, most healthcare institutions and insurance companies developed their own hospice facilities.

- Should healthcare institutions be able to profit of a patient's death?
- What do you think about for-profit end of life services?

TABLE 11-1

With the Two Different Types of Euthanasia, There are Four Possibilities:

	Active	Passive
Voluntary	The patient consents to taking measures that will end life.	The patient consents to not receiving treatment should he or she expire.
Involuntary	Measures are taken to cause the patient's death without the patient's consent.	Without the patient's consent, no action is taken to save the patient's life, although action is required.

Laurin Rinder/Shutterstock

📍 Understanding Your State

Some states have passed laws allowing physician assisted suicide; others have decriminalized certain actions. To find out what your state requires, check out the companion website.

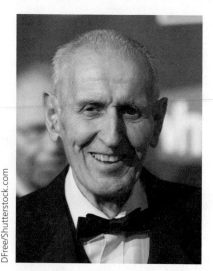

DFree/Shutterstock.com

Fig. 11-2. Dr. Jack Kevorkian, who passed away on June 3, 2011, was an advocate for physician-assisted suicide and death with dignity. Dr. Kevorkian admitted to helping 130 patients end their lives.

grief: bereavement; an emotional response to loss

Voluntary and Involuntary Euthanasia

Sometimes patients will request healthcare workers to perform euthanasia, by either providing them with lethal doses of medication or turning off alarms. The focus of voluntary and involuntary euthanasia is whether the patient consents to the euthanasia or not. With voluntary euthanasia, the patient is consenting to euthanasia. With involuntary euthanasia, the patient is not consenting to euthanasia.

Death With Dignity Laws

While many states have tried to pass euthanasia laws, only two have been successful, Oregon and Washington. These two states allow a physician to prescribe medications for their patients to take that will end their life (see Fig. 11-2). But before a physician can prescribe the medication, specific criteria must be met. The person requesting physician assisted suicide must be:

- at least 18 years of age.
- a resident of the state (something that requires a minimum of living in the state for at least six months).
- able to make healthcare decisions for themselves. (This requirement sometimes requires a psychiatric examination in order to be sure that a patient is competent to make decisions.)
- diagnosed with a terminal condition that will cause death within six months.

Even though some states have not passed Death With Dignity laws, some have decriminalized certain types of euthanasia when it is performed in specific situations. In other states, participating in euthanasia in any form is considered a felony and punishable by the state's criminal statutes.

The Grieving Process

In her 1969 book *On Death and Dying*, Dr. Elisabeth Kübler-Ross identified five different emotional stages that people undergo as they cope with the dying process. By identifying the five different stages of **grief**, healthcare providers

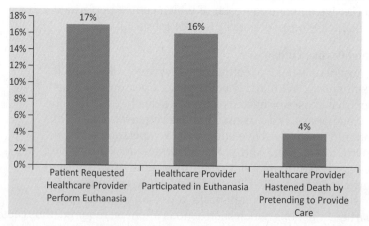

Graph 11-3. In 1996, Dr. David Ash mailed surveys to 1,600 critical care nurses; 852 responded stating that they worked in adult critical care. Of those surveyed: 141 reported that they had received requests to perform euthanasia, 129 reported that they had participated in euthanasia (active), and 35 reported that they had hastened a patient's death by only pretending to provide life-saving measures (passive).

Court Case

People v. Gregory Messenger

No. 9467694FH Ingham County Circuit Court (1995)

FACTS: On February 8, 1994, Traci Messenger went into labor. At only 25 weeks gestation Traci was taken to the local hospital, where doctors administered medication to halt her labor so that the child would not be born prematurely. Neonatologist Dr Padmani Karna was called in for a consultation. Dr Karna informed the Messengers that if the child were to be born at 25 weeks, that it had a 30–50 percent chance of survival, and if the child did survive, it had a 90 percent chance of having some degree of mental retardation and physical impairment.

The Messengers testified that they informed Dr. Karna that if the child was born, they did not want resuscitative measures performed, nor did they want the child placed on life support. Dr. Karna testified that she told the Messengers that if the child was born, that it was better to evaluate the child first to determine if any defects existed before making any decisions regarding resuscitation and life support.

Later that evening, Traci had a reaction to one of the medications that she had received to halt her labor. When the medication was stopped, Traci's labor began to advance again. Traci was rushed to surgery, where a baby boy was delivered by cesarean section at 11:38 p.m.

A NICU physician's assistant, who was present in the operating room, testified that she was instructed By Dr. Karna not to initiate resuscitation unless the child looked "vigorous." That because the child "appeared a deep purple color and limp" that she initiated resuscitative measures. The child was brought to the NICU on a ventilator. At 12:10 am, when Gregory Messenger arrived at the hospital, he was surprised to learn that, against his and his wife's wishes, that their child had been placed on life support. Dr. Karna arrived at the hospital at 12:20 a.m., and performed a series of test to determine the lung function of the child. Dr. Karna testified that at that time the child was pink and that the baby looked good.

When Traci Messenger returned from the recovery room, she and her husband requested some time alone with their child. Shortly afterward, Gregory Messenger unhooked the ventilator and placed their child in his wife's arms. Despite the ventilator alarming, no NICU staff intervened. The child died shortly thereafter.

Upon investigating the incident, Ingham County Prosecutors decided to charge Gregory Messenger with manslaughter.

ISSUE: Did Gregory Messenger commit manslaughter by removing his child from life support, allowing him to die?

RULE: Gregory Messenger was acquitted (found not guilty) of manslaughter charges. (The Messengers filed a civil lawsuit claiming negligence against the hospital and doctors. The jury returned a verdict of not guilty in that case as well.)

EMPHASIS: This interesting court case presents several different issues. One of the more interesting facts of this case, which adds a different dynamic, is that Gregory Messenger is not only a caring husband and father, but he is also a medical doctor. Dr. Gregory Messenger holds a license to practice medicine in the state of Michigan, and works as a dermatologist.

can offer the assistance that patients and their family members need when dealing with the grieving process.

The five stages of grief identified by Dr. Kübler-Ross are: denial, anger, bargaining, depression, and acceptance (see Fig. 11-3). By coming to terms with their grief, Dr. Kübler-Ross believes patients can lead more fulfilling lives, even if only for a short period of time. (Although the stages of grief were initially associated with the dying process, it has since been adopted for any form of stress or loss that a person may be undergoing.)

Denial

The initial stage of grief exhibited by people coping with loss is the denial phase. In the denial phase, people psychologically try to block the stressor. They are denying the existence of the stressor, hoping to remove it. In the case

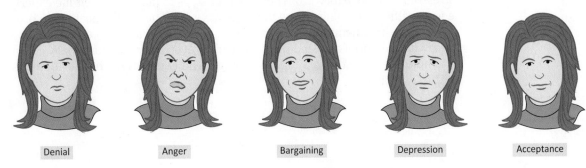

Denial   Anger   Bargaining   Depression   Acceptance

Fig. 11-3. The five stages of grief are denial, anger, bargaining, depression, and acceptance.

of terminal illness, a person might dispute a diagnosis or the accuracy of the test results. Another example is a parent who, not wanting to deal with the issue, disregards evidence that his or her child might be a homosexual. For the most part, the denial phase is short-lived, as evidence of the stressor remains despite the person's attempt to remove it.

Anger

The anger stage of grief is directly correlated to the impact the stressor has on the person. But instead of dealing with it internally, the emotion is expressed outwardly toward other people or objects. By expressing anger, the person is attempting to remove the stressor in hopes of eliminating grief. Because the expression of anger does not remove the grief or stressor, the person may become stuck in this phase. The person may direct his or her anger to other things or people, hoping to find the right avenue to release pent-up grief. For healthcare providers, this stage can be especially difficult because they may be the recipient of a patients' anger. But knowing that it exists and how to identify it will help us to respond to this stage appropriately.

Bargaining

The bargaining stage of grief is a person's attempt to find a way out. In the bargaining phase, a person will give something up (such as smoking or eating chocolate) in exchange for removal of the stressor. A common example is someone praying, "If you take this cancer away, I'll start going to church every Sunday." The problem that people encounter with bargaining is that even when they give something up, the grief or stressor remains. This may cause the patient to regress into the anger phase of grief, because the bargaining did not work. Or people may get stuck in the bargaining phase as they try giving up several different things in hopes of finding the one thing that will remove the stressor. But typically, after a few attempts, people realize that regardless of their behavior, the grief or stressor remains.

Depression

As the realization of the stressor, and the inability to remove it, starts to sink in, people enter the depression stage. This is the one stage that most people have difficulty escaping, and the one that causes the most concern. When entering the depression phase, people are coming to the realization that there is nothing that they can do to remove the stressor. The realization of the inevitable leads some people to believe that there is no hope. Of main concern for healthcare providers, regarding patients in the depression phase, is to monitor for signs of suicidal ideation. This is because as patients realize that the grief or stressor is not going to go away, they may try to take steps to end their suffering early.

Acceptance

The acceptance stage of grief is achieved when people are able to accept their stressors and move forward. They will take steps to maximize their life experiences, with the remaining time that they have left. The goal of healthcare providers is help patients move toward acceptance, so that they can adequately deal with their grief and lead productive lives, even if they are terminally ill. An example of acceptance is a cancer survivor who educates the public about his or her experiences.

Make FALSE statements TRUE.

Rewrite the false statements below by replacing the bolded, italicized, and underlined word(s) to make it a true statement.

1. The key difference between actual death and clinical death is whether there is ***treatable*** cessation of circulatory, respiratory, or brain function.

    _____

2. The Uniform Anatomical Gift Act, among other things, provides a list of people who can make decisions regarding ***who a patient's healthcare proxy will be.***

    _____

3. A living will is a type of ***DNR order.***

    _____

4. Under hospice, a patient is provided with ***curative*** care.

    _____

5. The stage of grief that raises a concern about suicide is ***bargaining***.

    _____

Circle Exercise

Circle the correct word from the choices given.

1. In (**clinical death, euthanasia, actual death**) the body has ceased to function.

2. To combat some of the growing ethical issues related to organ donation, Congress passed (**NOTA, UNOS, OPTN**).

3. Utilizing the law of intestacy, a patient's (**children, spouse, parents**) are given first priority.

4. There are four different types of (**living wills, euthanasia, DNR orders**).

5. Some states that do not have Death with Dignity laws consider euthanasia as a (**felony, misdemeanor, civil law**).

Matching

Match the numbered term to its lettered definition.

1. _____ advance directives
2. _____ DNR
3. _____ euthanasia
4. _____ grief
5. _____ healthcare proxy
6. _____ hospice
7. _____ intestacy
8. _____ living will
9. _____ palliative

A. the division of property by descent and distribution, for individuals who die without a will.

B. any document that provides instructions for patient care that is made by a patient before he or she becomes incapacitated.

C. a document detailing the situations and type of medical care a patient desires.

D. a person designated to make medical decisions for someone who is incapacitated.

E. an order written by the physician which indicates what medical treatments or procedures are not to be performed.

F. an ideology related to caring for patients and their families when facing the end of life.

G. an approach to patient care where comfort measures and pain relief are provided instead of trying to cure a patient's disease or medical condition.

H. the ending of person's life either voluntarily or involuntary, by taking measures to end that person's life or not performing measures that would save a person's life.

I. bereavement; an emotional response to loss.

Deliberations: Critical Thinking Questions

Question 1: Martha is a patient who has multiple medical problems. She has already received a kidney transplant, but is now in need of a liver transplant. Because Martha has already received one transplant organ, should she be able to receive another organ? Or, because she has received one organ already, should she be placed behind patients on the list who have not yet received an organ? Explain your answer.

Question 2: Robert accepted a job in a large corporation. As part of his benefits, he received free legal advice, which included drafting a living will. In the living will, Robert named his parents as his healthcare proxy. Years later, Robert got married and started to raise a family, but he never got around to changing his living will. Robert is involved in a car accident and has entered a persistent vegetative state. His parents and wife disagree about whether life support should be removed. Who should the court and healthcare team choose to make the medical decisions; Robert's parents or his wife? Explain your answer.

Question 3: Lance Armstrong is a cyclist who has won the Tour de France a record seven times. In 1996 Lance was diagnosed with testicular cancer that had metastasized to his brain and lungs. He underwent aggressive chemotherapy and treatment, and is now a cancer survivor. Go through the stages of grief and speculate as to how Lance may have dealt with each of the different phases of grief when dealing with his cancer diagnosis.

Question 4: In some states, if a person has been diagnosed with a terminal disease, a patient can be declared dead by registered nurses. In other states, only medical doctors are allowed to make the determination that someone has expired. What do you think? Should a registered nurse be allowed to declare someone dead? Why or why not? Explain your answer.

Question 5: A patient who has been diagnosed with a terminal illness has decided to enter hospice. Currently, as part of her treatment, she is receiving medications and intravenous fluids to support her blood pressure. Without these treatments, she would not remain conscious. While she has agreed to hospice, she has asked to have the IV fluids and medication continued, until her sister arrives from overseas so that she can say goodbye. Because the IV fluids and medication are considered curative, instead of palliative, the hospice facility declines to accept her. What are your thoughts? How are treatments categorized as curative and palliative? If you were the manager on this case, what would you do?

Closing Arguments: Case Analysis

Randy is a 42-year-old male who was diagnosed with HIV several years ago. He has been taking his medications, and his viral load is undetectable. But because of the medications, and combined kidney problems, Randy is now in need of a kidney transplant. Because of his HIV status and weakened immune system, Randy is not a candidate for a kidney transplant. But Randy has found a friend who is willing to donate a kidney to him.

Question 1: Should a living person who wants to donate an organ be able to decide whom that organ goes to? Or, when someone decides to make a living donation, should the organ go to the first person on the transplant list? Explain your answer.

Question 2: Due to an infection, Randy has been admitted to the hospital. Because of his condition, he has been talking to you about whether or not he should continue with his treatment. He asks that when you give him his medication, that you leave it on the bedside stand for him to take, instead of handing it to him directly. Is this a type of euthanasia, and if so what type? What stage of grief might Randy be in at this point?

Question 3: Randy's condition has gotten worse, and he has slipped into a coma. He continues to receive dialysis, but it is taking its toll on his body. Randy's partner of 15 years, Paul, arrives at the hospital with a copy of Randy's living will naming Paul as his healthcare proxy. Paul would like to stop the dialysis and allow Randy to die in peace. But Wanda, who Randy married right out of college and fathered a child with, arrives at the hospital. While Randy and Wanda have not lived together for 20 years, they were never legally separated or got a divorce. Wanda wants to continue dialysis and all other medical treatment. Who should be able to decide Randy's course of treatment? Explain your answer.

The Briefcase

This section repeats the objectives from the beginning of the chapter and provides a summary of the most important concepts for each objective. Use this section as a quick review and to check your understanding of the chapter key points.

Objective 1: Describe the difference between clinical death and actual death.

- Actual Death is the cessation of breathing, heartbeat, or brain activity.

- Clinical Death when the cessation of a patient's breathing, heartbeat, or brain activity is irreversible.

Objective 2: Explain how organ donation allocation works.
- A medical determination is made identifying a patient who needs an organ.
- The patient's application is given to the transplant team and if approved is provided to UNOS.
- UNOS adds the patient's name to a waiting list.
- If an organ becomes available, UNOS will determine what patients can receive that organ and notifies the hospital.

Objective 3: List the order of people that the courts use under the law of intestacy.
- See Figure 11-1 on pg. 174

Objective 4: Give an example of what an advance directive is.
- Living Will
- Healthcare Proxy
- DNR

Objective 5: Explain the difference between a living will and a healthcare proxy.
- A living will is a document, a healthcare proxy is a person.
- A living will describes what medical treatments will be provided and when they should not be provided. A healthcare proxy makes medical decision when a living will does not address issues or questions arise.
- A living will takes precedence over a healthcare proxy.

Objective 6: Determine what type of care will be provided when a doctor writes a DNR order.
- Typically excludes extraneous measures such as CPR, mechanical ventilation, and defibrillation.
- Does not mean Do Not Treat.
- Provides pain medication and comfort measures.

Objective 7: Describe the type of care a patient who enters hospice will receive.
- Hospice is a philosophy geared toward the patient and the patient's family.
- The goal of hospice is toward palliative care, focusing on pain and comfort instead of a cure.

Objective 8: Provide an example of the four different types of euthanasia.
- Active Voluntary Euthanasia
- Active Involuntary Euthanasia
- Passive Voluntary Euthanasia
- Passive Involuntary Euthanasia

Objective 9: List the stages of grief as identified by Dr. Kübler-Ross.
- Denial
- Anger
- Bargaining
- Depression
- Acceptance

Maximize Your Success with the Companion Website

The Companion Website to this textbook contains materials that can help you better understand the concepts presented in this chapter. Go to MyHealthProfessionsKit to access:

- Sample Quizzes
- Web Links
- Games
- and more…

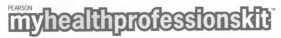

PEARSON
myhealthprofessionskit™

12 Uniqueness and Individuality

When taking care of patients, it helps sometimes to look at things from their perspective. There may be things that are important to them, that you may not be aware of until you place yourself in their shoes. In this chapter, we will discuss some of the unique components that make people individuals and how that uniqueness may impact the healthcare that you provide. Understanding what makes different people unique will help you to put your patient first.

MEASURE YOUR PROGRESS: LEARNING OBJECTIVES

After studying this chapter, you will be able to:

- Explain why it is important to understand the different healthcare needs of a diverse community.

- Identify the unique healthcare needs of a particular ethnic group.

- Describe some of the unique healthcare considerations of ethnic groups related to pregnancy and childbirth.

- Give an example of some of the philosophies concerning death and dying for particular ethnic groups.

- Identify the unique healthcare needs of a particular cultural group.

- Describe some of the unique healthcare considerations of different cultures related to pregnancy and childbirth.

- Give an example of some of the philosophies concerning death and dying for particular cultural groups.

- Identify the unique healthcare needs of different religions.

- Describe some of the unique healthcare considerations of different religions.

KEY TERMS

culture
ethnic
heritage
patriarchal
religion
shaman
talisman
wuzho / marime
yin yang

PROFESSIONAL HIGHLIGHT

Paul is a social worker at the local hospital in a large metropolitan city. A large percentage of the patient population at Paul's hospital is minorities, some of whom speak little to no English. In addition to the language barrier, some minorities have different approaches to healthcare. In order to provide the assistance that these patients need, and the healthcare professionals to provide that care, Paul needs to have an understanding of the different cultures and ethnicities that exist within his community.

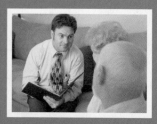

Lisa F. Young/Shutterstock

The world that we live in is a very diverse place. The United States developed from a melting pot of different people, which still continues today. There are a variety of different populations and groups, and subpopulations and subgroups, living throughout the United States. While each of these groups contribute to the diversity that makes up the United States, some groups have unique healthcare needs; or they may require different approaches to the delivery of healthcare than we are familiar with or normally provide. To further understand some of the unique needs of our diverse community, we can examine their needs based on three different, distinct categories: ethnicity, culture, and religion.

> I have heard that there are some religious groups that refuse certain medical treatments. Why would they rather die than receive medical care?

Ethnic Groups

One of the largest categories that make up the diverse world we live in are the different **ethnic** groups that make up the American population.

ethnic: a class or group of people that share a common race, nationality, culture, or religion

There are numerous ethnic groups around the world, far too many to discuss in this text. But there are some major ethnic groups that exist in the United States that you may encounter in your healthcare careers. Some members of these ethnic groups have unique healthcare considerations, views, and needs.

Native American

Throughout the United States and Canada, there are many different Native Americans. Some members of these groups do not classify themselves as Native Americans; instead they prefer to be called by their tribal name. There are currently over 700 different tribes in North America; the most populous are: Algonquian, Apache, Cherokee, Hopi, Iroquois, Lakota, Navajo, Pueblo, and Seminole.

Communication

There are some unique characteristics that you need to be aware of when communicating with some Native Americans. Any time that you address someone as a patient, you should do so by the name that they provide. While all Native Americans have a birth name, most also have a tribal name. If the patient provides a tribal name, then that is how you should refer to him or her. However, if a Native American patient does not offer a tribal name, it can be considered rude to ask for it.

While eye contact in Western civilization is considered proper etiquette, in some Native American cultures it can be an indication of aggression or disrespect. Therefore eye contact should be avoided when speaking to Native Americans, especially to members of the opposite sex.

While most Native Americans speak English, some do not. If you need an interpreter, you should always use a member of the same sex; even if that means going outside of the family circle.

> **Ethics Alert!** An inherent problem associated with the use of interpreters is whether a person is giving actual consent or not. The first step that you have to take when using an interpreter is to ensure that the patient is giving consent to the use of an interpreter. Most healthcare institutions have specific policies regarding the use of interpreters and who can serve as an interpreter. There are also paid services available where an interpreter for any language can be obtained at any time during the day, typically through telephone services.

Patient Care

Native American tribes have a long history of tradition, which includes a variety of different ceremonies. Some tribes have specific ceremonies and rituals that are performed when any body part or tissue is removed. This can include amputated extremities, organs (such as a gallbladder or appendix), products of conception (afterbirth), or even hair. If anything is going to be removed from the body of a Native American patient, you should ask the patient if they want those items returned to them—if you are medically allowed to do so—before such items are discarded. As an example of an important keepsake, some Native American women will place their child's dried umbilical cord in a

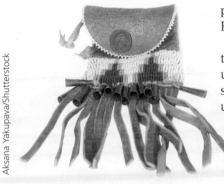

Fig. 12-1. A Native American amulet. It is filled with items that hold unique and/or special meanings to the person wearing it, thought to ward off evils spirits and bring good luck.

talisman: an object, usually worn around the neck, that is believed to contain spirits or mystical or supernatural powers

shaman: a medical and spiritual advisor and mediator between the human world and spirit world

pouch that they wear around their neck, known as an amulet or **talisman** (see Fig. 12-1).

Talismans are thought to provide guidance to an individual's spirit and protection from evil. Talismans should not be removed from Native Americans unless it is absolutely necessary. If removal is medically required, the patient should be informed beforehand, as he or she may want to designate a person, usually an elder, who will hold it until it can be returned.

Pain management can be difficult for some Native American patients. Since pain can be seen as a sign of weakness, some Native Americans will not admit that they are having pain—even if they are asked about it directly. Instead of admitting pain, they may tell a story about a friend, neighbor, or animal that experienced pain during battle or on a hunt. This may be an indirect way of informing healthcare providers that they are experiencing pain themselves.

Planning medical care for some Native Americans can present unique problems as well. In the healthcare environment, we typically utilize specific time frames to provide care; for example, taking medication every eight hours, or three times a day. Some Native Americans do not utilize the same concept of time that Western civilization does, and may not wear watches or own clocks. For this reason, special planning may need to be implemented for Native American patients. For example, telling a patient to take their medication at sunrise, when the sun reaches the high point in the sky, and when the sun sets, rather than at specified hours, will satisfy the medical need to take medications on a certain schedule.

Many Native Americans do not make medical decisions without first consulting their **shaman**.

A shaman is a medical and spiritual advisor that acts as a mediator between the human world and spirit world. If a patient consults with a shaman, the shaman may want to perform ceremonies or rituals for the patient. These ceremonies may include the use of herbs, roots, or the burning of incense. While we want to allow what ceremonies we can, we have to be cautious about how they will affect the medical care that we provide and the environment in which they are performed. For example, we cannot allow the burning of incense in a patient's room because of the existence of oxygen and other flammable materials. But is there a way to remove the patient from that environment to one where incense can be burned? Additionally, if herbs or roots are to be ingested as part of a ceremony, we may need to check to see if there will be any interaction with the medication that a patient may be taking.

Pregnancy and Childbirth

In the 1970s, the department of Indian Health Services received complaints about Native American women who had been sterilized against their will. Because of this fear some Native American women are reluctant to undergo any type of surgery involving the abdominal cavity, especially Cesarean sections. In addition, because of the fear of forced sterilization, some Native America women prefer to deliver their children at home instead of at a hospital.

According to some Native American customs, the mother and child should remain indoors until the child's umbilical cord falls off. Having the umbilical cord still attached is thought to provide an entryway for evil spirits to enter the body. After the umbilical cord falls off, it should be given to the mother, because it is thought to have special spiritual value and is typically placed in the woman's amulet. The umbilical cord should never be discarded without a mother's permission.

Death and Dying

The attitudes toward death and dying of Native Americans have traditionally centered on their close relationship with nature and their strong belief in the

Aksana Yakupava/Shutterstock

Ethics Case

Department of Indian Health Services and Forced Sterilization

United States (1960s–1970s)

FACTS: In the early 1970s, the department of Indian Health Services (IHS) received complaints that Native American women were being sterilized without their consent or knowledge. One complaint detailed a 26-year-old Native American woman who had entered the office of Dr. Pinkerton-Uri requesting a "womb transplant." The woman stated that she had received a complete hysterectomy six years earlier when she was being treated for alcoholism, but was told that the procedure was reversible. Another complaint was received indicating that two young Native American women, who had undergone appendectomies, had tubal ligations performed as well without their knowledge or consent.

ISSUE: Were IHS physicians performing sterilization procedures on Native American women without their consent?

RULE: A final report on the investigation was issued in November 1976. The reported detailed that their investigation was unable to verify that forced sterilization had occurred. The report did discover that IHS had not followed the appropriate procedures for obtaining consent and the forms that were being used to obtain consent did not adhere to the Department of Health, Education and Welfare standards.

EMPHASIS: When the final report was published it was highly criticized. The main focus of criticism focused on how information was gathered. At one IHS hospital, sterilization procedures were contracted to outside resources. Therefore, the number of sterilization cases reported for that hospital was zero, which critics claim impacted the statistics and altered the final numbers and outcome. The investigation and report remain controversial.

---

spirit world. Accordingly, members of many Native American tribes perform elaborate ceremonies upon death to help the body's spirit ascend into the spirit world. But members of some Native American tribes, such as the Apache and Navajo of the Southwest, fear death and view spirits as ghosts, something that should be avoided. For those tribe members, if they are notified that a person has died or that death is imminent, they do not console or visit the patient and will abruptly leave the area. While this avoidance may seem cold and callous to Western civilization, some tribes believe that if they are present when the spirit leaves the body that spirit might follow and haunt them.

Hispanic

The word *Hispanic* is used to describe an individual with Mexican, Cuban, Central American, or Puerto Rican heritage.

In many of the native countries that contribute to the Hispanic population, there is a definitive separation of socioeconomic classes. In most Hispanic countries the largest portion of the population lives at or below the poverty level. Living at this socioeconomic level, most cannot afford traditional medical care, which may have contributed to some of the special attitudes and beliefs that some Hispanics have toward healthcare.

heritage: attributes that are inherited or passed on from previous generations

Communication

One of the major influences in the Hispanic population is the strong sense of respect (*respeto*) for authority. This is thought to have arisen from the great disparity between the socioeconomic class structures. Any time that they interact with strangers or authority figures, they adhere to strict social etiquette, such as standing up when a person enters the room, preferring formal introductions using the proper title (*Senor, Senora,* or *Senorita*), and perhaps avoiding direct eye contact so as not to appear confrontational or intrusive. While handshaking is a welcome sign of respect, touching by strangers is unwelcome and can cause stress, discomfort, and embarrassment to some.

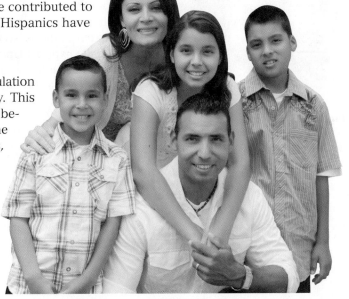

© Andy Dean/Alamy

Patient Care

Some Hispanics have a unique and interesting view of health and disease, which can directly affect the delivery of patient care. Following a belief with origins in folk medicine, some Hispanics believe that diseases fall into one of two categories, either hot or cold. It is thought that this belief stems from natural forces whereby heat (such as a fever) can be balanced by something cold (such as water). If a disease has been classified as a hot disease, it requires a cold treatment. Similarly, a disease thought of as being a cold disease requires a hot treatment in order to bring balance to the body.

The difficulty for healthcare providers occurs when medical treatments are contrary to this temperature classification. For example, pneumonia is thought of as a cold disease and therefore requires a hot treatment. But medical treatments for pneumonia, such as liquid medications, intravenous fluids, or increased fluid intake are seen as cold treatments. Therefore, some Hispanic patients may suspect that these cold treatments will not work in resolving their cold disease. This viewpoint can not only lead to noncompliance with medical treatment, but also to a negative perception about the competency of the healthcare worker who is providing care.

Pregnancy and Childbirth

Not all Hispanics have view pregnancy and childbirth as something that requires medical care. While the importance of prenatal care is growing within the Hispanic population, it is typically done through a community midwife or with a known healthcare provider (such as a general practitioner instead of an obstetrician or gynecologist).

During pregnancy, many Hispanic women remain very active. Part of this belief stems from an old Hispanic wives' tale that inactivity may cause the child to stick to internal organs. By remaining active, the mother may believe the child is allowed to move freely in the amniotic fluid and will not adhere to her insides. While activity in pregnancy is encouraged, we also have to be concerned about overactivity and potential harm to the fetus. Some Hispanic women will try to remain active even during the onset of labor and may have difficulty lying in a hospital bed to deliver their child.

Death and Dying

In most Hispanic populations, death is a very spiritual time. Many Hispanics prefer to die at home, rather than in a hospital. Part of this belief comes from the desire to be around extended family that can help care for the dying patient. In addition, it is believed that a person needs to die in familiar surroundings, so that their soul does not become lost when the patient actually expires. Upon death, the body is respected and must remain intact. Although attitudes are changing within Hispanic cultures, some do not allow organ donation or cremation. In addition, some family members view autopsies as intruding on the body and may disagree with one being performed.

Asian

As with Hispanic heritage, many different countries contribute to Asian heritage, including China, Japan, Korea, Vietnam, and other nations that make up Southeast Asia. These countries are some of the oldest civilizations in the history of the world. One underlying principle seen throughout Asian countries is the concept of **yin yang** (commonly referred to in Western society as yin and yang; see Fig. 12-2).

Yin yang is an expression of opposites, but also how those opposites are intertwined and closely related to each other throughout all aspects of nature,

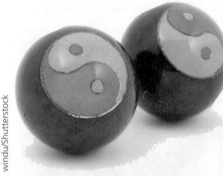

windu/Shutterstock

Fig. 12-2. Boading balls with an image of yin yang on them. Boading balls are also referred to as medicine balls or meditation balls.

yin yang: a belief in how opposites are related to and dependent on each other in all aspects of life

life, and philosophy. When disease or illness occurs, it is thought to be an imbalance of yin yang. Restoring the balance of yin yang lies at the heart of some traditional Asian medical thoughts and practices.

Communication

Eye contact and touching is very common among family members, but not with strangers. While some Asians may appear shy, especially at first; this shyness is really a sign of respect that is given to complete strangers. When talking with someone new they may not only avoid direct eye contact, but will typically keep a slight distance so as not to intrude into a person's personal space. Once properly introduced, the amount of eye contact will increase and the amount of distance will decrease as the stranger becomes more familiar and comfortable.

Patient Care

As in Hispanic cultures, respect for others is revered among individuals of Asian heritage. This respect is not only given to others but something that is expected in return. Showing respect toward people of Asian heritage can present problems during healthcare examinations because they may view too many questions as being intrusive and a sign of disrespect. In addition, physical examinations need to be performed with as much dignity and privacy as possible. Individuals of Asian heritage may be reluctant to discuss potentially embarrassing bodily functions or problems. Because of this, talking to other family members may be necessary in order to find out what symptoms a patient has. Because of the patients' modesty, the use of interpreters should be limited to family members if at all possible, instead of using strangers.

Pregnancy and Childbirth

Stemming from long tradition, contemporary Asians still follow some age-old customs associated with pregnancy. For example, some Asian women avoid animals while pregnant based on fear that their child will be born looking like any animal they encounter.

Asian women were traditionally expected to be stoic and complacent. This behavior may still be expected of many women of Asian heritage today, especially those who follow older, traditional customs and practices. However, childbirth is an exception whereby women are allowed to outwardly express their emotions. Being allowed to do so, some may have an augmented expression of pain, giving the indication that that they are either in a lot of pain or have a low pain threshold during childbirth.

Asian men do not traditionally play a role in the delivery process; instead female members of the extended family often tend to the mother and child.

Death and Dying

There are different attitudes toward death and dying in the Asian culture. Some believe that death should occur in a hospital so as not to infect the home. Others believe that death should occur at home so that the spirit is not lost. But despite this difference, there are some common beliefs following death shared by most Asians. After an Asian patient has passed, family members (mostly the women) will bathe the body after death. This practice is seen as restoring the yin yang of the body before it transcends into the afterlife. In addition, some Asian people believe that the body must remain intact after death and are strongly opposed to having an autopsy performed or discussing organ donation.

Romani/Gypsy

The Romani people are widely scattered throughout North America and Europe. While there exact origin is unknown, they are thought to have evolved from Romania via migration from medieval India. They are commonly referred to as Gypsies, a name that comes from the Greek word *gifti*. Even though the name Gypsy can carry negative or prejudicial connotations, many refer to themselves as Gypsies instead of Romani.

The traditional family structure of Gypsies is fluid, whereby children belong to the group and not necessarily to an individual mother or father. These groups are commonly referred to as clans and can encompass what Western society would classify as a nuclear family. Gypsy cultures have a **patriarchal** system, with a central male figure. The patriarch is usually the oldest male in the group, and serves as the clan's elder, father, and unofficial leader.

The word *patriarch* is a combination of the Greek word *pater* (meaning father) and *archon* (meaning leader).

In Gypsy culture, girls are often married at a very young age, either to young boys or even older men. Women's roles within the Gypsy culture are typically subservient, limited to tending to children and taking care of the men's needs. Most Gypsies typically live a nomadic life, traveling throughout the country visiting different areas and other Gypsy clans (see Fig. 12-3).

Communication

Most Gypsies are very dynamic people, and have what can appear to be an almost exaggerated communication style. While this style may appear to be aggressive or confrontational, to Gypsies, shouting is often used as a form of affection. They believe that the strength of the display of their emotion is as equally important as what is said.

Because of the strong patriarchal family unit, the oldest male usually speaks for everyone in the clan, especially when interacting with outsiders. This male leader will typically be consulted prior to anyone making any decisions, and his wishes are usually followed or the others face ostracism from the clan. Of concern for healthcare providers is whether an elder is making a decision that may be contrary to what the patient wants or what is in the patient's best interest. As healthcare workers, therefore, we have to be cautious about decisions that are made and ensure that we are upholding the wishes of the patient without violating their social structure.

Patient Care

Gypsies also have a unique view of the world, which has a direct impact on patient care. Gypsies view things as being either pure (which they call **wuzho**) or impure (referred to as **marime**).

This expression of pure and impure affects every aspect of life for Gypsies, including the body and bodily functions. For example, anything related to the upper body is considered pure—wuzho; and anything related to the lower body is considered impure—marime. Because the upper body is considered pure, Gypsies, men and women alike, tend not to be bashful about exposing their torso. Bodily functions that originate from the upper body, such as vomiting and spitting, are not something they are ashamed of or embarrassed by because it comes from the wuzho. In contrast, anything related to the lower body, such as urination, defecation, or reproduction, is considered impure—marime—which they are very modest and shameful about. Any examination of the lower body or discussion of physiology related to the lower body should only be done by a member of the same sex, if possible.

Like some Native Americans, some Gypsies will wear an amulet or talisman. Gypsies believe that these amulets protect them from evil and disease and bring them good luck. While amulets can be removed, they should be kept close to the patient's head and never below the waist (because of the separation of the wuzho and marime). It is believed by some that by

---

patriarchal: a society or group, usually of an extended family, that is led by a dominant male

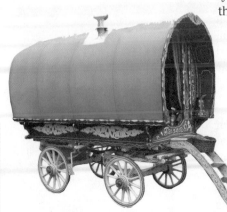

daseaford/Shutterstock

Fig. 12-3. A traditional, horse-drawn, Gypsy trailer. Early Gypsy travel consisted of multiple trailers, in a type of caravan. Although Gypsies still travel in large groups, today they utilize motor homes and recreational vehicles.

wuzho / marime: belief that things are pure or impure

Sidebar

Some Gypsies take the separation of purity and wuzho / marime very seriously. Clothes worn on the upper body are never washed together with clothes from the lower body in the same container or machine at the same time. In addition, men's clothes are usually not washed together with women's clothes and children's clothes are washed separately from adult clothes.

placing an amulet at the feet, or at the foot of the bed, will cause it to become impure and therefore lose its significance.

Because of their communication style, Gypsies are not shy about expressing pain. It is common for Gypsy patients to moan out loud with even the slightest amount of pain. The volume and amount of moaning will increase as the pain increases. This presents a unique challenge for healthcare professionals in regard to providing adequate pain control. Gypsies may be seen as needing large amounts of pain medication for what might be considered minor pain.

Pregnancy and Childbirth

At one time, Gypsies were reluctant to seek prenatal care with medical practitioners, utilizing instead Gypsy midwives. But with the increasing number of women doctors available to examine the expectant mother, that is rapidly changing.

When Gypsy women deliver their child, they are considered impure, because they have come in contact with bodily fluids from the lower half of the body. (Note: The child is not impure because it is carried above the waist—or in the wuzho portion of the body.) After childbirth, the mother will remain impure for nine days following the delivery and cannot have contact with men, or be involved in food preparation or cleaning. Gypsies have increasingly preferred hospital births because the hospital disposes of unclean materials and frequently changes linens, shortening the impure period following delivery.

While most families celebrate a delivery and invite friends and loved ones to see the child, Gypsies believe that children are very vulnerable to evil spirits, specifically what is sometimes referred as the "evil eye," or a glance thought capable of inflicting harm. Therefore, Gypsies rarely want anyone to look at their newborn and may ask that the child's face be covered by a cloth during their stay in the hospital, and that the cloth should only be removed by the mother.

Death and Dying

Just prior to a person's death is an important time for Gypsies, because their beliefs require that certain actions be carried out. When a person is thought to be dying, some Gypsies will place a guard at the window to chase away evil spirits. Usually this task falls to the older women of the clan who take turns guarding the window 24 hours a day until death occurs. The guards will remain after death until a cleansing ritual has been performed on the body.

During the dying process, friends and family members will typically gather and watch the person die with very little interaction. Some Gypsies believe that a person's last actions and words hold special meaning, and can provide insight as to what will happen to the dying person's spirit. Once a person has passed away, the deceased's family typically wants the body embalmed immediately, as the process of embalming is seen as cleansing of the blood and can help chase away any evil spirits. Because they believe that evil spirits can remain with the body until it is cleansed, Gypsies are typically not open to discussions about organ donation and are rarely themselves the recipients of organ donations.

Amish

Over disagreement with the Mennonite church, Jakob Ammann established the Amish church in 1693. The descendants of those that followed Jakob make up the Amish population that, for the most part, live in North America. The Amish lead a very simple life, and are reluctant to adopt "modern" ways of living. They do not have electricity, drive cars, or have other modern

Sidebar

The terms transgender and transsexual are often confused or used interchangeably; either of which can be correct. Typically, however, the word transsexual is used for a person who is undergoing or has undergone the surgery needed to change their sex. The word transgender is used for a person who does not wish to, or has not yet, had the sex reassignment surgery.

Sidebar
In 2010, President Barack Obama signed an executive order requiring all healthcare institutions that receive Medicare or Medicaid to have a policy in place whereby gay and lesbian patients are allowed to determine who can visit them in the hospital and receive medical information.

culture: a group of people that share common beliefs, traits, race, values, goals, or attitudes

Fig. 12-4. John Cameron Mitchell wrote a successful off-Broadway musical (later made into a feature film) called *Hedwig and the Angry Inch*. The title comes from a botched sex-change operation the main character Hedwig underwent, leaving her with a one-inch mound of flesh as her genitals.

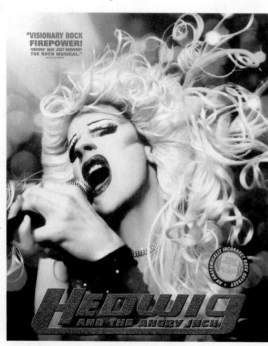

conveniences. There is usually only one phone, typically located at the community church, which only elders can use if communication with the outside world is necessary. The church is the center of the Amish community, and any contact with the outside world requires permission from the church elders.

The Amish believe that God is a healer and rarely seek outside medical assistance. The Amish do not believe in birth control, and will generally have large families. The Amish also prefer to die at home rather than bringing sick loved ones to a hospital.

Culture

The notion of **culture** differs from that of ethnicity, in that culture relates to a social group rather than a geographical classification.

While ethnic groups may share a similar culture, there are many subcultures that exist across ethnic groups. For example, homosexuality is a distinct culture that is seen in a small percentage of every ethnic group.

Lesbian, Gay, Bisexual, and Transgender (LGBT)

Although an exact figure is hard to obtain, some reports say that the LGBT community makes up 10 percent of the U.S. population. Part of the difficulty in coming up with an exact number relates to the fact that some may not want to openly admit that they are lesbian, gay, or bisexual, especially when asked by strangers.

Communication

Depending on the facet of the LGBT community you are dealing with, there are distinct communication practices that you need to be aware of. Most gays and lesbians who are in committed relationships refer to their loved one as their partner. Or if they are married—even though that marriage may not be recognized—they might refer to their loved one as their spouse. (Gay men will refer to their spouse as their husband and lesbian females will refer to their spouse as their wife. It is considered inappropriate to refer to a male as a wife or a female as a husband.)

Another communication concern relates to transgender patients. Transgendered persons believe that they are psychologically the opposite of what their anatomical gender is. Transgender people may prefer to be addressed, not by their anatomical gender, but what they consider to be their psychological gender. An anatomical male who lives as a female may prefer to be called Ms. instead of Mr., and may give a female name instead of a birth name (see Fig. 12-4).

Patient Care

Even though some states have approved same-sex marriages, or an equivalent to marriage known as a civil union; same-sex marriages are not legally recognized in all states or by the federal government. It is the legality of these relationships that lies at the heart of patient care concerns of the LGBT community.

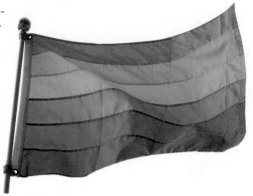

Any time that patients are unable to make medical decisions themselves, the law is very specific about who can make medical decisions for them. Only legally recognized individuals, such as a spouse, parent, or sibling, are allowed to intervene on the patient's behalf and make medical decisions. But for LGBT people, this presents unique problems. For example, suppose a lesbian woman is involved in a car accident and is in a coma. The woman's partner of 10 years arrives at the hospital and requests visitation and information. Since some LGBT people do not have a legally recognized relationship, can hospital personnel deny her visitation rights and refuse to tell her anything about her partner's medical condition? While attitudes have changed in recent years, in the past, members of the LGBT community experienced great difficulty in visiting loved ones in the hospital or ascertaining information.

Pregnancy and Childbirth

Many gay and lesbian couples desire to have children, but some states do not allow unmarried people to adopt children. Some states even go as far as to specifically forbid gay and lesbians the right to adopt. For those who desired to have biological children of their own, it was common to work within the LGBT community. For example, gay men would enter into surrogacy contracts with lesbian women, and lesbian women would obtain sperm donation from gay men. But with growing acceptance and tolerance, this practice is not as common as it once was.

Death and Dying

The main issue that arises for the LGBT community related to death and dying has to do with the legality of same-sex relationships. In states that do not recognize same-sex marriages, a homosexual partner has no legal standing to make medical decisions on behalf of his or her partner. If a person becomes incapacitated, and a person has no advance directives, the law of intestacy is used, which does not include LGBT relationships.

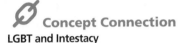

Concept Connection

LGBT and Intestacy

The law of intestacy creates unique problems for the LGBT community. Understanding what the law of intestacy is and how it works helps to shed light on why it creates problems for members of the LGBT community.

Court Case

Lofton v. Secretary of the Department of Children and Family Services

358 F.3d 804 U.S. Court of Appeals, Eleventh Circuit (2004)

FACTS: Steve Lofton and Roger Croteau are a homosexual couple that have been in a committed relationship for over 25 years. Both Steve and Roger are pediatric nurses and have cared for many children born with HIV throughout their career and at their home. One child, who is known as Bert, was a 9-week-old, HIV positive infant, who was abandoned at a Florida hospital under the Safe Haven law. Because Bert was HIV positive, the state of Florida did not consider him a candidate for adoption, and he was instead placed in foster care. Steve and Roger, who had previously been approved as foster parents in the state of Florida, asked to care for Bert in their home.

After Bert's tenth birthday, doctors discovered that Bert no longer tested positive for HIV. When tests confirmed that Bert was no longer HIV positive, the state of Florida determined that Bert was now a suitable candidate for adoption. When Steve and Roger applied to adopt Bert, the state of Florida denied their

application. Florida's adoption law, at the time, said, "No person eligible to adopt under this statute may adopt if that person is a homosexual."

After their story made the news, talk show host Rosie O'Donnell contacted Steve and Roger offering assistance. Along with the American Civil Liberties Union, Steve and Roger sued the State of Florida.

ISSUE: The question before the court was, "Why can homosexuals serve as foster parents to society's unwanted children, but not as adoptive parents?"

RULE: An appellate court, using the Best Interest of the Child standard, found that the Florida law barring homosexuals from adopting was unconstitutional. While the State of Florida submitted a certiorari petition to the U.S. Supreme Court, that petition was denied, ending the legal battle. Steve and Roger adopted Bert; they currently live in Vancouver, British Columbia, Canada, where same-sex marriages are legal.

EMPHASIS: LGBT legal rights have been in the news recently, identifying some of the unique struggles that LGBT community members have suffered with for many years.

Religion

religion: a set of beliefs, based on established doctrine, that typically involves worship, devotion, and the adherence to certain practices

In addition to the culture and ethnic diversity we share, there are several different **religions** practiced in the United States (see Graph 12-1).

Before we get into a discussion about the unique healthcare concerns that some religions have, it is important to note: as healthcare providers, we do not want to question a person's religion, their faith, or why they believe in or are against certain practices. All religious beliefs are based on religious doctrine and worship, which should not be questioned. While we may not agree with a particular belief or religion, understanding where those beliefs come from may help us to provide the special medical care that some religious groups require.

According to the 2010 Census report, when people were asked what religion they practiced, over 75 different religions were mentioned. The most common religion practiced in the United States is Christianity. More people in the United States practice Christianity than practice all the other religions combined. While there are many different types of Christian religions practiced in the United States, (see Graph 12-2) not all of them have unique healthcare requirements. For example, some Christians believe in circumcision, others do

Graph 12-1. The most prevalent religions practiced in the United States.

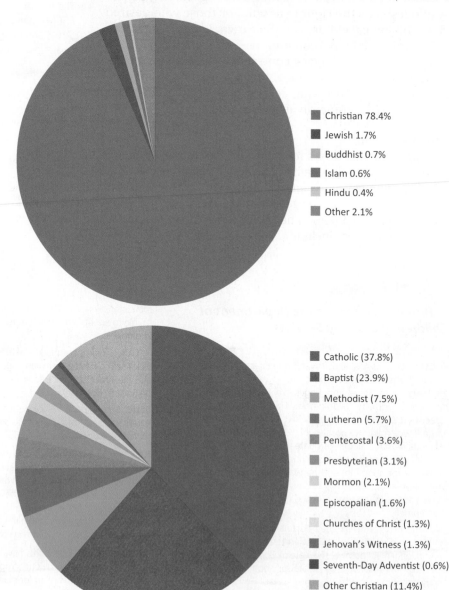

- Christian 78.4%
- Jewish 1.7%
- Buddhist 0.7%
- Islam 0.6%
- Hindu 0.4%
- Other 2.1%

Graph 12-2. The most prevalent Christian religions practiced in the United States.

- Catholic (37.8%)
- Baptist (23.9%)
- Methodist (7.5%)
- Lutheran (5.7%)
- Pentecostal (3.6%)
- Presbyterian (3.1%)
- Mormon (2.1%)
- Episcopalian (1.6%)
- Churches of Christ (1.3%)
- Jehovah's Witness (1.3%)
- Seventh-Day Adventist (0.6%)
- Other Christian (11.4%)

not. Some Christians believe in abortion, while others do not. But even though the Christian religion, as a whole, does not have unique healthcare considerations, there are some Christian religions that do.

Mormons

The Mormons, also known as the Latter Day Saints, follow the teachings of Joseph Smith. Part of the Mormon belief is that the physical body is an essential part of the gospel.

Patient Care

Some Mormons, who have undergone the Endowment Ceremony, will wear a special type of underwear, known as a temple garment (see Fig. 12-5). This garment serves several different purposes to believers of the Mormon faith and is viewed as sacred. Temple garments should not be removed unless medically necessary, and if removed should be put back on as soon as possible. Part of what makes temple garments sacred are the special symbols that are embroidered into the garment. For that reason, if a temple garment must be destroyed or thrown away, the symbols should be removed first and offered to the person before it is destroyed or discarded. The public display of temple garments is considered sacrilegious, so those wearing them may be modest about undressing or having others view these garments.

Pregnancy and Childbirth

Mormons have a strong sense of family and the family unit, and typically have large families. As part of this belief, most Mormons believe that abortion is one of the most sinful practices that can be performed. While Mormons allow artificial insemination to be performed, only a married woman can be inseminated using the sperm of her husband.

Death and Dying

Mormons do not hold any special beliefs regarding death and dying. While cremation is usually avoided, it is allowed. And while euthanasia is not specifically forbidden, most Mormons do not believe in the practice of assisted suicide.

Jehovah's Witnesses

Probably the best-known religious healthcare consideration has to do with Jehovah's Witnesses. Most Jehovah's Witnesses do not receive blood transfusions. This belief stems from a passage in Acts 15:29 that states "you should abstain from blood." There are additional passages in the Bible (Genesis 9:3–4; Leviticus 7:26–27; Leviticus 17:1, 2,10–12; and Deuteronomy 12:23–25) that also talk about abstaining from blood. Although not all Jehovah's Witnesses believe in the blood doctrine, and some will accept blood transfusions, the majority of Jehovah's Witnesses by far, will not accept blood transfusions or blood products. For those who do believe that receiving blood is wrong, the belief is so strong that they will refuse blood transfusions even in the face of death. There are many alternatives to receiving blood transfusions, which Jehovah's Witnesses are very knowledgeable about; such as auto-transfusion, cell-saver, volume expanders, blood substitutes, and the drug erythropoietin.

Christian Scientists

Christian scientists have a strong belief in the creation of the world by God. Everything that is created is done by God and in his image. As part of this belief, they view everything as having a spiritual existence instead of a material existence. What

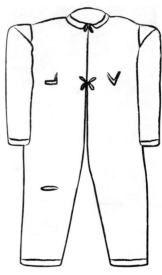

Fig. 12-5. An artist's rendition of a temple garment. Embroidered into the garment is a V-shaped symbol over the left breast, a reversed L-shaped symbol over the right breast, and horizontal rectangular symbols next to the navel and over the right knee. Each symbol holds specific meaning.

> ### ⇄ The Law of Ethics
> #### Court Overrides Parents
> The child of Christian Scientists is found to have appendicitis. But because of the parents' beliefs, they will not consent to surgery, opting to pray instead. In situations such as this, the courts may allow the medical team to perform surgery and provide medical treatment. This goes against the typical position of giving parents the right to decide what medical treatments their children will receive.
>
> - Why would the law go against a parent's wishes, especially in light of the religious implications involved?
> - Should the court have the authority to override a parent's wishes?

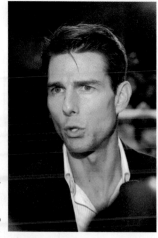

Fig. 12-6 In June 2005, while promoting a movie on the *Today Show*, the interview between Matt Lauer and Tom Cruise got heated and set off a media firestorm, when the issue of psychiatric medications was raised. Cruise, a member of the church of Scientology, spoke out against the use of psychiatric medications during the interview.

we perceive as material things, Christian Scientists believe, is only a distorted view of the spiritual existence. The only way to change our view of the material world, to clearly see the spiritual existence that God created, is through prayer. This differentiation between spirituality and material existence helps to explain the approach that some Christian Scientists have toward healing and medicine.

Some Christian Scientists believe that illness and disease exist when sin is affecting the spirit; that by removing the sin, which can only be accomplished through prayer, the spirit will be healed. Some wrongly assume that Christian Scientists do not believe in modern medicine, which is not true. What Christian Scientists believe is that modern medicine is only able to fix the material aspect of existence, and has no impact on the spiritual existence. Because the spiritual existence is their core belief, they do not see the use of modern medicine as the primary avenue to health.

Scientology

The religion of scientology follows the teachings of its founder L. Ron Hubbard. For the most part, scientologists do not have special healthcare considerations, except for when it comes to mental health. Scientologists do not believe in the use of psychologists, psychiatrists, or psychiatric medications (see Fig. 12-6). Instead of receiving mental health, scientologists undergo a procedure known as an Introspection Rundown. What the procedure involves or how it is performed is unknown to those outside of scientology, but is thought to include isolation where the person reflects inwardly. The views

Court Case

Ethics Case: Lisa McPherson

Clearwater, Florida (1995)

FACTS: In 1994 Lisa McPherson joined the church of Scientology at the age of 18. In November 18, 1995, Lisa was involved in a minor car accident. She was initially cleared by paramedics, but after she was seen disrobing at the scene of the accident, it was felt that she needed to be seen by medical professionals to be cleared both medically and psychologically. After being evaluated, it was suggested that she stay for observation, but congregation members from the local church of Scientology intervened and she opted to sign out of the hospital. Lisa was taken to a hotel by congregation members, where it is suspected she underwent an Introspection Rundown. An Introspection Rundown is a procedure created by church founder L. Ron Hubbard that is used for psychological problems. The person is placed in isolation and asked to reflect on their life and identify what might be causing their psychological problem. They have no interaction with the outside world, except through notes written by the procedure supervisor. When the supervisor is satisfied that the person has resolved their problem, they are let out of the isolation room.

On December 5, 1995, Lisa was taken by Scientology members to a hospital in critical condition, where she was later pronounced dead. Because of the suspicious death, an autopsy was performed where it was determined that Lisa had died of a thromboembolism (blood clot) of the pulmonary artery caused by bed rest and severe dehydration. The autopsy report also indicated that Lisa had multiple bruises and abrasions, with several lesions consistent with insect bites. Shortly following the autopsy, Lisa's body was cremated.

Because of the suspicious death, criminal charges were brought against some church leaders. Those charges included abuse or neglect of a disabled adult and the unauthorized practice of medicine. Following these charges, church leaders provided prosecutors with patient care logs that had been written during Lisa's stay at the hotel. But they readily admitted that the last three days of her care logs had been shredded after a summary report had been written. In addition, the Church of Scientology hired its own forensic pathologist to review the autopsy report and medical findings. The church's pathologist determined that the thromboembolism came from a knee injury sustained in the car accident, and not from dehydration, therefore clearing the church from any wrongdoing in her death. After reviewing the church's pathologist report, the state pathologist changed his findings, determining that the cause of death was an accident.

ISSUE: Was the church of Scientology responsible for Lisa's death?

RULE: Because the state pathologist changed his original findings, and determined that the cause of death was accidental, prosecutors did not believe that they would be able to prove their case. All criminal charges were dropped. However, Lisa's parents brought a civil suit against the church and several church leaders for wrongful death and false imprisonment. The civil suit was settled out of court and its terms were not disclosed publicly.

EMPHASIS: When writing about the Introspective Rundown, L. Ron Hubbard was quoted as saying, "This means the last reason to have psychiatry around is gone. I have made a technical breakthrough which possibly ranks with the major discoveries of the Twentieth Century. Its results are nothing short of miraculous." This quote demonstrates Scientology's views on psychiatry.

on mental health by scientologists were brought to light following the Lisa McPherson case.

Judaism

Part of Judaism's teaching is that life is a blessing and a gift from God. The belief that each person was created *b'tselem elohim* (in God's image) helps us to understand some of the special considerations healthcare professionals have to think about when taking care of Jewish patients.

Patient Care

Most Jewish people have a strong belief that people are descended from a single person. Because of this belief, they view the taking of a single life as equivalent to destroying an entire population. In addition, saving a single life is equivalent to saving an entire population.

Pregnancy and Childbirth

Jews believe that the human soul exists before birth. Therefore, most are against all forms of abortion, except to save the life of the mother. Eight days after the birth of a male, a *brit milah* (often referred to as a *bris*) is performed, part of which is a circumcision.

Death and Dying

Because of their views concerning the origins of life from one person, most Jewish people are adamantly opposed to euthanasia. But they do approve of the use of advance directives, allowing a person to die with dignity.

Most Jewish people consider exposing the body after death as disrespectful, so the body is typically covered with a cloth. In addition, a *shomerim* (guard) will remain with the body until after burial. Because viewing the body is considered disrespectful, Jewish funerals do not allow for open caskets.

Islam

While a majority of Muslims practice the religion of Islam, the word *Muslim* is used to identify the people as a cultural group. The religion of Islam is based on the Qur'an and the Sunnah. It is believed that the Qur'an, which was given to the prophet Muhammad directly from God, is the verbatim word of God. The Sunnah contains teachings of the prophet Muhammad. The Qur'an, often referred to by followers as a book of healing, and the Sunnah, teach its followers how to live physically, mentally, and morally fit lives. Both the Qur'an and Sunnah specifically address medicine, health, and disease. Most followers of traditional Islam view illness, disease, and suffering as necessary aspects of atonement for their sins (see Fig. 12-7).

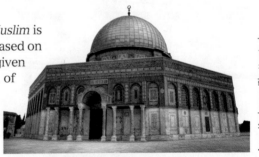

Fig. 12-7. Dome of the Rock (Al Aqsa Mosque), an Islamic shrine located on the Temple Mount in Jerusalem, Israel.

Anna Kucherova/Shutterstock

Patient Care

Most Islamic followers have no restrictions on receiving medical care, with the exception of gender roles. Male healthcare providers should only take care of male patients, and female healthcare providers should only take care of female patients. If a female patient must be cared for by a male healthcare provider, she may prefer that another female be present in the room.

A basic duty of all Islamic followers is to visit the sick, even those outside of their close friends and families. It is not uncommon for a follower of Islam to go to the hospital and ask to visit with Islam patients who are complete strangers.

Pregnancy and Childbirth

The Qur'an is very specific about gender roles; males serve as the dominant gender and women are subservient to males. As part of that belief, no males—other than the husband—are allowed in the delivery room when a child is born.

Court Case

Lirjie Juseinoski v New York Hospital Medical Center of Queens

No. 28516/98, 2004 NY Slip Op 50441(U) Supreme Court, Kings County (2004)

FACTS: On September 1, 1996, 47-year-old Elmaz Juseinoski collapsed at work. He was rushed to New York Hospital Medical Center of Queens (NYHMCQ), where resuscitative measures were unsuccessful. Juseinoski's medical records show his cause of death as cardiac arrest. When the Juseinoski family arrived at the emergency room, they were told by the ER physician, Dr. Sha, that Juseinoski had expired. According to testimony, Juseinoski family members notified hospital personnel that they were Muslim, and that according to their faith Elmaz's body needed to be taken to a mosque. They were told to return in the morning to recover the body. However, upon their return they learned that Juseinoski's body had been transferred to the NYC Medical Examiner's Office, where an autopsy had been performed. Mr. Juseinoski's family

filed suit against NYHMCQ and Dr. Sha, alleging that the hospital failed to notify them that an autopsy would be performed. They sued for the intentional infliction of emotional distress. The hospital contended that they were not informed that an autopsy was not allowed. That they were only told that they were Muslim and requested to take the body to a mosque.

ISSUE: Because of the possibility of religions objections, is there an affirmative duty to notify family members that an autopsy is going to be performed, prior to its performance?

RULE: Citing New York Public Health Law §4214(1) honoring religious objections to autopsies, the court agreed with Mr. Juseinoski's family, ruling in their favor.

EMPHASIS: In this case, the cause of death was not attributable to a crime. Therefore, performing an autopsy was against the religious beliefs of the decedent. This case emphasizes how important it is to know about what different religions and cultures will not allow.

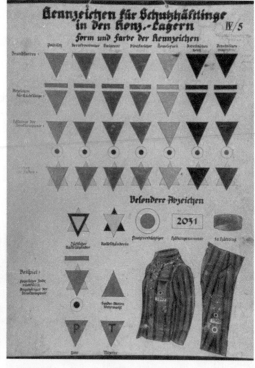

United States Holocaust Museum

Fig. 12-8. A poster, designating the color and symbols that were sewn onto the uniforms of concentration camp prisoners. Two yellow triangles together, one upside down, represented the Star of David, the designation for Jewish people. Upside-down pink triangles designated sexual deviants, mostly homosexual men. Upside-down brown was for Gypsies and upside-down purple triangles were for Jehovah's Witnesses.

Followers of Islam prefer that a female nurse midwife rather than a male doctor deliver children.

Death and Dying

Followers of Islam receive all illness and death with prayer. It is commonplace for followers of Islam to enter into prayer throughout the dying process. They consider death as the final journey to meet Allah. Because this is a journey, it should not be hastened, as no soul will die unless permitted by Allah. Followers of Islam have a strong believe that humans should not play God, and therefore euthanasia and assisted suicide is not allowed. In addition, most followers of Islam do not believe in advance directives, as they view the journey of death as determinable only by Allah. If that journey is altered, they risk upsetting Allah.

Followers of Islam are taught to treat the body with respect, therefore cremation is not allowed. Burials should take place as soon as possible after death occurs. For this reason, autopsies are not performed unless required by law.

Genocide

Throughout civilized history, many ethnic groups, cultures, and religions have been the target of prejudice and persecution through ethnic cleansing and genocide. One of the most recent examples of ethnic cleansing occurred during the Yugoslav War (1991–1995). The most horrific form of ethnic cleansing is through genocide, the intentional murder of distinct group members. It is estimated that 11 million people either died or were killed in Nazi concentration camps throughout occupied Germany during World War II. While the largest number of people murdered, by far, were Jewish, other ethnicities, cultures, and religions were targeted and killed as well; including some of the groups that we have discussed in this chapter. To identify which group a person belonged to, colored patches were sewn onto the uniforms of prisoners (see Fig. 12-8).

Make FALSE statements TRUE.

Rewrite the false statements below by replacing the bolded, italicized, and underlined word(s) to make it a true statement.

1. Some ***Asian cultures*** have specific ceremonies and rituals that are performed when any body parts or tissue is removed.

    _____

2. Some ***Gypsies*** believe that diseases fall into one of two categories, either hot or cold.

    _____

3. One underlying principle seen throughout the orient is the concept of ***wuzho / marime***.

    _____

4. Because of their communication style, the ***Amish*** are not shy about expressing pain.

    _____

5. It is not uncommon for ***Christian Scientists*** to go to the hospital and ask to visit with other ***Christian Scientists*** who are complete strangers.

    _____

Circle Exercise

Circle the correct word from the choices given.

1. Amulets, or talismans, are worn by (**Native Americans, Hispanics, Asians**).

2. Because of their modesty (**Gypsies, Amish, Asians**) the use of interpreters should be limited to family members if at all possible, instead of using strangers.

3. The traditional family structure of (**Christian Scientists, Gypsies, Hispanics**) is fluid, whereby children belong to the group and not necessarily to an individual mother or father.

4. Because of the law of intestacy, members of (**Jehovah's Witnesses, LGBT, Asians**) face difficulty.

5. The (**Amish, Mormons, Scientologists**) wear special garments that should not be removed unless absolutely necessary.

Matching

Match the numbered term to its lettered definition.

1. _____ culture

2. _____ ethnic

3. _____ heritage

4. _____ patriarchal

5. _____ religion

6. _____ shaman

7. _____ talisman

8. _____ wuzho / marime

9. _____ yin yang

A. a belief that things are either pure or impure.

B. a class or group of people that share a common race, nationality, culture, or religion.

C. a group of people that share common beliefs, traits, race, values, goals, or attitudes.

D. a medical and spiritual advisor and mediator between the human world and spirit world.

E. a set of beliefs based on established doctrine, that typically involves worship, devotion, and the adherence to certain practices.

F. a society or group, usually of an extended family, that is led by a dominant male.

G. an Asian belief in how opposites are related to and dependent on each other in all aspects of life.

H. an object, usually worn around the neck, that is believed to contain spirits or mystical or supernatural powers.

I. attributes that are inherited or passed on from previous generations.

Deliberations: Critical Thinking Questions

Question 1: A Native American woman was involved in an accident, injuring her neck. The patient is in the intensive care unit on life support, recovering from her surgery. The tribe's shaman and other members begin to perform a ceremony. As part of this ceremony herbs have been brought in that need to be burned so that she can inhale the smoke. Afterward, the herbs should be given to her to ingest. But because of her medical condition, she is unable to inhale the smoke, and concern has been raised about what the herbs are and how they might interact with her medication. What should you do? Explain your answer.

Question 2: The emergency room has notified you that a patient needs to be admitted to your floor for observation and treatment. The patient is a transgender, anatomical male living as a female, who appears as, speaks as, and dresses as a woman but has not yet had gender reassignment surgery. There are only semi-private rooms available, and the patient has requested to be placed in a room with another female. What should you do? Explain your answer.

Question 3: Mrs. Pearson is 63-year-old patient who was diagnosed with pancreatic cancer. She has advance directives that state no extraneous medical procedures or treatments are to be performed. One evening Dr. Aboo, who is a follower of Islam and does not believe in advance directives, is making rounds and finds Mrs. Pearson unresponsive. He starts to perform CPR and yells for you to bring the crash cart. What should you do? Explain your answer.

Question 4: A Native American woman is in the hospital to give birth. She asks that after the child is born, that the afterbirth be saved so that she can take it to the desert, bury it, and perform a ceremony. What do you do? Would there be any concerns over burying human tissue? Explain your answer.

Question 5: An elderly Asian woman comes to the doctor's office. Because of her complaints, the doctor needs to perform a pelvic exam. However, the patient refuses because the doctor is male. The patient requests that the nursing assistant, who is female, perform the procedure instead. While the nursing assistant cannot perform the procedure, what should you do? How would you resolve this issue?

Closing Arguments: Case Analysis

Two days ago, paramedics brought in two patients who were in a car that had driven over a cliff. The driver is 16-year-old female named Sally, who is unconscious and in critical condition. A young child, presumed to be only a few weeks old, was found strapped in a car seat and does not appear to be injured, but is being monitored in the hospital.

Question 1: The following day, a large group of Gypsies arrive at the hospital asking about the patients. An elderly man approaches, who appears to be in his late seventies, and asks to see his wife and child and inquires about their condition. What should you do? Should you give out patient information and allow him to see his wife and child? Explain your answer.

Question 2: Police have been unable to explain why the accident occurred, and speculate that it might have been a suicide attempt.

Investigators talked to a young woman in the clan, who told them that our patient had talked about leaving the clan and taking her child with her. Does this information change what information you will release to the family and who can visit her in the hospital? Explain your answer.

Question 3: The doctors have determined that Sally's condition is grave, and she has only a few days to live. Sally's extended family has gathered around her bedside to hold vigil over her and to watch her die. During the evening, Sally's husband arrives with six children, all under the age ten, to visit Sally. Your department manager feels that it is inappropriate that young children be exposed to this environment and also complains about the number of visitors in the room. She has asked you to inform Sally's husband that the children are not allowed to visit Sally and that the clan should limit their visitation to two people at a time. How would you respond? Explain your answer.

The Briefcase

This section repeats the objectives from the beginning of the chapter and provides a summary of the most important concepts for each objective. Use this section as a quick review and to check your understanding of the chapter key points.

Objective 1: Explain why it is important to understand the different healthcare needs of a diverse community.

- Different groups may have unique healthcare needs that differ from our own.
- Some groups require different procedures than what we may be used to.

Objective 2: Identify the unique healthcare needs of a particular ethnic group.

- Native Americans
  - Removal of body parts and tissue
  - Difficulty with pain management
- Hispanic: Diseases and treatments are either hot or cold
- Asian
  - Yin yang an essential part of their ethnicity and life
  - Shy and modest
- Gypsies
  - Exaggerated conversation style
  - Refer to things as either pure or impure
- Amish: Simple life, with rare interaction with the outside world

Objective 3: Describe some of the unique healthcare considerations of ethnic groups related to pregnancy and childbirth.

- Native Americans
  - Fear of forced sterilization
  - May prefer to deliver child at home
  - Mother remains indoors until umbilical cord falls off
- Hispanics: women remain active throughout pregnancy
- Asian
  - expression of pain during childbirth allowed
  - Men do not typically play a role in delivery
- Gypsies
  - After delivering, women are considered impure for up to nine days
  - Children should not be looked at by strangers

Objective 4: Give an example of some of the philosophies concerning death and dying for particular ethnic groups.

- Native Americans: Close relationship with nature, and strong belief in the spirit world
  - Some bury their dead, others might leave them open to nature
  - Some fear a dead person's spirit
- Hispanics
  - Prefer to die at home
  - View autopsies as intrusive
- Asian
  - Some believe that death should occur in a hospital so the home is not infected with the person's spirit
  - Some believe that death should occur at home in familiar surroundings
- Gypsies: may gather and quietly watch a person die

Objective 5: Identify the unique healthcare needs of a particular cultural group.

- LGBT
  - Address a gay man's spouse as his husband (not as a wife) and a lesbian woman's spouse as her wife (not as a husband).
  - Refer to transgendered individuals, as their preference, as male or female

Objective 6: Describe some of the unique healthcare considerations of different cultures related to pregnancy and childbirth.

- LGBT
  - in vitro fertilization
  - surrogacy

Objective 7: Give an example of some of the philosophies concerning death and dying for particular cultural groups.

- LGBT
  - Legality of same-sex couples
  - Advances Directives
  - Healthcare proxies
  - Law of intestacy

Objective 8: Identify the unique healthcare needs of different religions.

- Judaism: strong belief that people originate from one person.
- Islam: strict gender roles
- Mormons: wear temple garments
- Jehovah's Witnesses: do not receive blood transfusions
- Scientology: disbelieve psychology and psychiatry as a science or medicine

Objective 9: Identify the unique healthcare needs of a particular religion.

- Judaism:
  - some do not believe in abortion
  - some oppose euthanasia
- Islam:
  - only women should care for pregnant women
  - do not believe in advance directives
- Mormons:
  - do not believe in abortion
  - do not utilize assisted suicide

Maximize Your Success with the Companion Website

The Companion Website to this textbook contains materials that can help you better understand the concepts presented in this chapter. Go to MyHealthProfessionsKit to access:

- Learning Tools, Games, and more
- Sample Quizzes
- Related Links
- Understanding Your State

PEARSON
myhealthprofessionskit™

13 Bioethics

The topic of bioethics, which deals with the ethical issues related to life, is always controversial because it involves the ethics of life. People will have differing opinions about life: not only when life begins, but also whether we should be interfering with life at all. In this chapter, we will review some of the ethical situations that arise in medical bioethics that address issues that may affect other people and other things.

MEASURE YOUR PROGRESS: LEARNING OBJECTIVES

After studying this chapter, you will be able to:

- Explain why the National Research Act was passed.

- Identify the three main ethical principles used in medical research.

- Describe the clinical trial process

- Give an explanation of why stem cell research is controversial.

- Explain why anencephaly creates difficult situations for healthcare.

- Identify the reason some critics are against fetal reduction.

- Describe the ethical controversies surrounding conjoined twin separation surgery.

- Explain why cloning is being investigated by scientists.

- Give a reason some would be opposed to xenotransplantation.

KEY TERMS

anencephaly

clinical trail

cloning

cryonics

double-blind

fetal reduction

pluripotent

research

xenotransplantation

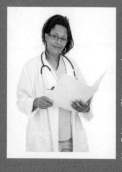
et alia (et al.) { And other things; and other people.

Part of the confusion related to testing and experimentation is that they mean two different things. Testing is performed to measure what knowledge we already have. For example, taking a test for a class is a measurement of the knowledge you have about a particular subject. **Research**, on the other hand, is performed to obtain new knowledge.

To add to the confusion, there are additional words, such as studying and experimentation, which add to the confusion about bioethics, what is ethical, and what the law regulates.

National Research Act

As a result of the Tuskegee Syphilis Experiment (see the Ethics Case on the next page), Congress enacted the National Research Act. The National Research Act created the National Commission for the Protection of Human Subjects of Biomedical and Behavioral Research. This commission was given the responsibility of developing rules and regulations regarding the use of human subjects in research and testing.

One of the first tasks undertaken by the commission was to identify the basic ethical principles that should be utilized in biomedical and behavioral research when human subjects are used. Once the committee identified the ethical principles, those principles would be used to write policies and procedures regarding the use of humans in research. The three ethical principles initially identified by the commission were justice, autonomy, and beneficence.

Justice
The ethical principle of justice addresses what is right and wrong by looking at fairness. What is fair is right and what is not fair is wrong. The commission identified the ethical principle of justice to addresses *how research should be performed*. If human participants are going to be used, the research should:

1. be based on sound scientific principles,
2. have a goal that is well thought out and not based on conjecture, and
3. have a clear and identifiable indication of what the research is trying to achieve.

Autonomy
The ethical principle of autonomy when used in relation to research, addresses *how the research subjects should be treated*.
One of the ethical issues involving the Tuskegee Experiment was that participants were not told the purpose of the study; nor that they had contracted a disease. By using the ethical principle of autonomy, all research subjects will be treated with the respect and dignity that all human beings deserve.

To ensure that a patient's autonomy is being upheld, research participants are required to provide informed consent before being enrolled in a research project. Informed consent can only come from providing them with truthful information regarding the study, what the study is purported to reveal, and what the pros and cons are regarding participation.

Beneficence
The ethical principle of beneficence addresses one of the most difficult aspects of research: whether research should be performed, and if so, how it should proceed. Beneficence is the ethical principle that centers on *how research should help others*.

> Isn't the testing of new medications and procedures on human beings experimentation? I thought that was against the law.

research: a process that is used to obtain new knowledge, usually based on scientific principles

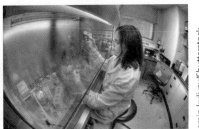
emin kuliyev/Shutterstock

⌀ Concept Connection
Bioethics and Ethical Principles
One of the first things that the National Commission for the Protection of Human Subjects of Biomedical and Behavioral Research did, was to look at the list of all of the basic ethical principles, that have been identified. Some basic principles did not apply to research, but it was worthwhile to look at them first to make that determination.

TABLE 13-1
Knowledge Techniques
research: a process that is used to obtain new knowledge
experimentation: a process used to verify if knowledge is accurate or correct
studying: processes that are used to incorporate knowledge
testing: performed to measure knowledge we already have

Michelle Marsan/Shutterstock

Ethics Case

Tuskegee Syphilis Research

Macon, Alabama (1930–1972)

FACTS: In 1932, a research project was commissioned by the U.S. Public Health Service to study the long-term effects of syphilis. Researches focused their attention in Macon, Alabama, where a large number of syphilis cases had been reported. They started testing sharecroppers for syphilis to determine whether they would qualify to participate in the research. Those in whom a syphilis diagnosis was confirmed were enrolled in the research project. In all, 399 African American sharecroppers were enrolled in the study. But what made this study controversial was that participants were not informed that they had syphilis. Instead, when enrolled in the study, they were only told that they had "bad blood," which could have included any number of different diseases. Researchers defended this decision by claiming that had participants known they had syphilis, they could have sought treatment, which would have defeated the purpose of the study.

The study continued for over ten years, despite the discovery, in the interim, of penicillin as a cure for syphilis.

ISSUE: Because the study was initiated to understand the long-term effects of syphilis, participants were not provided with a treatment. Again, researchers argued that treating the participants would alter the outcome of the study.

RULE: When information regarding the study was released to the press in 1972, it prompted public outcry over the ethics of the medical research. The study was quickly abolished, and medical treatment was provided for those participants that remained.

EMPHASIS: In all, 28 participants died of syphilis, 100 died of complications related to syphilis, 40 participants' wives were infected with syphilis, and 19 children were born with congenital syphilis. When Dr. John Heller, one of the project researchers, was asked about the ethics of the study, he was quoted as saying, "The men's status did not warrant ethical debate. They were subjects, not patients; clinical material, not sick people."

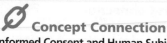

TABLE 13-2

Ethical Principles and Research

justice: how research should be performed

autonomy: how research subjects should be treated

beneficence: how research should help others

This can be difficult to determine because of how research works, utilizing a test group and a control group. In order to understand the role that beneficence plays in medical research, we need to review how medical research is performed.

Medical Research

Any time that a new drug or piece of medical equipment is developed, before it is approved for general use, it must undergo vigorous experiments and testing. The initial stage of laboratory testing helps to determine what the drug or equipment is supposed to do. Once the company determines that they have enough information to proceed, it applies for a **clinical trial**.

The Department of Health and Human Services (HHS), the Food and Drug Administration (FDA), and the Office of Human Research Protections (OHRP) oversee clinical trials in the United States. The clinical trial process is lengthy, involving numerous regulatory controls and oversight throughout.

Ⓧ Concept Connection

Informed Consent and Human Subjects

There are requirements for what needs to be included in informed consent. The emphasis of "informed" consent is that the person giving the consent has been informed by providing them with the information that they need to make a decision.

clinical trial: a research process using humans to test medication, equipment, or procedures

Clinical Trials

Once a company has performed all of the tests that it can in a laboratory, the next step is to start testing on humans. But before a company can start testing on humans, it has to submit an application to an Institutional Review Board (IRB).

Initially most IRBs were located at institutions of higher learning, but some commercial IRBs have surfaced lately. In order to qualify as an IRB, the board must meet the requirements set forth in the National Research Act. To be qualified as an IRB:

1. Boards must have a minimum of five members, and the group should be as diverse as possible.

2. One member of the IRB must be a nonscientist, and one member cannot be affiliated with the

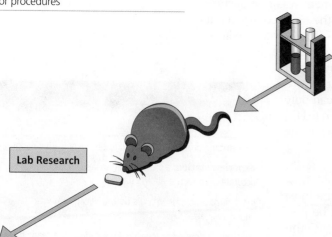

Lab Research

institution or be a relative of someone affiliated with the institution. (The non-affiliated member of the IRB is commonly referred to as the community liaison, as he or she is supposed to be representing the interests of the community.) It is permissible for the nonscientist requirement and community liaison requirement to be filled by one person, if that one person meets both criteria.

3. All remaining members of the IRB must have experience and expertise in medical research. (This requirement ensures that the research is ethical, that informed consent is sufficient, and that appropriate protocols and safeguards have been established.)

4. All members of the IRB cannot be of the same profession. (For example, the IRB cannot be made up only of doctors; rather, its membership must represent multiple professions.)

Once an application for clinical trials has been received and reviewed, the IRB votes on the application. In order for an application to be approved, a majority of *all* board members must vote in favor of the application. (The rules governing IRBs are clear; a majority vote is based on the number of board members that make up the IRB, and not the members who are currently present at the time the vote occurs.) If a majority of board members do not approve the application, the application is denied. An application that has been denied can be reintroduced some other time, when changes have been made to the application or the board members change. If a clinical trial application is approved, then the clinical trial process begins. There are three different phases involved in clinical trials.

Phase 1 Clinical Trials: Pilot Study

The initial phase, commonly referred to as the pilot study, is limited to 10 to 100 human participants. Participants who are enrolled in Phase 1 clinical trials must be healthy and cannot have any current medical conditions, nor can they be taking any medications—either prescription or over-the-counter. Approved participants are enrolled in the study and are provided with the medication or treatment. Part of why participants need to be healthy for this phase, is to ensure that any preexisting medical conditions or medications a participant is taking will not skew the results.

Medical examinations are performed to determine how the medication or treatment has affected the participant. Participants are monitored throughout Phase 1 clinical trials, and typically keep a detailed log that includes a variety of different information, such as elimination habits, appetite, sleep habits, moods, feelings, and emotions. After all of the information has been received, tabulated, and correlated, the Phase 1 final report is submitted to the IRB for review. When submitting the Phase 1 repot to the IRB, the company will typically attach to the report an application for a Phase 2 Clinical Trial.

Phase 2 Clinical Trials: Clinical Trial Protocol

If a Phase 2 Clinical Trial is approved, a new set of participants is obtained. At this stage, anywhere from 50 to 500 participants are enrolled. But, unlike the participants who are enrolled in Phase 1, Phase 2 participants must suffer from the disease or condition that the drug, medication, or equipment is suppose to benefit. For example, if a new medication is being researched for the treatment of high blood pressure, a person enrolled as a Phase 2 participant must currently have high blood pressure.

Participants who are enrolled in a Phase 2 clinical trial will take part in a **double-blind** study (See Fig 13-1).

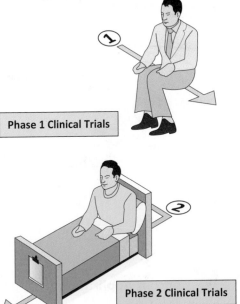

Phase 1 Clinical Trials

Phase 2 Clinical Trials

double-blind: a research process where a test group and a control group are used and then compared

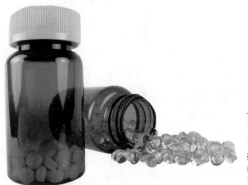

Kellis/Shutterstock

Fig. 13-1 In a double-blind study, both groups receive pills to take. However, when participants are assigned a number, the researcher will be told which bottle to give the patient. Neither the participant nor the researcher knows which is the medicine and which is the placebo. That information cannot be obtained until the study is finished.

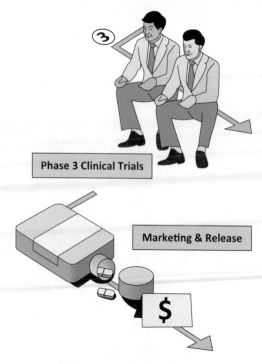

Phase 3 Clinical Trials

Marketing & Release

A Phase 2 clinical trial participant, once identified, is assigned a number. Neither the researchers nor the study participants know whether they are being enrolled in the test group or the control group, as the assignment is anonymously and randomly assigned by number. Members who are enrolled in the test group are given the medication, and members enrolled in the control group are given a placebo.

Once the study is completed, information obtained from both groups is compared. This comparison allows researchers to determine the effectiveness of the medication or treatment. (Theoretically, members of the test group should demonstrate what the research is trying to ascertain, such as a decrease in blood pressure., while those in the control group experience no change in medical condition.) Once the Phase 2 study has been completed, a final report is submitted to the IRB. If the results are deemed favorable, an application to proceed on to a Phase 3 clinical trial will be completed as well.

Phase 3 Clinical Trials: Expanded Enrollment

In Phase 3, anywhere from hundreds to thousands of participants are enrolled. As with Phase 2, in the third phase all participants who are enrolled must be diagnosed with the disease or condition the medication or treatment is intended to help. But this time, there is no test group or control group. Instead, all participants receive the medication or treatment. Information regarding the effectiveness of the medication or treatment is not the only information obtained. Throughout the

---

Concept Application

Clinical Trials: Phase 3

In 1997, the diet drug Fen-Phen was voluntarily removed from the market when it was discovered that some people had developed heart valve disease after taking the medication. Even though the drug had been through all three phases of clinical trials, heart valve disease had not presented itself as a side effect or complication during the clinical trials. It was not until the drug was released to the general public that information regarding heart valve disease first surfaced. After further studies were performed, Fen-Phen was rereleased in the marketplace with added warnings to prescribers concerning heart valve disease. It is currently available as a prescription, and classified as a Schedule IV drug in the United States.

Sidebar

Even successful completion of all three phases of the clinical trials is not a guarantee of final approval. Of all the new drug applications that are submitted to the FDA, only about 20 percent are given final approved.

Ethics Case

azidothymidine (AZT)

United States (1990s)

FACTS: In the early 1990s, the drug AZT (azidothymidine) was undergoing clinical trials as a treatment for patients with HIV and AIDS. During the Phase 2 clinical trials, the response by participants enrolled in the test group—the group that was actually receiving the medication—were dramatic. Because of the potential life-saving impact that the drug had, the clinical trial process was accelerated and the medication released to the general public before the clinical trial process was complete.

ISSUE: Critics complained that by accelerating the clinical trials, information regarding side effects, contra-indications, and complications might be missed.

RULE: Regulators felt that because of the devastating impact of the disease (at that time), the risks of withholding the medication

to complete the study far outweighed the information that might be obtained. By not releasing the mediation to the general public, researchers felt that they would be providing more harm to patients infected with HIV than if the study continued. This rationale is an example of beneficence that clinical research is built on.

EMPHASIS: Although there is a specific process for clinical trials, which must be followed, as we saw in the law, there are always exceptions. In this case, regulators and researchers struggled with whether it was better to gather information or try to save people's lives. Fortunately, the incorporation of AZT into treatment protocols for patients with HIV drastically changed the life expectancy of people living with HIV. It is theorized that AZT changed what was once an almost certain death sentence into a disease that could be managed with medication.

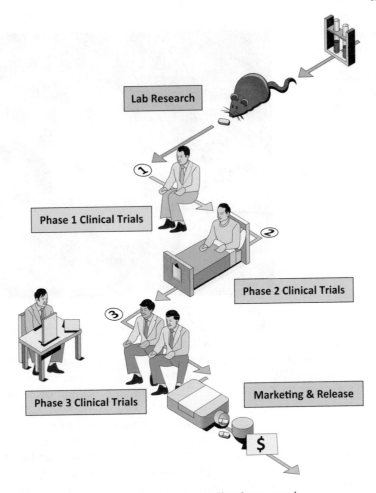

clinical trial process, side effects, complication, or contra-indications can be obtained as well. For example, if a significant number of participants indicated that they had a dry mouth while enrolled in the study, then dry mouth may be listed as a complication or side effect of taking the medication.

Once the Phase 3 trial has been completed, reports are again submitted to the IRB for a final recommendation. If the IRB gives their approval, the company will submit an application to the Food and Drug Administration. If that application is approved by the FDA, physicians will now be able to prescribe the medication to the general public.

Stem Cell Research

Another area of research that has garnered a lot of controversy over the past few years is stem cell research. The main issue surrounding the controversy relates to where stems cells are obtained. Embryonic stem cells are **pluripotent**, having the potential to differentiate into any of the three different layers of tissue.

pluripotent: the ability to differentiate into many different layers of tissue

The three layers that an embryonic stem cell can develop into are:

- endoderm, which creates the interior stomach lining, gastrointestinal tract, and the lungs;
- mesoderm, which creates the muscles, bones, blood, and urogenital tissue; and
- ectoderm, which creates the epidermal tissue and nervous tissue.

Because of the potential to differentiate into different tissue, embryonic stem cells can be used to grow new tissue or possibly even complete organs. The controversy over stem cell research is not with the research or the results that they hope to obtain. The controversy exists because when

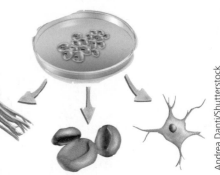

Andrea Danti/Shutterstock

Fig. 13-2. Many believe that with stem cell research, a cure for Parkinson's disease can be found. Michael J. Fox, who suffers from Parkinson's disease, testified before Congress concerning stem cell research and the need for additional funding.

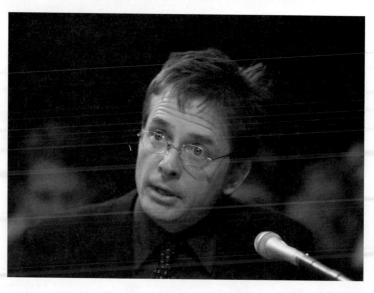

© Danita Delimont/Alamy

Sidebar

An article written by J. Timson, and published in the journal *Genetica*, states that about 1 in 150,000 to 200,000 children are born with anencephaly.

The Law of Ethics

Anencephalic Children

Any time that a child is born, parents have the right to view the child. Some parents may want to view their stillborn child while others may not. What role should healthcare professionals take in this decision?

- If a child is stillborn, should we encourage or discourage a parent from viewing their child?
- What psychological effects can you think of in regards to a parent viewing or not viewing their stillborn child?
- What if a stillborn child is disfigured (anencephaly or is a molar [hydatidiform] birth)? Should we encourage or discourage a parent from viewing the child?

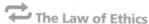

anencephaly: a medical condition that occurs when the brain does not develop

stem cells are harvested from embryos, the embryo is destroyed. With some believing that life begins at conception, they believe that killing an embryo is not something that we should do to advance medical science (See Fig 13-2).

Due to budget cuts and the controversy surrounding the use of embryonic stem cells, researchers are starting to look at other avenues, such as using adult stem cells. But adult stem cells do not have the pluripotent abilities that embryonic stem cells do, so their use is limited. One of the more promising areas of research that is being investigated involves the harvesting of stem cells from umbilical cord blood. Because stems cells exist in the umbilical cord, and are not embryos, they could hold the key that scientists are looking for, while satisfying some of the critics' responses about destroying life. Because the use of umbilical cord blood holds promise for researchers, after a child is born parents may be asked to donate the umbilical cord blood. The donation of umbilical cord blood, however, is not the only time when parents might be asked about donation after a child is born.

Anencephaly

There is an unfortunate and rare medical condition, known as **anencephaly**, that creates difficult bioethical issues, not only for healthcare providers, but for new parents as well.

Anencephaly is a central nervous system disorder whereby the cephalic portion of the brain does not form. While most anencephalic children are stillborn, of the few that are born alive, only their brain stems have formed. The brain stem, responsible for cardiac and pulmonary function, meet the clinical criteria for life. But, with the absence of the cephalic portion of the brain, responsible for cognitive functions, interpretation of pain, and the expression of moods or feelings, the child is essentially born in a comatose state. The longest an anencephalic child has survived was two months, during which time the child required aggressive medical treatment and life support.

If an anencephalic child is born alive, because their brain stem is functioning they do not meet the legal criteria for clinical death established by the Uniform Determination of Death Act (UDDA). However, there are some who believe that an anencephalic exception should be written into the law. With thousands of children on the waiting list to receive organs, such as those born with congenital heart defects, anencephalic babies might be able to serve as organ donors. While medical researchers at Loma Linda University attempted to research the possibilities of utilizing anencephalic organs for transplants, citing ethical concerns they suspended their anencephalic transplant program. Of concern were how the possible benefits that could be obtained weighed against the need to respect the child as a human being. A hospital in Canada is the only reported case of a successful heart transplant from an anencephalic child.

Fetal Reduction

Due to advances in medical imaging, most cases of anencephaly can be identified early in the pregnancy. Routine sonograms performed between the first and second trimester, or 10–14 weeks gestation, have been able to identify cases of anencephaly and other birth defects. But identifying problems at this critical juncture can result in legal issues, depending on which state you live in.

If a mother decides to terminate a pregnancy, the type of procedure performed depends on the gestational age of the fetus. Certain abortion procedures are only available during certain trimesters. But what if a woman is pregnant with twins or multiple births, and only one child has anencephaly? Depending on when the condition is identified, performing certain types of abortions would terminate all pregnancies. But with a procedure known as **fetal reduction**, one or more fetuses in a multiple pregnancy can be removed, leaving other fetuses in the womb.

With the increased number of children a woman carries come inherent risks. Multiple-birth children have an increased risk for birth defects and cerebral palsy, and some if not all may be stillborn.

In order to address some of the problems that result from a multiple pregnancy, fetal reduction can be performed on one or more of the fetuses, allowing the others to remain. The difficulty however, and why this procedure is controversial, is how fetuses are chosen for reduction. While sometimes the choice is made based on a medical condition of the child, such as a child with anencephaly, other times decisions are not as clear-cut. For example, suppose that a woman who is small in statute is pregnant with four children. Doctors have determined that she will be unable to carry all four fetuses to term without serious consequences to the health of the children and herself. Doctors have recommended that she undergo fetal reduction to remove two of the fetuses. But which two? What if the woman and her spouse already have a girl from a previous pregnancy, so they decide to keep the male fetuses and select the female fetuses for reduction? It is these types of situations that have raised ethical concerns about fetal reduction and have led some to call for strict guidelines and policies regarding the procedure's use.

Conjoined Twins

Conjoined twins, previously known as Siamese twins, occur when identical twins join together in utero. The condition is rare, estimated to occur only once in every 50,000 to 100,000 births.

While there are many different types of conjoined twins, the eight most common are:

- cephalopagus: two faces on opposite sides of a joined head. They typically share cerebral vascular anatomy.
- craniopagus: two bodies are joined at any point on the skull, except for the face.

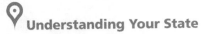

Understanding Your State

To determine what your state requirements are for obtaining abortions, check out the interactive map on the companion website.

Sidebar

The most children born during a single pregnancy is nine—known as nonuplets—which has occurred only twice in recorded history. Some of the children were stillborn, but of the few that were delivered alive, none survived longer than six hours.

fetal reduction: a procedure used in multiple pregnancies where only a portion of the embryos are aborted

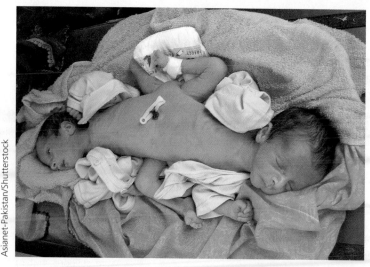

Asianet-Pakistan/Shutterstock

Fig. 13-3 Conjoined twins.

- ischipagus: two bodies joined at the lower half, with their spines conjoined. They typically have one anus and one set of genitalia.
- parapagus: two bodies joined at and share a single pelvis.
- synecephalus: two lower bodies form, but with only a single head.
- thoraco-omphalopagus: two bodies joined at the chest. They typically share one heart.
- thoracopagus: two bodies joined together from the chest to the abdomen. They share one heart.
- xiphopagus: two bodies joined from the lower chest to the mid abdomen. They commonly share a single liver.

Surgery to separate conjoined twins, such as craniopagus twins for example, usually results in the death of one or both of the twins. Some have raised ethical concerns over whether conjoined twins should be separated at all, regardless of the medical risks. Some even argue that even if the patients consent, it is a form of suicide because the surgery is rarely successful.

Separation surgery for certain types of conjoined twins is usually performed only if one of the twins has a parasitic relationship with the other

Ethics Case

Jodie and Mary

Great Britain (2007)

FACTS: On November 7, 2000, in Great Britain, surgery was performed on xiphopagus conjoined twins who were named Jodie and Mary. Jodie was the stronger of the two, with Mary having an underdeveloped brain and limited functioning of her heart and lungs. Mary was relying on Jodie's cardiopulmonary system to survive; but the strain was starting to take its toll on Jodie. Doctors determined that it was inevitable that Mary would expire, and became concerned about how they could save Jodie. Without performing separation surgery, neither Mary nor Jodie would survive.

The children's parents strongly objected to the performance of the separation surgery. They opted instead, based on religious reasons, to let nature take its course. Doctors disagreed and petitioned the court to have the surgery performed.

ISSUE: The question that the court struggled with was "whether it was lawful to kill one twin (Mary) in order to save the other (Jodie)?"

RULE: Following a three-month legal battle, the court gave approval for doctors to proceed with the separation surgery.

EMPHASIS: During the separation surgery, Mary passed away, but Jodie survived. Following her recovery, Jodie and her parents moved back to their native island country of Gozo, in the Mediterranean Sea, where they buried Mary.

and without surgery could cause the death of both. Consider the following ethics case:

Cloning

The mere mentioning of the word **cloning** can stir up dramatic controversies and debates.

cloning: a medical procedure that creates an exact duplicate of a living organism

The idea that science can create an exact duplicate of another living organism raises a variety of different ethical concerns. The arguments against cloning focus on whether scientists are playing God. That creating life is not something that scientist should do—or even be allowed to do.

This naturally begs the question, why are scientist interested in cloning in the first place?

Part of the reason for investigating cloning possibilities had to do with the possibility of creating human tissue or even complete organs. Cloned tissue could be used to treat diseases, such as Parkinson's or Alzheimer's. Or, if cloning entire organs becomes possible, people in need of transplants could have their own organs cloned instead of having to wait for a donor organ. Even though the cloning of an entire human being is not medically possible, most countries in the world have specifically outlawed the practice, including the United States.

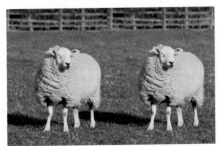

Jason Bennee/Shutterstock

Fig 13-4. On July 5, 1996, Dolly the sheep was born. Dolly was the first mammal to be successfully cloned and born. The news set off a flurry of ethical debates within the scientific community and politics across the world. Dolly lived for six years before she was euthanized because of a medical condition.

Xenotransplantation

An unfortunate reality is that a large number of people die while on the waiting list for organs. According to the FDA, 10 people die each day while awaiting transplants. To combat this shortage, scientists have been researching whether animal organs can be used in humans, in a technique known as **xenotransplantation**.

xenotransplantation: the use of animal tissue or organs in humans

But even from the original conception of the idea, scientists were faced with both medical and ethical hurdles they will have to overcome before it can be successful.

Initially, scientists looked at using chimpanzees and baboons as donors, because of their relatively close genetic structure to humans. But because both species have since became endangered, scientists have had to look at other species to provide donated organs. Current research is investigating the use of pig tissue and organs for xenotranplantation, but effectiveness and feasibility questions remain. Pigs only live for 15 years, which may limit the length of time pig organs can be used in humans. In addition, pigs' body temperature is higher than that of humans, which might create difficulty when the animals organs are transplanted into humans because of how the organ functions in a lower temperature setting and with different physiology. But perhaps the most important concern over xenotransplantation is with xenozoonosis.

With xenozoonosis, infectious agents are transmitted from one species to another. Even though xenozoonosis is extremely rare, due to changes in viral morphology its occurrence has increased over the years. The latest example is the avian influenza that moved from poultry to humans, causing an epidemic in recent years. If xenotransplantation is performed, scientists are concerned that incidences of xenozoonosis will also increase, causing diseases and illness that have not been encountered in humans before.

From an ethical standpoint, xenotransplantation has animal rights activists upset, because they do not believe that animals should be sacrificed for use in humans. Another concern relates to the use of pigs as tissue, especially for those religions that do not allow the eating of pork. Would transplanting pig tissue violate such religious restrictions, creating religious discrimination in the arena of transplantation?

Ethics Case

Baby Fae
California (1984)

FACTS: On October 14, 1984, Baby Fae was born two weeks premature, with hypoplastic left heart syndrome (a condition that at the time was 100 percent fatal). Baby Fae's mother, Teresa Beauclair, was presented with two options; keep the child in the hospital or take the child home. Teresa opted to take the child home, and was preparing to go through the dying process until Dr. Leonard Bailey presented her with a third option. The highly experimental surgery involved replacing Baby Fae's heart with that of a baboon. Dr. Bailey had been investigating the possibility of cross-species transplantation and discussed his research with Teresa, gaining her consent to the operation.

ISSUE: When news of the medical procedure broke, it set off a media frenzy. Many medical ethicists raised concern over the experimental nature of the procedure. In addition, animal rights activists were outraged because of the preference that was given to human life.

RULE: Due in part to the ethical controversies raised by the xenotransplantation procedure, and concerns over infection, cross-species transplantations are no longer performed. But research continues in the arena of xenotransplantation.

EMPASIS: While initially, the operation appeared to be successful, Baby Fae's organs started to fail, leading to her death 21 days after the transplant surgery was performed. In announcing her death at a press conference, Dr. Bailey stated, "Infants with heart disease yet to be born will someday soon have the opportunity to live, thanks to the courage of this infant and her parents." One year later, the first human to human heart transplant was performed in a child. Dr. Bailey credits the success, in part, to the information and experience that was gained by performing the xenotransplant procedure.

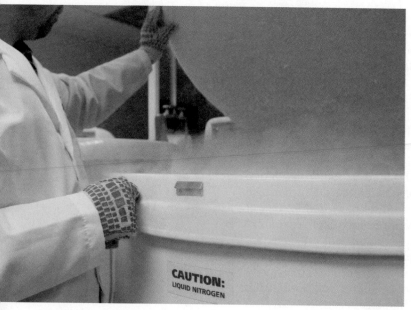

© Huntstock, Inc/Alamy

---

cryonics: the freezing of humans at death for revival in the future

---

Xenotransplantation surgery has been performed in the past, but without long-term success. Most patients who have received animal tissue or organs have died shortly after receiving the transplant.

Cryonics

Some people believe that being pronounced dead does not necessarily have to mean the end of life. As technology evolves in the field of **cryonics**, so do the number of people who are contemplating the procedure.

The idea behind cryonics is a novel one. A patient who has been pronounced dead or has been diagnosed with a fatal disease is placed in cryostasis. A substance is injected to prevent ice formation in tissue, and then the body placed in liquid nitrogen. The patient is kept in a state of deep freeze until medical science is able to discover and/or perfect a cure. When that occurs, the theory is that the patient can be thawed and receive life-saving treatment. Cryonics has also been suggested for use in organ transplantation whereby a person can be thawed if a compatible organ because available.

But regardless of the theory, cryostasis reversal is not yet possible as it has not yet been successfully performed in humans. That fact has not stopped some people from undergoing the procedure. According to the website of the Cryonics Institute, located in Clinton Township, Michigan, as of 2011, they have placed over 100 patients in cryostasis.

Because of the theory behind cryonics, placing someone in cryosuspension should optimally occur before human tissue has died. But the law only allows cryosuspension to be performed on patients who have been declared legally dead, using the criteria established by the UDDA. Supporters of cryonics hope to change that, but until advances in science make suspension reversal a possibility, it is unlikely that an exception to the UDDA will be implemented.

Make FALSE statements TRUE.

Rewrite the false statements below by replacing the bolded, italicized, and underlined word(s) to make it a true statement.

1. The ethical principle of ***justice*** is used to determine how research subjects should be treated.

    _____

2. The medical research process demonstrates the ethical principle of ***autonomy***.

    _____

3. An IRB must be made up of a minimum of ***ten*** members.

    _____

4. The use of a test group and a control group occurs during ***Phase 1*** clinical trials.

    _____

5. Part of the reason embryonic stem cells are used, is because they are ***anencephalic***.

    _____

Circle Exercise

Circle the correct word from the choices given.

1. (**Testing, Studying, Experimentation**) is used to measure knowledge that we already have.

2. In (**Phase 1, Phase 2, Phase 3**) only healthy participants are enrolled.

3. In (**cryonics, fetal reduction, anencephaly**) only a portion of multiple birth children are aborted.

4. The use of (**cloning, xenotransplantation, stem cells**) might allow for duplicate tissue to be created for transplantation.

5. Ultimately, (**cryonics, xenotransplantation, stem cells**) should be performed while the patient is still alive, but the law does not currently allow it.

Matching

Match the numbered term to its lettered definition.

1. _____ anencephaly

2. _____ clinical trials

3. _____ cloning

4. _____ cryonics

5. _____ double-blind

6. _____ fetal reduction

7. _____ pluripotent

8. _____ research

9. _____ xenotransplantation

A. a medical condition that occurs when the brain does not develop.

B. a medical procedure that creates an exact duplicate of a living organism.

C. a procedure used in multiple pregnancies where only a portion of the embryos are aborted.

D. a process that is used to obtain new knowledge, usually based on scientific principles.

E. a research process using humans to test medication, equipment, or procedures.

F. a research process where a test group and a control group are used and then compared.

G. the ability to differentiate into many different layers of tissue.

H. the freezing of humans at death for revival in the future.

I. the use of animal tissue or organs in humans.

Deliberations: Critical Thinking Questions

Question 1: A new medication used for depression has been approved by the FDA. One of the side effects discovered during the clinical trial process was weight loss, but the FDA has only provided approval for the drug in treating depression. A medication sales representative has come to your office, and is marketing the drug as a weight-loss drug. Should doctors be able to prescribe medications for their side effects, instead of the purpose the drug was tested for? Explain your answer.

Question 2: After a series of ultrasounds and other diagnostic tests, it is discovered that the child a woman is carrying has anencephaly. Because of religious reasons, she did not have an abortion. She is in active labor and asks that if the child is born alive, that the child be resuscitated for possible organ donation. But her husband, and the child's father, disagrees and does not want resuscitative measures performed. What should you do?

Question 3: Your sister is pregnant with triplet embryos. Because of her small frame, she has been advised that she will be unable to carry all three children to term and has to undergo a fetal reduction to remove at least one of the children. At this point in the pregnancy, doctors have not yet determined what

the sex of the three different children are. Your sister asks you your advice on how to choose which one should be reduced. How would you respond?

Question 4: A prominent and well-respected pharmaceutical company has discovered a new drug that it believes can cure sudden infant death syndrome (SIDS). All of the laboratory results have been overwhelmingly favorable, and the company has been given quick approval to start clinical trials on humans. However, because the medication can only be given to newborn children, the company has had difficulty getting enough participants to enroll in the study. What do you think about testing new medications on children? How else could the pharmaceutical company determine whether the medication is affective and/or safe in children?

Question 5: Your spouse has been asked to sit on an IRB as the community liaison. Even though you work in a doctor's office, there is no conflict of interest. After several meetings, your spouse complains to you that the other committees are constantly overruling his suggestions and comments. He asks for your input about what he should do. What suggestions do you have for him?

Closing Arguments: Case Analysis

Acme Medication Company has developed a drug designed to decrease the chances of miscarriages in pregnant woman. It has completed the first phase of clinical trials, and no problems have been identified by healthy participants. Acme has now submitted an application to the IRB to move on to Phase 2 clinical trials.

Question 1: Because Phase 2 clinical trials require that patients have the medical condition the drug is targeted for, only women who are currently pregnant can be enrolled. Some of the members of the IRB have expressed concern over enrolling pregnant women in a study, especially since we do not know what affect the drug will have on the fetus. What are your thoughts? Should we allow pregnant woman to participate in clinical trials? Explain your answer.

Question 2: Even though enrollment in the Phase 2 clinical trials has been low, the results of the test group have been dramatic. None of

the participants enrolled in the test group have had a miscarriage. Acme Medication Company would like to accelerate the clinical trial process, because of the potential life-saving affects the medication could have. Should there be specific guidelines for accelerated clinical trials, or should it be handled on a case by case basis? Explain your answer.

Question 3: During the medical examinations related to clinical trials, it is discovered that one of the pregnant women has a child with anencephaly. The child's parents are firm believers in cryonics, and want to have the child delivered and immediately frozen so that later on when science finds a cure they will be able to save their child. Since the law allows a person to be frozen only if he or has been declared legally dead, there is nothing stating that the procedure cannot be performed. What are your thoughts?

The Briefcase

This section repeats the objectives from the beginning of the chapter and provides a summary of the most important concepts for each objective. Use this section as a quick review and to check your understanding of the chapter key points.

Objective 1: Explain why the National Research Act was passed.
- Tuskegee Syphilis Study
- Provide guidelines for the use of human subjects in research.

Objective 2: Identify the three main ethical principles used in medical research.

- Justice: how research should be performed.
- Autonomy: how research subjects should be treated.
- Beneficence: how research should help others.

Objective 3: Describe the clinical trial process.
- Investigational Review Boards (IRB)
- Phase 1: Limited healthy participants.
- Phase 2: Limited sick participants.
- Phase 3: Expanded sick participants.

Objective 4: Give an example of why stem cell research is controversial.
- Embryos are destroyed when stem cells are harvested.
- Embryos should not be used in scientific research.

Objective 5: Explain why anencephaly creates difficult situations for healthcare.
- Children are born without the cephalic portion of their brain.
- Children can be resuscitated, but may not live long.
- Organs can be used for transplantation.

Objective 6: Identify the reasons some critics are against fetal reduction.
- A form of abortion.
- Being able to choose one child over the other.
- Could be used for esthetic, not medical reasons.

Objective 7: Describe the ethical controversies surrounding conjoined twin separation surgery.
- Interfering with nature.
- Could be a form of suicide.
- Some separation surgery results in the death of both twins.

Objective 8: Explain why cloning is being investigated by scientists.
- To grow tissue to treat and cure diseases.
- To grow organs for transplantation.

Objective 9: Give a reason some would be opposed to xenotransplantation.
- Use of animals in humans.
- Fear of how animal parts might function in humans.

Maximize Your Success with the Companion Website

The Companion Website to this textbook contains materials that can help you better understand the concepts presented in this chapter. Go to MyHealthProfessionsKit to access:

- Learning Tools, Games, and more
- Sample Quizzes
- Related Links
- Understanding Your State

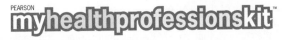

14 The Future of Healthcare

The more things change, the more they remain the same; or so the saying goes. While thought provoking, there is some truth to it. Healthcare will continue to evolve to meet the changing needs that society has. But even though the delivery of healthcare may change, some of the core concepts will not. Even though laws may be passed that relate to healthcare, the process of law will remain the same. And, when scientists develop new techniques or advances in medicine, it will ultimately reveal new ethical issues that we had not thought of before. While we can only speculate as to what the future of healthcare holds, in this chapter we will discuss some issues that have come up recently that may impact the future of healthcare in the United States.

MEASURE YOUR PROGRESS: LEARNING OBJECTIVES

After studying this chapter, you will be able to:

- Give an example of some of the medical issues we will face in the healthcare of the future.

- Explain how the global burden of disease is used to adjust the life expectancy age.

- Describe the purpose of the PPACA.

- List some of the changes that the PPACA has on insurance companies.

- Give an example of how the PPACA has changed Medicare and Medicaid.

- Provide a reason staffing ratio and physician hour laws might be used.

- Explain the rationale behind lawmakers' attempting to pass Healthcare Conscientious Objector Bills.

- Describe how nanotechnology and robotics could be used in healthcare.

- Give an example of some of the questions medicine in space is attempting to address.

KEY TERMS

conscientious objector

global burden of disease

individual mandate

life expectancy

lifetime dollar limits

nanomedicine

premium

robotics

socialized medicine

PROFESSIONAL HIGHLIGHT

Lucinde is a political advisor who works for the U.S. legislature. Because of her medical background, Lucinde focuses her time on identifying issues related to healthcare. Her main responsibility is to provide information to legislatures to let them know about current healthcare trends that are facing the nation. She writes reports and advisory opinions so that lawmakers can make a determination if healthcare laws need to be passed to address some of the problem areas she has identified. In order to keep the legislature up to date, Lucinde needs to have a thorough understanding of what the future holds for healthcare.

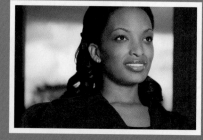

Part of the reason healthcare issues seem to be constantly in the news is because of the constant change in our society and the advances in the field of science and medicine. And now that you have had a chance to review some of the basics related to healthcare law and medical ethics, you can apply those basics to more advanced healthcare laws and medical ethical issues that you might face in the future.

Legal Future of Healthcare

In the United States, we have the best and latest medical equipment that the world has to offer. In addition, we have the best trained and the most experienced medical team in the world. But when it comes to the impact that best and most experienced healthcare has, the United States is almost last among industrialized nations.

The World Health Organization (WHO) provides statistics that measure the impact of healthcare around the world. Some of the measurements that it uses to assess healthcare are **life expectancy**, infant mortality, and **Global Burden of Disease** statistics (GBD).

The life expectancy gives an average number of years that a person can expect to live. The GBD utilizes information about diseases and injuries to demonstrate how certain diseases or injuries impact lives and life expectancy. To measure that impact, WHO researchers utilize statistics to determine if any changes occur in the life expectancy. Any changes that result from incorporating the GBD statistics demonstrates the impact of disease. For example, in 1990, the life expectancy for healthy people living in South Africa was 61 years. But, when information regarding people infected with HIV was entered into the statistical formula, the life expectancy dropped to 24 years. Interpreting the data, it meant that HIV was shortening the lives of people in South Africa by 37 years. In comparison, the life expectancy in the United States in 1990 was 74 years old, but with GBD statistics for HIV included the life expectancy dropped to 32 years (see Graph 14-1).

Healthcare Reform

One contributing factor to the United States being last in some areas of healthcare may be the number of people living in the United States who are not covered by health insurance. According to information provided by the Centers for Disease Control and Prevention's National Center for Health Statistics, the number of

> It seems that healthcare issues are constantly in the news. Why is that? When are we going to be able to come to some sort of resolution about healthcare in the United States?

life expectancy: the average number of years a person is expected to live, based on diseases and mortality

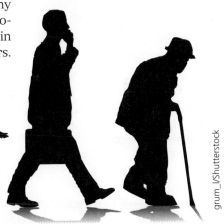

grum_l/Shutterstock

global burden of disease: the loss of health due to disease, injuries, and risk factors

Graph 14-1 Life Expectancy in the United States, United Kingdom, and Canada.

Legend: 1960, 1970, 1980, 1990, 2000

uninsured Americans has been increasing each year; the number of people covered by private health insurance has been drastically decreased; and the number of people covered by public health insurance (such as Medicaid and Medicare) has significantly increased. The results of this study indicate that more and more people are losing their private healthcare insurance and are either going without insurance or relying on public assistance. Unless drastic changes are implemented, analysts predict these trends will continue to worsen.

Healthcare reform has been a topic of national debate for several decades, but until recently, politicians have been unsuccessful at making a significant impact. That changed on March 23, 2010, when President Barack Obama signed the Patient Protection and Affordable Care Act (PPACA) into law. In conjunction with the Health Care and Education Reconciliation Act of 2010, the PPACA provided sweeping healthcare reform measures in the United States. Some of the act's provisions took effect immediately upon singing; other provisions will take effect according a schedule outlined in the Act.

Beyond the Scope

Many of the provisions of the PPACA that we will discuss have variable effective dates. In order to facilitate discussion, language will be used in this section as if the provisions have already taken effect. For more detailed information regarding effective dates of certain provisions, the reader is directed to outside resources.

PPACA: Private Insurance Companies

The PPACA includes many different provisions, some of which are directly aimed at private health insurance companies. Some of the clauses in the PPACA that regulate private insurance companies are the focus of lawsuits currently before the court that are questioning the constitutionality of the PPACA.

Lifetime Dollar Limits for Private Insurance Payments

In the past, private insurance contracts contained a clause that capped the amount of money an insurance policy would pay. These caps are commonly referred to as **lifetime dollar limits** because they limit the amount of money an insurance company will pay for a medical condition over the course of a patient's lifetime.

lifetime dollar limits: the maximum amount of money an insurance company pays on an insurance policy over the course of a lifetime

For example, picking an arbitrary amount for discussion purposes, once an insurance company has paid out, say, $1 million for a patient, the insurance policy has been maximized and no further benefits would be provided. Lifetime dollar limits have caused many Americans with devastating and debilitating

TABLE 14-1			
Insurance in America from 1997 to 2006			
	Percent Uninsured	Percent with Public Health Coverage	Percent with Private Health Insurance
1997	15.6	13.6	70.8
1998	15.3	12.7	72.0
1999	14.5	12.4	73.1
2000	15.3	12.9	71.8
2001	14.8	13.6	71.6
2002	15.0	15.2	69.8
2003	15.8	16.0	68.2
2004	15.3	16.1	68.6
2005	14.8	16.8	68.4
2006	15.4	18.1	66.5

Andrei Marincas/Shutterstock

diseases to go without health insurance. Because they now have a pre-existing condition, many Americans are ineligible for an affordable health insurance policy with another company. With the PPACA, health insurance providers are no longer allowed to place caps on their insurance policies or drop a patient because of a medical condition, effectively eliminating the lifetime dollar limits.

Private Health Insurance Premiums

Prior to the enactment of the PPACA, insurance companies based **premiums** on information obtained on the application, such as age, sex, smoking history, diet, and pre-existing medical conditions.

The PPACA now requires that insurance companies offer the same premium to everyone, based only on age and sex (with some fluctuation allowed for geographical differences). For example, any male between 20 and 30 years of age will pay the same premium, regardless of any other factors or medical conditions they may have. Most importantly, this clause removes the use of pre-existing conditions to determine premiums.

premium: the amount of money a person pays for insurance coverage

PPACA: Medicaid Eligibility

There is an old saying that describes some people's financial situation: too rich to be poor, and too poor to be rich. Many Americans that do not have health insurance make too much money to qualify for Medicaid, but not enough to afford a private health insurance policy. Under the PPACA, eligibility for Medicaid will be increased to 133 percent of the poverty level (see Table 14-2).

Health Insurance Exchange

In addition to offering Medicaid for those who qualify, the PPACA mandates that each state create a Health Insurance Exchange. This exchange is essentially a store, where individuals and small businesses can comparatively shop for and purchase health insurance policies. Although the PPACA does not determine what insurance companies are listed, because the exchange will be run by the state, it is speculated that any insurance company that operates in a given state will have to be listed in the exchange.

For individuals who purchase insurance through the exchange, if they earn between 133 and 400 percent of the federal poverty guidelines, a sliding scale

TABLE 14-2

Federal Poverty Levels

Persons in Family	Poverty Level	133 percent of Poverty	400 percent of Poverty
1	$10,830	$14,404	$43,320
2	$14,570	$19,378	$58,280
3	$18,310	$24,352	$73,240
4	$22,050	$29,327	$88,200
5	$25,790	$34,301	$103,160
6	$29,530	$39,275	$118,120
7	$33,270	$44,249	$113,080
8	$37,010	$49,223	$148,040

2009 Poverty levels published in the Federal Register by the Department of Health and Human Services. For families with more than 8 persons add $3,740 for each additional person (133 percent equals $4,974 for each additional person; 400 percent equals $14,960). Note: This table only applies to residents of the 48 contiguous states and the District of Columbia. Alaska and Hawaii have their own federal poverty guideline table.)

Suzanne Tucker/Shutterstock

will be used to determine how much they will pay for their insurance policy. For businesses that have less than 25 employees, and purchase insurance through the exchange, subsidies are provided through tax credits based on calculations established in the act.

PPACA: Shared Responsibility Payment

With all of the clauses of the PPACA that we have discussed thus far, there is one common theme. One of the main reasons behind creating the PPACA was to create a program that would provide healthcare coverage for all Americans. The idea is that by including everyone in the healthcare equation, everyone can *share the responsibility* of healthcare equally. To accomplish that goal, under the PPACA everyone must be covered by some type of health insurance. That policy can be Medicare, Medicaid, employee-provided insurance, or a policy purchased through the state's insurance exchange. If a person does not carry health insurance, the Shared Responsibility clause, commonly referred to as the **individual mandate** clause, levies a fine against any individual who is not covered by a health insurance policy.

individual mandate: a clause in the PPACA that levies a fine against those who do not carry health insurance

Individuals and families who do not qualify for a public health insurance policy, such as Medicaid, or do not have employee health insurance, must purchase an individual insurance plan. (This plan can be purchased either privately or through the state's healthcare exchange.) Anyone who fails to be covered by an insurance policy will be assessed a "shared responsibility" fee. The shared responsibility clause applies not only to individuals but businesses as well. If the government subsidizes an employee's insurance because his or her employer does not offer them a health insurance policy (or their policy is inadequate or unaffordable), the employer is assessed a shared responsibility fee. (Shared responsibilities fees for both individuals and business are based on calculations included in the PPACA.)

Some believe that the federal government does not have the legal authority to mandate its citizens to purchase health insurance. Several states filed lawsuits against the federal government over the Shared Responsibility clause.

Court Case

U.S. Citizens Association et al. v. Kathleen Sebelius et al.

Case No. 5:10 CV 1065 RWS (2011) United States District Court Northern District of Ohio Eastern Division

FACTS: The individual mandate provision of the PPACA is schedule to take effect in 2014. Believing that the individual mandate clause of the PPACA is unconstitutional, a small advocacy group called U.S. Citizens Association filed a lawsuit. In their lawsuit the group claims the PPACA violates the Commerce Clause, freedom of expression and association, and due process of the U.S. Constitution, along with the constitutionally protected right to privacy. They request that the court declare the PPACA unconstitutional and enjoin (stop) the enforcement of the PPACA. The defendants moved to dismiss.

ISSUE: There are many issues raised by this lawsuit, some of which are based on constitutional law procedural issues. Does the plaintiff, as an association, have the legal authority to bring a lawsuit? Because cases can only be brought if there is an existing "case or controversy," is the plaintiff's lawsuit ripe? (If an issue is speculative or hypothetical, it is not considered ripe for judicial review by the courts. Meaning, you can't file suit against someone because they *might* break the law, but only when they actually do.)

RULE: Citing similar cases in other parts of the country, the judge stated, "The results in other United States District Courts to date, in responding to motions to dismiss, have been mixed." The judge also wrote that "the controversy ignited by the passage of the legislation at issue in this case will eventually require a decision by the Supreme Court after the above-described litigation works its way through the various circuit courts."

EMPHASIS: Courts across the country have issued conflicting rulings over the constitutionality of the PPACA. As the judge in this case noted, and many political and legal analysts believe, this issue will ultimately be presented before the U.S. Supreme Court for a final decision. This case demonstrates how the court system and appeals work, using a healthcare law as an example. In regards to the future of healthcare, new laws will be written regarding healthcare, which can always be subjected to lawsuits and court scrutiny.

PPACA: Medicare

There are two aspects of the PPACA that directly affect Medicare. The first is an expanded and improved prescription drug coverage program for Medicare Part D; the second restructures reimbursement under Medicare. Medicare reimbursement in the past was based on a fee-for-service (ICD-9) or a lump sum (DRG) payment structure. But the PPACA changes that structure to a bundled payment system.

Under DRGs, a hospital is paid a lump sum for a diagnosis, which is paid to the hospital upon the patient's discharge. Not being paid until discharge has caused some hospitals to discharge their patients early, either to a nursing home, rehabilitation facilities, or home to receive home healthcare. The problem, however, is that most of these services are not covered by typical health insurance policies, which leaves the burden of payment on the patient. While the bundled payment system is similar to DRGs, it takes it one step further.

With a bundled payment structure, all medical treatments that relate to a patient's condition are lumped together, regardless of who provides services. For example, assume that a patient suffers a fractured hip, requiring surgery. Following a hospitalization, the patient is transferred to a nursing facility to receive physical therapy and other rehabilitation measures. After being discharged home, the patient will require follow-ups with the orthopedic surgeon. Under the bundled payment structure, all of the entities: the hospital, the rehab facility, and the doctor's office visits, will share a single lump-sum payment.

There are some details that have not yet been worked out with this system, such as the amount or percentage each party will receive; or if one person will receive the entire bundled payment and be expected to pay the other parties. The implementation of this provision will not take effect until 2013 as a pilot program, to be expanded in 2016. This timeframe will allow healthcare facilities and medical providers time to form relationships and develop contracts with one another, so that the necessary mechanisms can be in place when the payment structure is implemented.

PPACA: Additional Provisions

The provisions and clauses that we have discussed so far, are only a part of the sweeping changes regarding healthcare reform established by the PPACA. Below is a summary of some of the additional programs and clauses included in the PPACA.

1. The creation of a voluntary insurance policy that will provide for assisted living facilities, nursing homes, and home healthcare.

2. Additional funding will be provided for medical research and the National Institutes of Health.

3. The enrollment process for the Child Health Insurance Program (CHIP) and Medicaid will be simplified.

4. Families can keep children on their insurance policy until they reach their twenty-sixth birthday. (There are no longer any requirements that a child be enrolled in college, be an income tax dependent on the parent's IRS return, or even living in the parent's home.)

Universal Healthcare

There are some who believe that the PPACA is the first step toward universal healthcare coverage in the United States, which some refer to as **socialized medicine**.

 Sidebar

The state of Virginia filed a motion with the U.S. Supreme Court asking for a review of the state's lawsuit questioning the constitutionality of the PPACA. The state of Virginia argued that because the case would eventually end up before the Supreme Court, that the court allow the state of Virginia to bypass the normal appeals process. On April 26, 2011, the U.S. Supreme Court rejected the State of Virginia's request, without comment or written opinion.

 Concept Connection

PPACA and ICD-9/DRG

The system of reimbursement based on ICD-9 and DRG codes is what most insurance companies including Medicare and Medicaid use for reimbursement. This payment structure will change under the PPACA.

Sidebar

When Medicare introduced the ICD-9 and DRG payment system, private health insurance companies quickly followed suit. What will be interesting to watch over the next few years is how private insurance companies will respond to the changes in Medicare reimbursement and the PPACA.

socialized medicine: a healthcare system that is publicly financed and administered by the government

The term *socialized medicine* is commonly used to describe universal healthcare, because when initially introduced to the American public critics associated it with socialism. While some countries that have universal healthcare are socialist countries, there are some democratic countries that have universal healthcare, like England and Canada.

When discounting the universal healthcare system, many critics point to the issues that countries with universal healthcare coverage face. For example, one of the most common problems mentioned about Canada's universal healthcare system is the long wait time patients must endure in order to see a healthcare provider or have a procedure performed. Health Canada, the Canadian equivalent to the U.S. Department of Health and Human Services, publishes reports regarding healthcare services. In the latest report released by Health Canada, the average wait time to see a physician specialist was a little over four weeks. In comparison, a report released by Merritt Hawkins, a private consulting and healthcare recruiting firm in the United States, found that the average wait time to see a physician specialist in the United States was three weeks.

While the arguments over the PPACA, universal healthcare, and healthcare reform will continue, healthcare strategists and policy advisors agree that the argument over healthcare boils down to one basic issue. Is healthcare a right or a privilege? Prior to the PPACA, only a small percentage of Americans were covered by health insurance. While that system was not perfect, and had multiple problems, there are those that believe universal healthcare is not the way to go. Opponents agree that the PPACA is not going to be perfect, and readily admit that there will be problems. But they argue that is better to try to create a new system where everyone is covered by health insurance, instead of trying to fix the old system, where only a fraction of people are.

Staffing Ratios

Having health insurance is only one of the problems that we face with healthcare in the United States. By increasing the number of people who will access healthcare, are we going to over-burden an already short-staffed healthcare system? For example, one of the problems that we are currently facing in this country is the nursing shortage. Nurses are leaving the profession in greater numbers than those that are entering the profession. With the current trend, hospitals are finding it difficult to provide enough staff members to treat their patients. In some nursing units, one nurse can be responsible for taking care of 10–15 patients. With that many patients to provide care to, nurses are concerned about the quality of care that they provide. To combat this growing problem, some nurses and nursing organizations are asking the legislature to create staffing ratio laws. Staffing ratio laws take one of three different approaches:

1. Require that healthcare institutions have a staffing committee, which is nursing driven, and that staffing decisions be made based on patient need (such as acuity).
2. Mandate reporting by healthcare facilities to publicly disclose staffing levels to the public and regulatory agencies.
3. Mandate specific nurse-to-patient ratios.

It is the last approach, mandating specific ratios, that has created the most discussion. Critics of staffing ratio laws have expressed concern that mandating specific numbers will allow patients to go without receiving care. For example, if the ratio is set at 10 patients to one nurse, and there are two nurses on a floor with 28 patients, what happens to the eight patients who do not have a nurse? Will nurses not provide them with medical care, or will care be provided by unlicensed personnel? Supporters of staffing ratio laws are quick to point out that the reason and purpose of the laws is directed at management, not the nurses themselves. That if nurses are placed in above-quota situations, they will not be held accountable for any lapses in patient care. The difficulty management and administration point out, is that patient census fluctuates and is not something that they can control. Because hospitals cannot turn patients away, and in the face of a nursing shortage, staffing ratio laws do not address the problem. Some critics to the staffing ratio laws do not believe that they are laws at all, because they have no substance or teeth when it comes to violations of the laws. Penalties for violating staffing ratio laws vary from notification to state health departments to monetary fines levied against the institution.

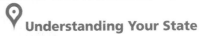

Understanding Your State

To see whether your state has a staffing ratio law, or proposed law, check out the interactive U.S. Map on the companion website.

Physician Hours

Both the airline and trucking industries in the United States are highly regulated. There are very specific laws that indicate the number of hours an airline pilot can work before being required to take time off, or that truckers are allowed to drive before they have to stop. The obvious reason is because we do not want a pilot or a trucker falling asleep while working, because if they do, the result would be catastrophic. But even though there are strict requirements over the number of hours a pilot or trucker can work, the same does not hold true for doctors.

It is not uncommon for medical residents and interns to stay awake for 36 to 48 hours at a time. Staying awake for longer periods of time has become standard in medical training, with some believing that it is an essential part of a doctor's training. But questions have been raised regarding how effective a doctor can be if they have been awake for long periods of time.

While there are no laws that limit the number of hours a doctor can work without taking time off, some professional organizations have developed standards. The Accreditation Council for Graduate Medical Education (ACGME) is responsible for "setting standards, monitoring and accrediting medical residency programs throughout the U.S." The council, in 2011, issued new and updated guidelines for work limits of resident physicians.

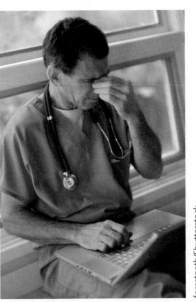

forestpath/Shutterstock

Court Case

Ricky Wyatt et al. v. Charles Fetner et al.

92 F.3d 1074 (1996) U.S. Court of Appeals, Eleventh Circuit

FACTS: Bryce State Hospital in Tuscaloosa, Alabama, is a state-run mental health and mental retardation center. In the 1970s, a tax, specifically earmarked for mental health services, was cut. This cut in funding caused Bryce to lay off staff including 20 healthcare professionals. After the layoffs, staffing ratios consisted of one physician per 350 patients, one nurse per 250 patients, and one psychiatrist per 1,700 patients. The staffing ratios at the other state-run mental health facilities, Searcy Hospital and Camp Partlow, were not much better. Many of the 5,200 patients at Bryce had been involuntary committed. Ricky Wyatt, a 15-year old labeled as a juvenile delinquent, was housed at Bryce. Wyatt and his aunt, W. C. Rawlins (who was also one of the laid-off employees) testified about the inhumane conditions and inadequate and improper treatment at Bryce. A class action lawsuit involving the patients at Bryce was filed against the state of Alabama and several state officials.

ISSUE: What minimal standards exist for the treatment of patients involuntary admitted to state institutions?

RULE: This case involved 33 years of litigation in the courts. The end result of this case is the Wyatt Standard, a nationwide model of four criteria used to evaluate the care of the mentally ill: 1) Humane psychological and physical environments, 2) Qualified and sufficient staff for administration of treatment, 3) Individualized treatment plans, and 4) Minimum restrictions of patient freedom.

EMPHASIS: While nursing staffing ratio laws are relatively new, they conform to an established ideology, the safe and adequate treatment of patients. The difference is that in this case, the lack of staff was within the government's control. Part of the appeals process for this case required the state to provide more staffing. (Supplementary reports estimate that the state of Alabama paid $15 million to settle this lawsuit.)

- Duty hours are limited to 80 hours per week (based on four-week period).
- Residents must have one scheduled day free of duty every week.
- First-year residents cannot work longer than 16 hours in duration. Second-year residents cannot work longer than 24 hours in duration.
- First-year residents must have eight hours off after a scheduled shifts. Second-year residents must have 14 hours off after a scheduled shift.

While some patient advocacy groups are lobbying lawmakers to write laws that will limit physician hours, legislatures are hopeful that the professional organizations will self-regulate and not require legislative intervention.

Ethical Future of Healthcare

Regardless of the changes and advances that are made in science and medicine, ethical issues will remain. While advances in science may resolve some of the current ethical issues, we will never be able to entirely rid ourselves of ethical debates associated with healthcare and medicine. And while most ethical issues center around a specific procedure or treatment, what about the ethics of the healthcare providers themselves?

Conscientious Objector Bill

Because of the evolving fields of medical technology, bioethics, and pharmacology, healthcare workers are being faced with an increased number of ethical complexities that we have not encountered before. Some have expressed concern over how healthcare professionals are being placed in ethically challenging situations that ask them to compromise their personal ethical standards or moral beliefs. There are some lawmakers who agree, and believe that healthcare workers should not be required to compromise their principles while on the job. Collectively referred to as **conscientious objector** bills, they would allow a healthcare provider to maintain their ethical principles and moral beliefs when providing patient care.

conscientious objector: a person who claims a right not to perform a specific action, usually for ethical or religious reasons

Essentially what conscientious objector bills attempt to do is protect healthcare workers from being fired from their jobs or discriminated on the job. In addition, some proposed bills provide healthcare workers with immunity from criminal prosecution and civil lawsuits, should such threats arise from actions workers take based on their moral beliefs.

Ethics Case

Eckerd Pharmacy

Denton, Texas (2004)

FACTS: In early 2004, a female teenager was the victim of a sexual assault. She was taken to the local hospital where she underwent examination and treatment. As part of her post-assault treatment, she was offered emergency contraception that would terminate pregnancy that may have occurred due to the assault. Because the rural hospital did not stock the medication, she was provided with a prescription to be filled at a pharmacy. (In order for emergency contraception to be effective, it must be taken within a specific postcoital time period.) The first two pharmacies that she visited did not stock the medication. At the third drug store, an Eckerd pharmacy, she was told that they did stock the medication. But, citing personal beliefs, all of the pharmacists on duty that evening declined to fill the prescription, considering it a violation of their personal morals. The prescription was returned to the patient, to be filled elsewhere.

ISSUE: Can a pharmacist refuse to fill a valid medical prescription, based on personal moral and ethical grounds? As licensed healthcare practitioners, would that refusal be a violation of their licensure requirements?

RULE: Because their actions violated Eckerd Pharmacy policy, the pharmacists working that evening were terminated. (The only laws, at the time, that would apply to this situation is tort law. But, because the victim was able to obtain the prescription at a competitor's pharmacy, the damage element for torts would be limited to emotional distress.)

EMPHASIS: This case was one of the early catalysts for creating conscientious objector bills. After this story hit the national news, similar occurrences occurred throughout the country. While legal issues are involved in situations such as this, there are ethical questions as well.

Most conscientious objector bills have complex exceptions written into the statute's language. To name a few:

- A healthcare worker has to provide notice to an employer about an ethical position beforehand and cannot make on-the-spot decisions.
- Ethical concerns cannot be based on constitutionally protected classes (i.e., age, race, gender).
- Emergency situations are not covered, which includes people working in emergency rooms or first responders, although accommodations should be made if staffing allows.
- While all attempts should be made to accommodate a person in a supervisory position, if no one else is available, a supervisor may be required to provide care.

Most healthcare professional organizations have spoken out against these bills. In addition, most healthcare professional organization's Code of Ethics have provisions that are contrary to what the legislature is attempting to do. The American Medical Association (AMA) is being proactive, working with state legislatures to quash these bills before they are passed.

Prescription Drug Advertising

If you watch television or surf the Internet for any length of time, you will inevitably run across an advertisement for prescription medication. For many years, pharmaceutical companies only advertised to healthcare providers. But pharmaceutical companies started to study the benefits that marketing directly to consumers might have, and petitioned the FDA to allow them to start advertising.

Sidebar
The Food and Drug Administration (FDA) provides strict guidelines about what information must be provided in a drug advertisement. For example, the disclosures of complications, side effects, or contraindications that you frequently hear during drug advertisements are part of the requirements imposed by the FDA.

While some would argue that marketing prescription drugs in itself is unethical, other issues have arisen that have changed the views on drug advertising. In recent years, pharmaceutical companies have spent billions of dollars on prescription drug advertising. This increase in advertising budgets occurs at a time when a large number of Americans are having difficulty paying for their prescription medications. Some critics have argued that the cost of advertising has directly contributed to the rising cost of prescription drugs.

Recently, the number of prescription drug advertisements has fallen slightly as pharmaceutical companies evaluate the cost/benefit of direct to consumer advertising. Part of that decrease has been attributed to the continuing decline in the U.S. economy. Another contributing factor is that some media outlets are decreasing the amount of time or space they attribute to drug advertising because consumers are growing weary of seeing advertisement after advertisement for prescription drugs.

The Scientific Future of Healthcare

A thorough review of the future of healthcare would not be complete without delving into some esoteric, if not existential, ideas. Indeed there are a few medical and scientific endeavors on the horizon that will impact healthcare, not in the near future, but far into the future.

Nanotechnology

Scientists have been utilizing and experimenting with nanotechnology for many years. Nanotechnology is the manipulation of matter on the atomic or molecular level. And while the initial use of nanotechnology was in the field of engineering, medical researchers have been investigating the impact that nanotechnology could have on the field of medicine. The application of nanotechnology in medicine is known as **nanomedicine**.

nanomedicine: the use of molecular technology for healthcare purposes

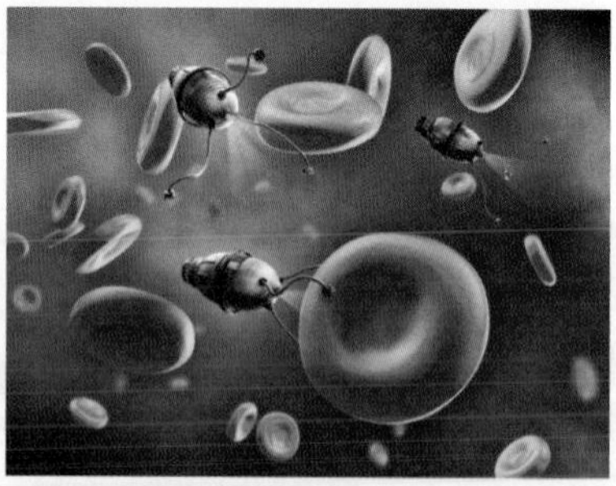

Andrea Danti/Shutterstock

Fig. 14-1. An artist's rendition of a nanotechnology concept used to monitor and treat blood cells.

The prefix *nano-*, meaning "one-billionth," as in the metric measurement nanometer, or one-billionth of a meter, comes from the Greek word *nanos*, for "dwarf." Science uses the nanometer to measure small things, such as the cells in the human body. While the field of nanomedicine is still in its infancy, medical researchers are excited about the possible uses nanotechnology has to offer to the field of medicine. One area that is currently being investigated is the use of nanotechnology in pharmacology. By delivering medication directly to the cells that need it, scientist speculate that they can diminish the complications and side effects that some medications have. In addition, nanotechnology can be used to monitor the body and deliver medication when it is needed. For example nanorobots can be implanted into the body to monitor blood glucose levels, and if levels reach a point where insulin is needed, they can release insulin into the bloodstream.

While scientist continue to investigate how nanotechnology and nanomedicine can be used, many are concerned about the lack of regulatory guidelines in the field of nanotechnology and its possible unintended consequences. Part of the debate is over who should be responsible for regulating the field. Should it be the Food and Drug Administration (FDA), the Environmental Protection Agency (EPA), Health and Human Services (HHS) or Occupational Safety and Health Administration (OSHA)?

Robotics

While the use of nanomedicine is pure speculation at this point, the use of **robotics** in the field of medicine is currently a reality (See Fig. 14-2).

Robots have been used for many years in the manufacturing industry, most often on assembly lines to build computers and cars for example. And while robotics has become an essential part of manufacturing, many other industries have been slow to adopt the technology for their use; healthcare is no exception. Robots are currently being used by pharmacies to fill hundreds of prescriptions per day, and have far less incidences

> ### Sidebar
> Ever heard of the term the Mad Hatter or Mad as a Hatter? It comes from an actual disease that was contracted by hat manufacturers in the 1800s. Part of the manufacturing process of turning fur into felt used to make hats included the use of mercury. Over the years, inhaling mercury particles caused mercury poisoning, which affects the nervous system, including the brain. Many hat manufacturers suffered psychological symptoms associated with mercury poisoning, which contributed to the term mad as a hatter.

robotics: the use of computers and machines to perform tasks, which often includes intelligence technology

Ethics Case

Silver Nanotechnology 1990s – Present

FACTS: Silver nanoparticles are included in many of the products that we use today. Computer equipment, cell phones, food storage containers, textiles, and even teddy bears contain silver nanoparticles. Because silver nanoparticles have antibacterial and odor-absorbing properties, their use in clothing has increased over recent years. Some manufacturers of socks have incorporated silver nanoparticles into their products to combat foot odor. Product researchers have tested socks after repeated washings to determine how long the silver remains in the sock and beneficial to consumers. Scientific and medical researchers were also interested in learning about silver nanoparticles, but for different reasons. When silver nanoparticle clothing is laundered, or food containers washed, some of those silver nanoparticles end up in the waste water and enter either water treatment or waste management facilities.

ISSUE: What impact do nanoparticles have when they enter the water table, the environment, and eventually humans?

RULE: Because of the properties of silver, when deposited into the environment it kills beneficial bacteria used in the management of waste. The sludge from waste management facilities is used to make fertilizer, commonly sold to farmers. Researchers have found small levels of silver nanoparticles in water tables, which can have a negative impact on the aquatic environment, as it kills many types of fish. Small amounts of silver entering the body cause few medical problems, mostly cosmetic, because it deposits in the skin. But researchers are quick to point out that only the impact of small amounts of silver ingestion are known; the impact of larger quantities of ingested silver has not been thoroughly studied.

EMPHASIS: Even though the use of nanoparticles and nanotechnology is relatively new, it can create unique, unintended, and unknown consequences. As the world becomes more environmentally conscious, concern is growing over the impact that scientific and medical advances might have on the environment. While beneficial in some respects, do the unintended consequences outweigh that benefit?

of errors in filling prescriptions than humans do. But part of the reason robotics has been slow to catch on in the healthcare arena is because many are concerned about using them on actual patients. In part, this concern is raised because of the possibility of mechanical failures that might occur during medical procedures.

Computer games currently exist where a player can perform mock surgery on a patient. Could a surgeon, through the combination of game consoles and technology, combined with virtual reality, perform surgery on a patient remotely? While the possibility does not currently exist, some researchers are intrigued by the idea that it presents.

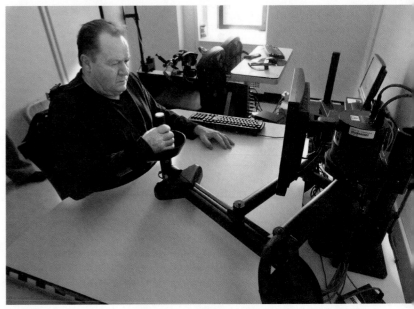

© Enigma/Alamy

Fig. 14-2. A man uses a computerized robot arm as part of his rehabilitation after a stroke. The robot can automatically measure and adjust settings, based on the user's response.

Medical Care in Space

The idea that humans will inhabit other planets is pure science fiction at this point. But with the creation of the space station MIR, astronauts are starting to live in space for extended periods of time. Medical science has already seen the impact that anti-gravity has on the human body. To combat muscle atrophy, astronauts stationed in MIR spend time on fitness bikes to prevent muscle atrophy and bone loss that is seen in astronauts who have spent extended time in zero gravity. And while astronauts undergo extensive medical tests before being launched into space to ensure that they are healthy, it is inevitable that medical care will need to be performed in space at some point.

There is a contingency of medical theorists who are studying how healthcare can be provided in space. They have raised interesting questions regarding some of the challenges that we will face as we look to the stars. For example:

- if surgery is performed in space, how will bodily fluids (such as blood) react in zero gravity when an incision is made?
- will we be able to maintain a sterile field in space?
- what effect will zero gravity have on wound healing?
- can we provide adequate long-term nutrition in space?
- what are some of the psychological effects of isolation and living in confined spaces?

While the concept of medicine in space may seem far-fetched, there is an organization dedicated to the study of medicine and medical treatment in space: the Space Nursing Society (SNS).

Sidebar

What happens if a person in zero gravity is injured by bouncing off the walls of a spacecraft? The creators of the ICD-9 Code are already prepared for that with the ICD-9 Code; E845—Accident Involving Spacecraft.

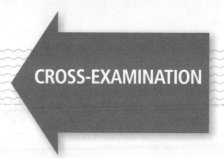

Make FALSE Statements TRUE.

Rewrite the false statements below by replacing the bolded, italicized, and underlined word(s) to make it a true statement.

1. The **_United Nations_** provides statistics that measure the impact of healthcare around the world.

_____

2. The abbreviation PPACA stands for **_Providing Patient Assurance and Care Act_**.

_____

3. Some lawmakers are concerned about healthcare workers who have to compromise their personal ethics, have tried to pass laws collectively known as **_Staffing Ratio Laws_**.

_____

4. Healthcare Reform and the PPACA have been associated by some critics as a form of **_capitalism_**.

_____

5. The Health Insurance Exchange, mandated by the PPACA, will be run by **_private insurance companies_**.

_____

Circle Exercise

Circle the correct word from the choices given.

1. The PPACA removes caps, also known as (**premiums, lifetime dollar limits, life expectancy**) on insurance companies.

2. To increase the number of people eligible for Medicaid, the PPACA increase eligibility to (**133%, 233%, 444%**) of the poverty guideline.

3. The Shared Responsibility clause of the PPACA is commonly referred to as the (**individual mandate, premium, GBD**) clause.

4. The use of computers to perform healthcare tasks is known as (**robotics, nanomedicine, conscientious**).

5. Of the professions listed, only (**pilots, truckers, doctors**) are not limited by law for the number of hours that they can work.

Matching

Match the numbered term to its lettered definition.

1. _____ conscientious objector

2. _____ global burden of disease

3. _____ individual mandate

4. _____ life expectancy

5. _____ lifetime dollar limits

6. _____ nanomedicine

7. _____ premium

8. _____ robotics

9. _____ socialized medicine

A. a clause in the PPACA that levies a fine against those who do not carry health insurance.

B. a healthcare system that is publicly financed and administered by the government.

C. a person who claims a right not to perform a specific action, usually for ethical or religious reasons.

D. the amount of money a person pays for insurance coverage.

E. the average number of years a person is expected to live, based on diseases and mortality.

F. the loss of health due to disease, injuries, and risk factors.

G. the maximum amount of money an insurance company pays on an insurance policy over the course of a lifetime.

H. the use of computers and machines to perform tasks, which often includes intelligence technology.

I. the use of molecular technology for healthcare purposes.

Deliberations: Critical Thinking Questions

Question 1: The PPACA sets a premium standard that all people of the same age and sex will pay. But what about people who smoke, do not exercise, or have other unhealthy habits. They will be paying the same premium as health-conscious people of the same age and sex. Should people who smoke pay a different premium than nonsmokers? What about those that do not eat healthily, or those that are overweight? Should they have to pay a different premium?

Question 2: Most employers only offer health insurance to full-time employees. Usually, part-time employees are not eligible for employee-provided health insurance. Some critics of the PPACA believe that in response companies are going to minimize the number of full-time employees so that they do not have to offer health insurance. Should the law require companies to provide health insurance to all employees, both full- and part-time? Explain the impact your position might have.

Question 3: Suppose that a robot has been developed that allows a physician to perform surgery remotely. Instead of going to a hospital, a surgeon can operate via a control panel in his or her office. This technology could allow a surgeon in Maine to perform surgery on a patient in California. Because each state provides healthcare licenses separately, where should this doctor be licensed; in Maine or California? What if the surgeon

commits an act of negligence; where should the negligence lawsuit be filed, in Maine or in California?

Question 4: Using nanotechnology, monitoring devices have been developed that monitor blood sugar levels in the bloodstream. Patients no longer needs to monitor their blood sugar or administer insulin injections, saving the patient from hundreds of needle sticks a month. These tiny robots are injected into the bloodstream, and can survive for a number of weeks before they are removed from the body through the urine. The downside is that patients cannot have an MRI or CT scan performed while the devices have been implanted. And, if the patient is sent home, he or she must strain all urine and return any collected devices back to the hospital for proper disposal. What are your thoughts? Do the benefits outweigh the other problems these devices create?

Question 5: NASA has decided to send a nurse to space, so that she can further her studies about space nursing. During her trip aboard the space shuttle, a crew member has an accident. The tip of his index finger was almost ripped off and is now hanging by a few tendons and ligaments. The nurse knows that the finger has to be cut off the rest of the way and the end bandaged. Even though she has seen similar procedures done, and she has the necessary tools, she is not licensed to perform this procedure. What should she do? Should she perform the procedure or not? Explain your answer.

 # Closing Arguments: Case Analysis

Mary is a medical assistant who has been working for Dr. Smith, an OB/GYN doctor for five years now. In addition to Mary, there are two other medical assistants, an office nurse, an office manager, a medical biller, and a receptionist working in Dr. Smith's office. A significant portion of Dr. Smith's practice involves performing abortions, on average 10 a week.

Last week, when Mary's sister had a miscarriage, she started to change her views on abortions. She is becoming increasingly opposed to abortions, and believes that they should not be performed. Assuming that a Healthcare Conscientious Objector bill has been passed in her state, Mary goes to Dr. Smith and makes her beliefs known and respectfully requests that she no longer be required to participate in abortion procedures or take care of patients who have had abortions.

Question 1: Because of Mary's objection to the performance of abortions, there are days when she has very little to do. Should the doctor be required to keep Mary on his payroll? What about making Mary take the day off unpaid?

Question 2: Assume that a staffing ratio law has been passed in your state. Since Mary objects to caring for abortion patients, the other medical assistants are now caring for more patients than the staffing ratio law allows. The doctor has already told you that hiring more staff is not financially possible. As the office manager, how would you handle this situation?

Question 3: At a staff meeting, Dr. Smith mentions that he is thinking about purchasing a robot that will assist him in performing simple laparoscopic procedures in his office. One thing he is concerned about is what would happen should the power go out and he is in the middle of a procedure. Dr. Smith is asking you to think about some of the other problems that might result from using robotics for procedures. What issues can you think of? Do you have any thoughts about how these problems should be handled?

The Briefcase

This section repeats the objectives from the beginning of the chapter and provides a summary of the most important concepts for each objective. Use this section as a quick review and to check your understanding of the chapter's key points.

Objective 1: Give an example of some of the medical issues we will face in the healthcare of the future.
- Legal Future of Healthcare
  - Patient Protection and Affordable Care Act
  - Universal Healthcare
  - Staffing Ratio Laws
  - Physician Hour Laws
- Ethical Future of Healthcare
  - Healthcare Conscientious Objector Bills
  - Prescription Drug Advertising
- Scientific Future of Healthcare
  - Nanotechnology
  - Robotics
  - Medicine in Space

Objective 2: Explain how the global burden of disease is used to adjust the life expectancy age.
- Takes into consideration disease and injury.
- Allows for adjustments based on how disease affects health.
- The gap between the GBD and life expectancy, demonstrates the health of the disease in that country.

Objective 3: Describe the purpose of the PPACA
- Increase health insurance to all citizens.
- Make health insurance affordable to all citizens.
- Provide incentives for business to offer insurance and individuals to purchase insurance.
- Making healthcare more affordable by sharing the burden of healthcare.

Objective 4: List some of the changes that the PPACA has on insurance coverage.
- Removes pre-existing conditions as a consideration for insurance.
- Removes capitations on lifetime dollar limits.

- Equalizes insurance premiums for similar people.
- Disallows insurance to be canceled due to a devastating or debilitating disease.

Objective 5: Give an example of how the PPACA has changed Medicare and/or Medicaid
- Increase eligibility for Medicaid.
- Increases the number of people who can obtain Medicaid.
- Changes the way that Medicare reimbursement will be made.
- Increases the proficiency and coverage of Medicare Part D.

Objective 6: Provide a reason staffing ratio and physician hour laws might be used.
- To provide guidelines on the number of patients a healthcare worker will be responsible for.
- To provide limits on the number of hours a healthcare worker is allowed to work at one time.

Objective 7: Explain the rationale behind lawmakers attempting to pass Healthcare Conscientious Objector Bills.
- To protect the ethics and morals of healthcare workers.
- To ensure that healthcare workers are not required to compromise their ethics or morals when providing patient care.

Objective 8: Describe how nanotechnology and robotics could be used in healthcare.
- Nanomedicine
  - Improve the delivery of medications
  - To determine how nanotechnology might affect healthcare
- Robotics
  - Increasing efficiency and productive in healthcare
  - To perform medical procedures

Objective 9: Give an example of some of the questions medicine in space is attempting to address.
- Determining the effect of zero gravity on:
  - surgery
  - sterile fields
  - wound healing
- Providing adequate nutrition.

Maximize Your Success with the Companion Website

The Companion Website to this textbook contains materials that can help you better understand the concepts presented in this chapter. Go to MyHealthProfessionsKit to access:

- Learning Tools, Games, and more
- Sample Quizzes
- Related Links
- Understanding Your State

Glossary

accountability: being held responsible; being required to answer to a situation

actuarial tables: a comprehensive list of statistical data; used most often by insurance companies to determine illness, disease, and accident projections

advance directives: any document that provides instructions for patient care that is made by a patient before he or she becomes incapacitated

altruism: concern for the welfare of others; an obligation to benefit others

anencephaly: a medical condition that occurs when the brain does not develop

apodictic: pertaining to an expression or statement of absolute certainty

applied ethics: a subcategory of ethics that uses ethical concepts and principles to reach an ethical decision

arbitration: a process using a neutral, unbiased third party to make a final decision about a dispute

artificial insemination: the placement of sperm into the female reproductive system by means other than sexual intercourse

autonomy: being independent, making your own decisions, the right of self-governance

beliefs: what a person holds to be true, or rules that are followed that are not based on tangible proof

beneficence: an action that is used to help other people

casuistry: a method of reasoning or legal analysis using conditions and results

certification: a credentialing process that confirms or guarantees that specific knowledge has been obtained or that a person has proven proficiency in a task or skill or demonstrated expertise in a particular area

chattels: a person's belongings, other than land

civil law: a law that covers the rights and remedies of individuals

clinical trial: a research process using humans to test medication, equipment, or procedures

cloning: a medical procedure that creates an exact duplicate of a living organism

code of ethics: written statements that detail the type of behavior a professional should strive toward when performing his or her professional duties

common law: law developed by judges through court decisions rather than through a legislature

compliance: the adherence to a policy or rule

conflict: when opposing forces of incompatibility exist at the same time or place

conscientious objector: a person who claims a right not to perform a specific action, usually for ethical or religious reasons

consequentialism: a decision-making process that uses the outcome to determine whether something is right or wrong

contract: an agreement between parties which the law will recognize

covered entity: an institution or group that is the subject of a regulation or law

credentialing: validation of an individual's background and qualifications, or fulfillment of the requirements established by the organization granting the verification

cryonics: the freezing of humans at death for revival in the future

culture: a group of people that share common beliefs, traits, race, values, goals, or attitudes

damages: a quantified amount of money used to demonstrate a loss or injury to a person or property

defendant: the person accused of wrongdoing in a civil case; or the person charged with a crime in criminal prosecutions

defensive medicine: the type of medical practice used by healthcare workers to protect themselves against potential lawsuits

de-identify: the process of removing any information from documents, or restricting electronic access to information, that a person is not authorized to receive

deontology: the use of duty and rules to determine an outcome

deposition: the taking of testimony of a witness, under oath, by an attorney before a trial

dilemma: a problem for which all outcomes are either equal or all outcomes are undesirable

DNR: an order written by the physician that indicates what medical treatments or procedures are not to be performed

double-blind: a research process where a test group and a control group are used and then compared

egoism: the use of individual self-interest

electroejaculation: a medical procedure whereby an electrical charge is applied to male reproductive organs to obtain a sperm sample

embryo: a fertilized ovum from 7 days after fertilization through 8 weeks gestation

endemic: a disease that is always present, to some degree, in a population or location

epidemic: the occurrence of disease in greater numbers than expected, or the development of disease in a shorter than normal time frame

epidemiology: the study of the characteristics, determination, frequency, and distribution of a disease

ethics: values that are used to determine moral conduct or beliefs

ethnic: a class or group of people that share a common race, nationality, culture, or religion

etiquette: the manner of behavior, determined by custom, that is used in social, official, or professional interactions

eugenics: the process of applying selective breeding to humans

euthanasia: the ending of a person's life either voluntarily or involuntary, by taking measures to end that person's life or not performing measures that would save the person's life

fertilization: conception; the uniting of a female gamete (called an ovum) and a male gamete (called a spermatozoon)

fetal reduction: a procedure used in multiple pregnancies where only a portion of the embryos are aborted

global burden of disease: the loss of health due to disease, injuries, and risk factors

grief: bereavement; an emotional response to loss

healthcare proxy: a person designated to make medical decisions for someone who is incapacitated

heritage: attributes that are inherited or passed on from previous generations

hospice: an ideology related to caring for patients and their family when facing the end of life

in vitro **fertilization:** the fertilization of an ovum outside of the womb

individual mandate: a clause in the PPACA that levies a fine against those who do not carry health insurance

insurance: the transfer of an obligation from one party to another, usually in exchange for a fee

interrogatories: a formal set of written questions provided to opposing parties in a lawsuit that help attorneys discover facts about the case

intestacy: the division of property by descent and distribution, for individuals who die without a will

isolation: the measures taken to prevent the spread of disease, either from patient to patient or from patient to healthcare worker

jurisdiction: the authority provided to a court to preside (exercise authority) over specific legal matters

jurisprudence: the theory, philosophy, science, or study of the law

law: standards of conduct or a system of rules established by an authority

legal document: any writing that provides information or ideas that can be attributed to the author

libel: the communication of a false or defamatory statement that is written or seen

licensure: a credentialing process where a person is granted the authority to perform particular tasks or skills, after demonstrating expertise

life expectancy: the average number of years a person is expected to live, based on diseases and mortality

lifetime dollar limits: the maximum amount of money an insurance company pays on an insurance policy over the course of a lifetime

limited data set: a document that has had some, or all, of the patient's private information removed

living will: a document detailing the situations and type of medical care a patient desires

malfeasance: the performance of an unlawful act through wrongdoing or misconduct

mediation: a process using a neutral party who gets the parties to work together to resolve their differences

medical examiner: a medical professional who's responsibility is to determine the cause of death and gather forensic evidence

medical practice acts: laws that a state has passed to determine the requirements for health care and healthcare professionals

meta-ethics: a subcategory of ethics that defines what ethics is and the contributing factors that define ethical principles

misfeasance: a lawful act, performed in a wrongful manner

mitigate: to lessen, make less severe or less intense

morals: the determination of right and wrong

nanomedicine: the use of molecular technology for healthcare purposes

negligence: when damages are caused by a breach of duty

neonate: a newborn from the time of birth until 1 year of age

nonfeasance: the failure to take action when action is required

normative ethics: a subcategory of ethics that defines how ethical decisions are made and the factors that contribute to ethical decision-making

palliative: an approach to patient care where comfort measures and pain relief are provided instead of trying to cure a patient's disease or medical condition

pandemic: the occurrence of disease in many different populations or geographical locations

parens patriae: Latin for "father of the people," a legal concept whereby the government takes on the role of parent

patriarchal: a society or group, usually of an extended family, that is led by a dominant male

perjury: intentionally lying under oath; a criminal offense for making a knowingly false statement under oath

plaintiff: the party who brings a civil claim of wrongdoing against another party, or the government in criminal prosecutions

pluripotent: the ability to differentiate into many different layers of tissue

portability: the ability of something to be moved or transported from one place to another

precedence: a decision by a court made in the past that is used to determine the outcome of a current court case

premium: the amount of money a person pays for insurance coverage

privacy: something that belongs to or is intended only for an individual or particular group

privileged communication: statements made in private, during the existence of certain relationships, that cannot be used as evidence in civil or criminal trials

professional: a person who earns a living through the expertise of his or her work

protocol: the manner of behavior, determined by authority, that is used in social, official, or professional interactions

quarantine: imposed isolation, most often used to contain individuals with highly contagious and/or deadly diseases

reasonable person standard: a legal standard used to determine whether the actions of a party are warranted

reciprocity: the requirements established for the exchange of credentials from one state to another

religion: a set of beliefs, based on established doctrine, that typically involves worship, devotion, and the adherence to certain practices

res ipsa loquitur: "the thing itself speaks"; a legal theory whereby the mere occurrence of an event infers causation

research: a process that is used to obtain new knowledge, usually based on scientific principles

respondeat superior: "let the master answer," a concept where the employer is responsible for the actions of its employees

robotics: the use of computers and machines to perform tasks, which often includes intelligence technology

shaman: a medical and spiritual advisor and mediator between the human world and spirit world

slander: the communication of a false or defamatory statement that is spoken or heard

socialized medicine: a healthcare system that is publicly financed and administered by the government

sovereign: having independent and supreme power and authority

standards of care: written requirements that detail the responsibilities a professional will be held accountable for in the performance of his or her duties

subpoena duces tecum: "bring with you under penalty of punishment," a requirement that documents be delivered to a court or brought with you to court

surrogate: a woman who carries and gives birth to another person's child

talisman: an object, usually worn around the neck, that is believed to contain spirits or mystical or supernatural powers

torts: the area of civil law that addresses the harms a person receives, except for harms arising out of contract

upcoding: using an incorrect ICD or CPT code to gain a larger insurance payment

utilitarianism: providing the greatest good

values: the measurement of worth or importance

vicarious liability: liability without fault; a person is held legally responsible for the actions of others even though they themselves did nothing wrong

virtue: the pursuit of moral excellence

vital statistics: the information gathered by governmental agencies related to births, marriages, divorces, and death that occur in a population

wuzho / marime: a belief that things are either pure or impure

xenotransplantation: the use of animal tissue or organs in humans

yin yang: a belief in how opposites are related to and dependent on each other in all aspects of life

zygote: a single cell that is produced by the union of an ovum and spermatozoon

Court Cases and
Ethical Case Studies Appendix

Court Cases

(Court citations are written according to legal writing standards: the name of the parties, the identification information, the year of the decisions, and the court that decided the case. The identification numbers used vary depending on the type of case and which jurisdiction the case comes from.)

Caruso v. Pine Manor Nursing Center 538 N.E.2d 722, 182 Ill.App. 3d 879 (1989) Appellate Court of Illinois, First District, Fifth Division	Pg. 59
Clyde F. Deal v. L. John Kearney 851 P.2d 1353 (1993) Supreme Court of Alaska	Pg. 106
Collins v. Park 621 A.2d 996, 423 Pa.Super. 601 (1993) Superior Court of Pennsylvania	Pg. 26
Corley v. State 749 So.2d 926 (La.App. Cir 2) (1999) Louisiana Court of Appeals	Pg. 41
Crabtree v. Dodd No. 01A01-9807-CH-00370 (Tenn.App. 08/17/1999) Tennessee Court of Appeals	Pg. 124
Edmund G. Brown Jr., Governor of California, et al., Appellants v. Marciano Plata et al. No. 09-1233 (October Term, 2010) Argued November 30, 2010. Decision May 23, 2011 Supreme Court of the United States	Pg. 135
Elodie Irvine v. Regents of the University of California 57 Cal.Rptr.3d 500, 149 Cal.App.4th 994 (2007) Court of Appeal State of California, Fourth Appellate District Division Three	Pg. 172
Guanzon v. State Medical Board of Ohio 123 Ohio App.3d 489 (1997) Court of Appeals of Ohio, County of Ohio, Tenth District, Franklin	Pg. 44
Hoffman v. Moore Regional Hospital Inc. 114 N.C.App. 248, 441 S.E.2d 567 (1994) Court of Appeals of North Carolina	Pg. 67
In Re Application of the Milton S. Hershey Medical Center of the Pennsylvania State University. Appeal of John Doe, M.D. in Re Application of the Harrisburg Hospital. Appeal of John Doe M.D. 595 A.2d 1290, 407 Pa.Super. 565 (1991) Superior Court of Pennsylvania	Pg. 82
In Re Eric Halko on Habeas Corpus 246 Cal. App.2d 553, 54 Cal.Rptr. 661 (1966) District Court of Appeal of California, Second Appellate District, Division Four	Pg. 123
Italo Falcone v. Middlesex County Medical Society 162 A.2d 324, 62 N.J.Super. 184, 1960 NJ 40212 New Jersey Superior Court, Law Division	Pg. 151
Jose N. Proenza Sanfiel, R.N. v. Department of Health 749 So.2d 525 (1999) Florida Court of Appeals	Pg. 80
Keene v. Brigham and Women's Hospital, Inc. 439 Mass. 223, 786 N.E.2d 824 (2003) Massachusetts Supreme Judicial Court	Pg. 61
Liebeck v. McDonald's Restaurants No. D-202 CV-93-02419, 1995 WL 360309 Bernalillo County, N.M. Dist Ct. (Aug. 18, 1994)	Pg. 93
Lirjie Juseinoski v New York Hospital Medical Center of Queens No. 28516/98, 2004 NY Slip Op 50441(U) Supreme Court, Kings County (2004)	Pg. 198
Lofton v. Secretary of the Department of Children and Family Services 358 F.3d 804 U.S. Court of Appeals, Eleventh Circuit (2004)	Pg. 193

Ethics Cases

(Ethics cases do not have specific citations rules as court cases do. The citation format provided is as close to the legal format as possible, when information is available, to provide continuity.)

Index